INTERNAL MEDICINE DIFFERENTIAL DIAGNOSES THROUGH ILLUSTRATIONS

Sinisa M. Trbovic, MD, PhD

Prof. Alexander M. Trbovich, MD, PhD

Table of Contents

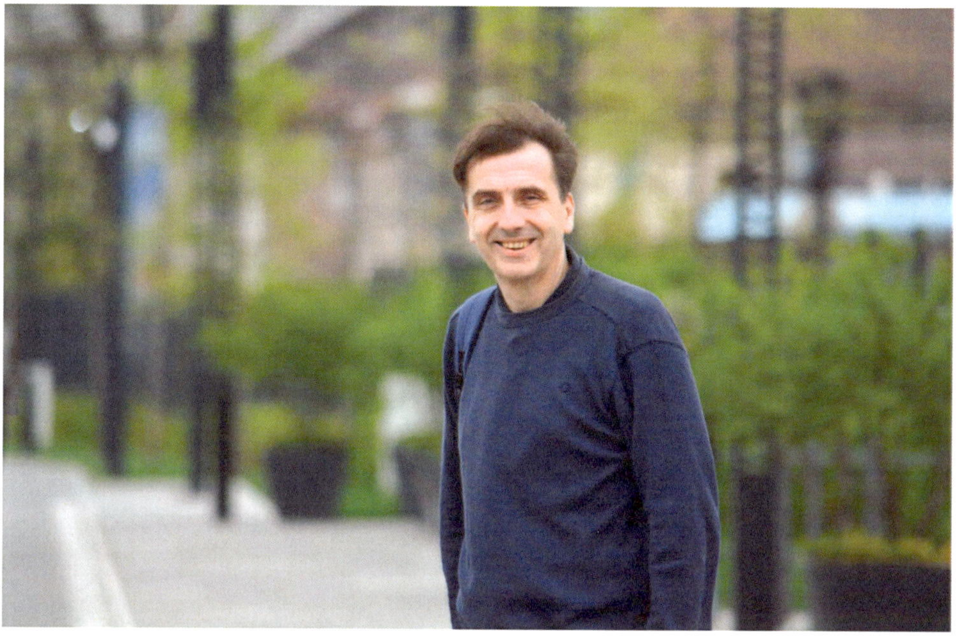

Dedicated to my brother Alexander, a coauthor of this book, who fell asleep just a few weeks before this book was sent for publication.

VISUALIZATION OF DATA

"The eye which is said to be the window of the soul, is the primary means by which understanding of the brain may most fully and magnificently contemplate the infinite works of nature, and the ear is the second, acquiring nobility through the recounting of that which the eye has seen... Oh excellent above all other things created by God...And it triumphs over nature..."

Leonardo da Vinci (1452 –1519) [Kemp, pp.51-52]

The use of illustrations in medical education has been heavily underutilized. Cognitive psychology tells us that 90% of information absorbed by the brain is visual. Approximately 5% is auditory, while the rest belongs to the other senses. In comparison to some animals, such as a dog with a refined sense of smell, or a bat with a refined sense of hearing, a human is 90% a visual being with respect to collection of external data.

George A. Miller, one of the founders of cognitive psychology, conducted experiments on short-term memory and published in 1956 a famous article entitled, *"The Magical Number Seven, Plus or Minus Two: Some Limits on Our Capacity for Processing Information"*.[1] This is one of the most frequently cited papers in psychology. His experiments led him to conclude that we can only retain 5 to 9 items in our short-term memory. However, the medical differential diagnoses frequently include more than 5, and sometimes more than 9 possibilities. Several other researchers have supported Miller's findings, including Lloyd and Margaret Paterson in 1959. Miller believed that our short-term memory stores "chunks" of information rather than individual numbers or letters.

The eye converts the external world into the internal one. The accompanying picture shows the difference between textual and visual presentations of data. For textual presentation, this written sentence needs to be read 2-3 times before it can be fully understood. By contrast, just a glance at the chart provides an instant understanding of the idea. The layperson's saying "a picture is worth a thousand words" captures this fact. The reading of the text goes to short-term memory, where 7 bits of information can be stored. Visual information goes to long-term memory and stays there permanently![2] Visual information is processed **60,000 times** faster than textual information, and visual information is easier to recall. Researchers claim that **people tend to remember only 20% of what they read**.

In addition to the limited capacity of the brain to retain the data in short-term memory, sleep deprivation also limits the ability of the brain to work efficiently. The medical profession, particularly during the time of residency, is notorious for insufficient amounts of sleep. A study has shown that 17 hours of sustained wakefulness leads to a decrease in performance equivalent to a blood alcohol level (BAL) of 0.05% **(two glasses of wine).** This is the legal drunk driving limit in the UK. A wakefulness of 24 hours is equivalent to a BAL of 0.1%, which is equal to being legally drunk in any country.[3] Sleep-deprived individuals often have difficulty in responding to rapidly changing situations and making rational judgments. Thus, the limited brain capacity for short-term memory in combination with sleep deprivation significantly compromises the care of patients. Therefore, there is a major need for help via visual, long-term memory.

VISUALIZATION OF DATA

I HEAR AND FORGET.
I SEE AND REMEMBER.
I DO AND I UNDERSTAND.
-CONFUCIUS

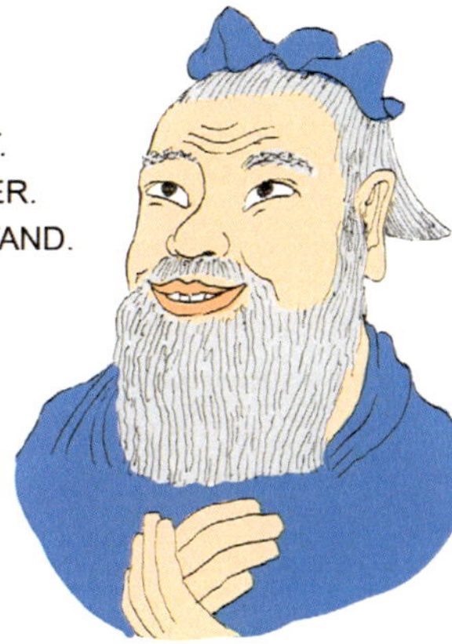

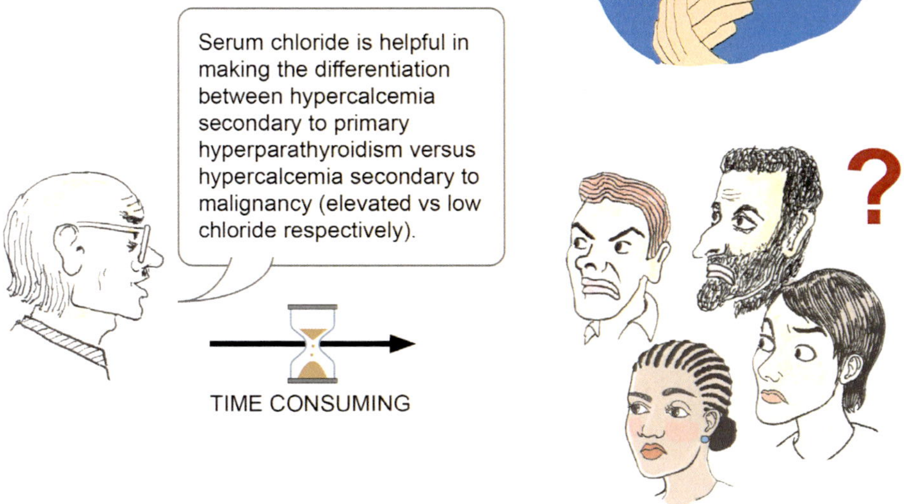

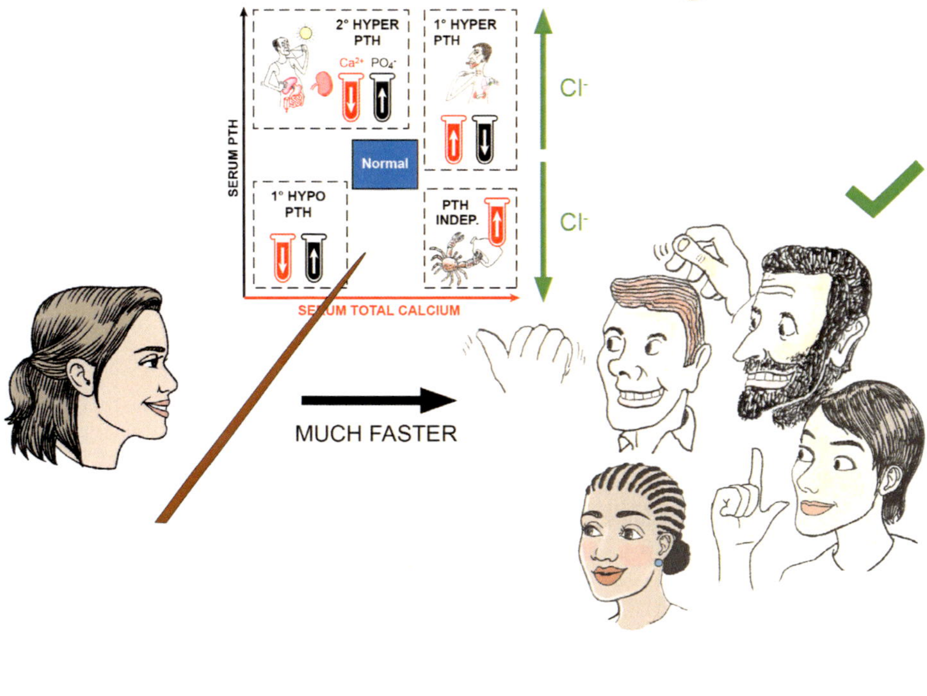

This book was inspired by a Japanese resident in one of the US residency training programs. His knowledge of medicine was legendary. Not only did he have sky-high scores on the annual In-Service exams, but even the attending physicians used to ask him occasionally for advice. When one of the attending physicians was asked to explain how a resident knew medicine so well, he answered: "He must have a system." However, his system was never revealed. This book is a humble attempt to provide a visual system in approaching the most common problems in internal medicine.

****

When, as a medical student, I admired the books of Prof. Radivoj V. Krstic, MD, Professor Emeritus of Histology and Embryology at the University of Lausanne, Switzerland, I could not have imagined that one day I would ask him to help illustrate my and my brother's book on internal medicine. Through his beautiful, self-taught scientific and medical drawings, he revealed to us an inner cosmos that had never been seen before (such as in the book: Krstic, R.V.; Human Microscopic Anatomy. An Atlas for Students of Medicine and Biology. Springer-Verlag Berlin Heidelberg New York London Paris Tokyo Hong Kong Barcelona Budapest, 1997).

As a resident of internal medicine, I thought how wonderful it would be if there were an internal medicine book drawn in the clear style of Prof. Krstic, in which one picture would summarize a differential diagnosis for a given symptom or sign. I mustered up the courage to ask him to transfer what he drew in the micro world to the macro clinical world. Prof. Krstic initially apologized that he was unable to help me because of his age (83). Nevertheless, he asked me to send him a rough draft of an illustration I had in mind so he could draw a couple of sketches. To my delight, Prof. Krstic embraced the idea of helping medical students and residents by illustrating our book. Because I really like his drawings, I asked him to help with an additional one. And then, like a child, when given a finger and reaches for the entire hand, with each new drawing, I asked for another one.

Little by little, the drawings accumulated over the course of four years. And when the illustrations were near completion, Prof. Krstic's health worsened, not only from his advanced age but also as a result of his constant eye strain working on different types of microscopes and hand tremors impacting his legendary accuracy. When he could no longer draw and revise his illustrations, I asked the talented Ms. Ellen Weiss to help Prof. Krstic complete the remaining drawings.

Any connection between the drawn characters and real people is unintentional and accidental, except for the first topic "Chest pain," where the figure depicts the illustrator of this book.

This book should not be used without exercising clinical judgment.

This book was created to educate those interested in the field of differential diagnoses and Dr. Trbovic encourages educators and students to use and adapt the illustrations in this book for educational purposes.

TOP 12 SYMPTOMS

1. CHEST PAIN
2. SHORTNESS OF BREATH
3. ACUTE GI HEMORRHAGE
4. ACUTE KIDNEY INJURY (AKI)
5. HYPERTENSION
6. HYPOTENSION
7. ABDOMINAL PAIN
8. ALTERED MENTAL STATUS
9. HEADACHE
10. FEVER
11. SYNCOPE
12. FALLS

CHEST PAIN

One of the most common reasons for visiting the emergency room (ER) for chest pain is panic attacks. However, "fast killers" should always be considered first: myocardial infarction (MI), pericardial tamponade, pulmonary embolus (PE), aortic dissection, pneumothorax and mediastinitis. Any abnormality in the vital signs is alarming, signaling that chest pain has a potentially serious cause.

Acute coronary syndrome results from hypoxia which leads to sudden chest pain. Angina pain (angina pectoris) is often described as tightness, squeezing, pressure, heaviness, or burning in the chest. Pain could spread to the arms, particularly to the left one, neck, jaw, shoulder, or back. **Stable** angina usually happens during exertion and disappears with rest or angina medications. The stable angina pain typically lasts five minutes or less. **Unstable** angina is unpredictable and occurs at rest. It is a medical emergency. It is typically severe and lasts longer than stable angina, often 20 minutes or longer. The pain does not go away with rest or the usual angina medications. **Variant angina** (**Prinz metal angina**) is not due to coronary artery disease, but rather due to spasms of the coronary arteries. It most often occurs in cycles, typically at rest and at night. The pain may be relieved by angina medications. Certain groups of people (patients with diabetes, women, and younger adults) may not have a classic chest pain but symptoms of dyspnea, weakness, nausea, vomiting, palpitations, or syncope.

Aortic dissection – Aortic dissection is rare but may be a surgical emergency. Patients with acute aortic dissection typically present with acute chest and back pain that is severe and sharp and may have a ripping or tearing quality. Pain can radiate anywhere in the chest or into the abdomen.

Cardiac tamponade symptoms are sudden and include chest pain, tachypnea, dyspnea, tachycardia with often muted heard sounds, jugular venous distension which could be associated with the venous distension in the forehead and scalp, and confusion.

Pulmonary embolism symptoms include dyspnea, chest pain, particularly upon inhalation and hemoptysis.

Aortic dissection symptoms may include sudden chest pain radiating to the neck (described as tearing), severe abdominal pain, dyspnea, paralysis of the leg and loss of consciousness.

Tension pneumothorax symptoms include sudden sharp chest pain, dyspnea, cyanosis, severe tachycardia and jugular vein distention. If left untreated, tension pneumothorax can rapidly progress to cardiovascular collapse (hypotension) and cardiac arrest.

Esophageal rupture, or perforation is associated with excruciating retrosternal chest pain. It can be caused by severe vomiting, foreign objects, corrosive substances, and surgical lesions. The patients with gastroesophageal reflux disease (GERD) or a hiatal hernia are at increased risk of esophageal tears.

If chest pain is elicited when pressing on the chest, this suggests **musculoskeletal etiology.** Chest pain due to **GERD** can mimic angina pectoris. (It can last from minutes to hours and resolves spontaneously or with antacids). Hypoxia due to anemia, such as from **sickle cell** disease can cause chest pain. **Takotsubo cardiomyopath**y (broken-heart syndrome) is a temporary condition characterized by a sudden enlargement of the heart muscles, usually caused by extreme emotional or physical stress. (For didactical reasons, the heart in the illustration is shifted to the right.)[1]

---

1 Abbreviations: COPD: chronic obstructive pulmonary disease. CAD: coronary artery disease. DZ: disease

CHEST PAIN

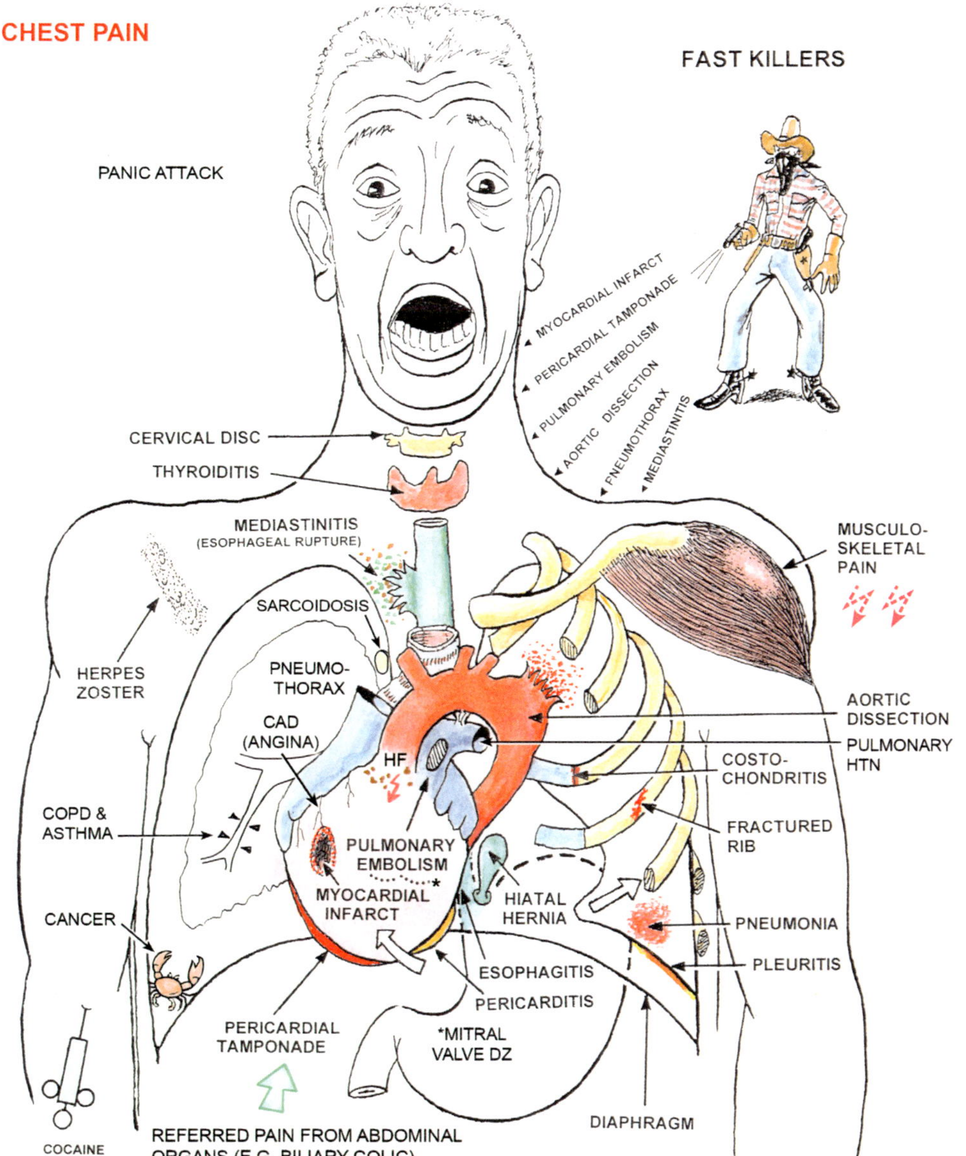

REFERRED PAIN FROM ABDOMINAL ORGANS (E.G. BILIARY COLIC) OR LIGAMENTS, MUSCLES AND PERIOSTEUM OF THE CERVICAL AND THORACIC SPINES

= STRESS (TAKOTSUBO) CARDIOMYOPATHY

= SICKLE CELL ANEMIA (ACUTE CHEST SYNDROME)

SHORTNESS OF BREATH

Normal oxygen saturation does not exclude the possibility of a serious disorder.

Central nervous system (CNS) disorders such as Amyotrophic lateral sclerosis (ALS) and multiple sclerosis (MS) can cause shortness of breath.

Restrictive lung disease (such as asbestosis, sarcoidosis or pulmonary fibrosis) are extrapulmonary, pleural, or parenchymal respiratory diseases that restrict lung expansion, due to a decrease in the elasticity of the lungs themselves, resulting in a decreased lung volume, an increased work of breathing, and inadequate ventilation and/or oxygenation.

Acute respiratory distress syndrome (ARDS) is a type of respiratory failure characterized by rapid onset of widespread inflammation in the lungs. Symptoms include dyspnea tachypnea and cyanosis.

The big "i" in the center of the picture represents myocardial infarction (MI).

Dyspnea in MI can occur in the absence of chest pain.

Pericardial tamponade should always be considered in a patient with right-sided heart failure without evidence of left-sided heart failure.

(The red arrows in the pulmonary artery represent increased pressure).

Audible stridor or wheezing can represent upper airway obstruction or severe bronchospasm, but congestive heart failure (CHF) could also cause wheezing.

Agitation, somnolence, or other alterations in mental status in the dyspneic patient suggests severe hypoxia or hypercarbia. Patients with a depressed mental status from carbon dioxide (CO_2) retention may look comfortable.

SHORTNESS OF BREATH

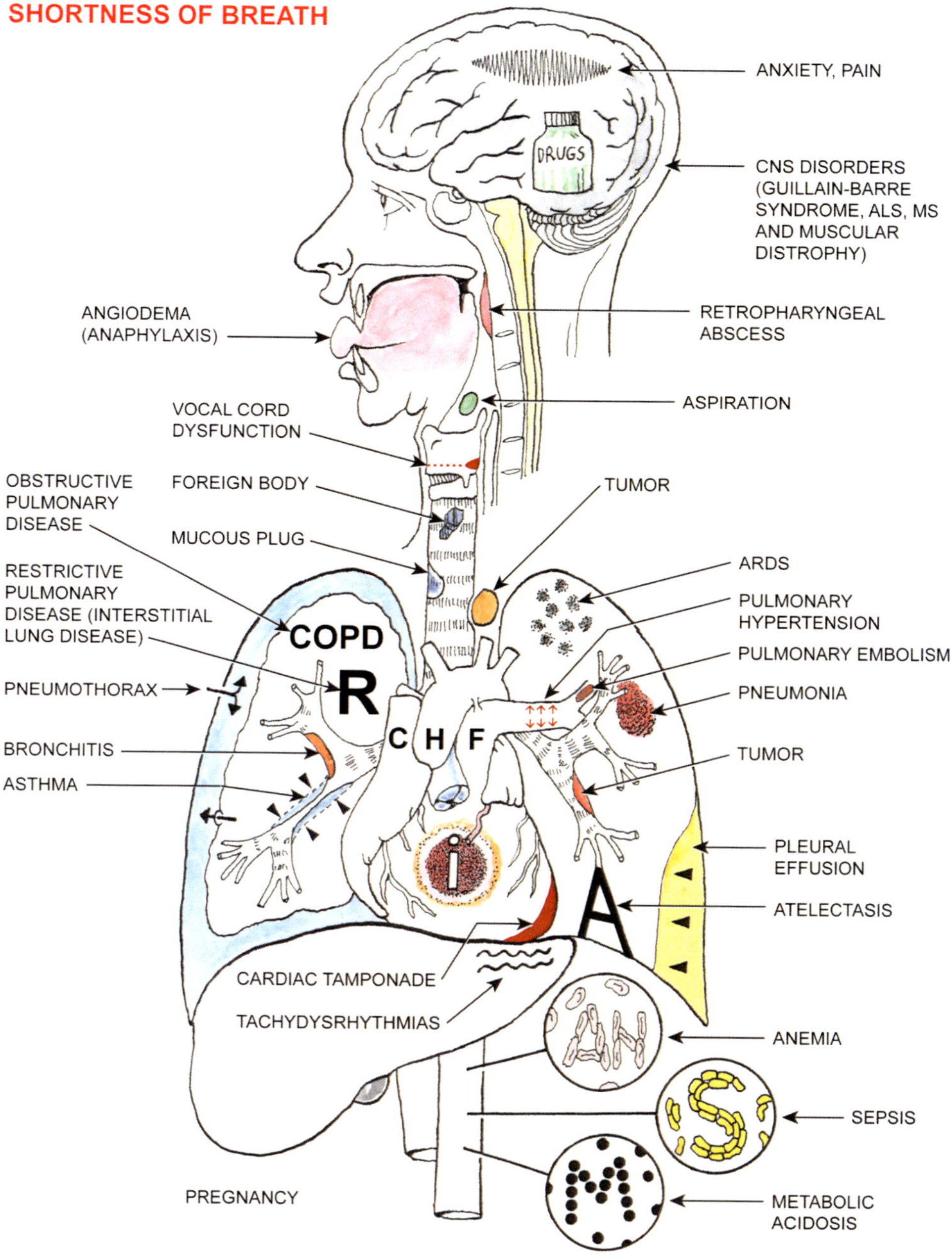

ACUTE GASTROINTESTINAL HEMORRHAGE

Hematemesis is blood in vomitus. It can also look like a "coffee ground." It represents an upper gastrointestinal (GI) hemorrhage.

Hematochezia is the blood in the stool. It is a consequence of a lower GI hemorrhage or a rapidly bleeding GI hemorrhage. In 10% of patients with hematochezia, the source is in the upper GI tract.

Melena is black-colored stool. It usually indicates upper GI hemorrhage, but small bowel and right-sided colonic hemorrhage can also produce it. Iron pills, spinach, blueberries, charcoal, and bismuth subsalicylate can produce melena.

Neovascularization (shown as NEO, NE in red, O in blue, representing newly formed arterial and venous vessels, respectively) in the GI tract can cause hemorrhage. **Ischemia** upregulates the vascular endothelial growth factor (VEGF) that stimulates neovascularization.

A patient on beta blockers might have a normal pulse regardless of a large volume loss. [2]

---

2 Abbreviations: ERCP: endoscopic retrograde cholangiopancreatography. NSAIDs: non-steroidal anti-inflammatory drugs

ACUTE GASTROINTESTINAL HEMORRHAGE

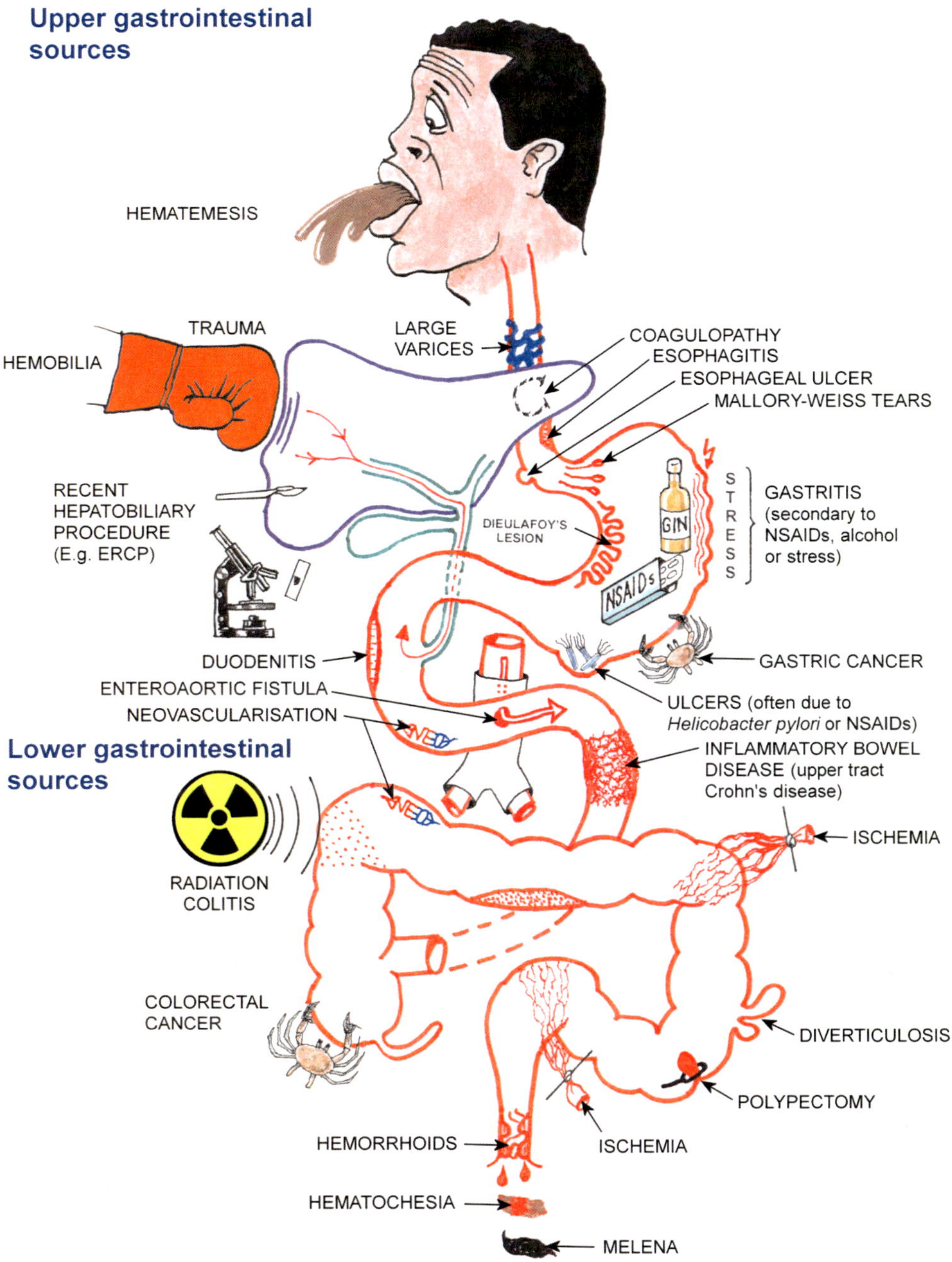

ACUTE KIDNEY INJURY (AKI)

AKI can result from several causes:

Prerenal causes ("pre-renal azotemia") are conditions that decrease effective blood flow to the kidney and cause a decrease in the glomerular filtration rate (GFR). They include aortic stenosis, right ventricular failure, mitral stenosis, decreased left ventricular function, hypotension, hypovolemia, renal artery stenosis, narrowing of the afferent arteriole, renal vein thrombosis, and end stage liver disease (ESLD). AKI is a frequent complication of ESLD, especially in those with acute-on-chronic liver failure, occurring in up to 50% of hospitalized patients with cirrhosis.

Renal causes include pathological processes which directly damage the kidney itself. Intrinsic AKI can be due to one or more of the kidney's structures including the glomeruli, kidney tubules, or the interstitium. Common causes of each are glomerulonephritis, acute tubular necrosis (ATN), and acute interstitial nephritis (AIN). Other causes of intrinsic AKI could be certain medication, rhabdomyolysis and tumor lysis syndrome.

Postrenal causes include disease conditions downstream of the kidney and most often occur as a consequence of urinary tract obstruction due to benign prostatic hyperplasia (BPH) renal stones, obstructed urinary catheter, or cancer of the bladder, ureters, or prostate.

The same disorder may cause more than one type of AKI. [3]

3 Abbreviations: MAHA: microangiopathic hemolytic anemia; NSAIDs: nonsteroidal anti-inflammatory drug; Uosm: urine osmolality; UNa: urine sodium concentration; FeNa: fractional excretion of sodium; BUN: blood urea nitrogen; Cr: creatinine.

ACUTE KIDNEY INJURY (AKI)

PRERENAL CAUSES
(60%-70% of AKI)

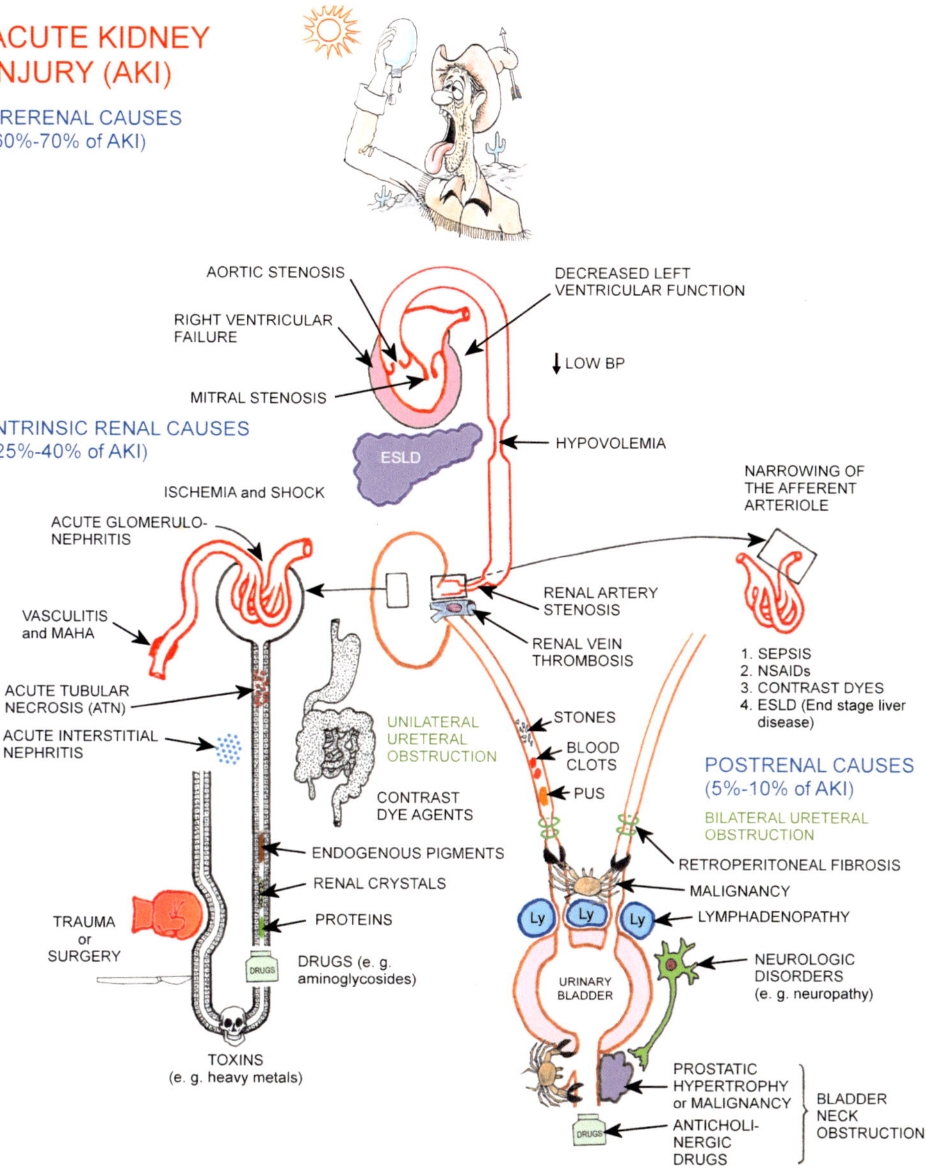

Classic laboratory findings in AKI				
Type	U_{Osm}	U_{Na}	Fe_{Na}	BUN/Cr
Prerenal	>500	<10	<1%	>20
Intrinsic	<350	>20	>2%	<15
Postrenal	<350	>40	>4%	>15

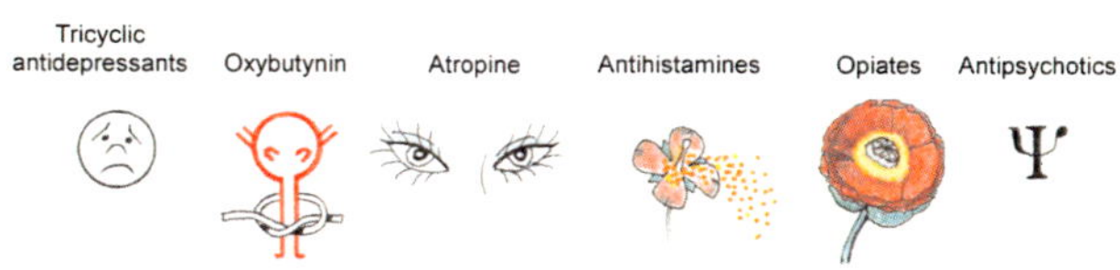

HYPERTENSION

Cushing's triad refers to a set of signs indicative of increased intracranial pressure and consists of bradycardia, irregular respirations, and hypertension.

Hutchinson's pupil is a clinical sign in which the pupil on the side of an intracranial mass lesion is dilated and unreactive to light, due to compression of the oculomotor nerve on that side.

The long bone (femur), rich in calcium, symbolizes hypercalcemia.

Renal artery stenosis as the cause of hypertension should be considered when a patient shows a dramatic increase in serum creatinine after starting angiotensin converting enzyme (ACE) inhibitor therapy.

Primary hyperaldosteronism should be suspected if a hypertensive patient is hypokalemic and not taking diuretics.

With respect to the picture of the family history of hypertension, it could be noticed one face in the family tree is very similar to the man who is eating in front of the TV. However, there are lots of slender patients with genetic predisposition to hypertension. [4]

4 Abbreviations: CPAP: continuous positive airway pressure.

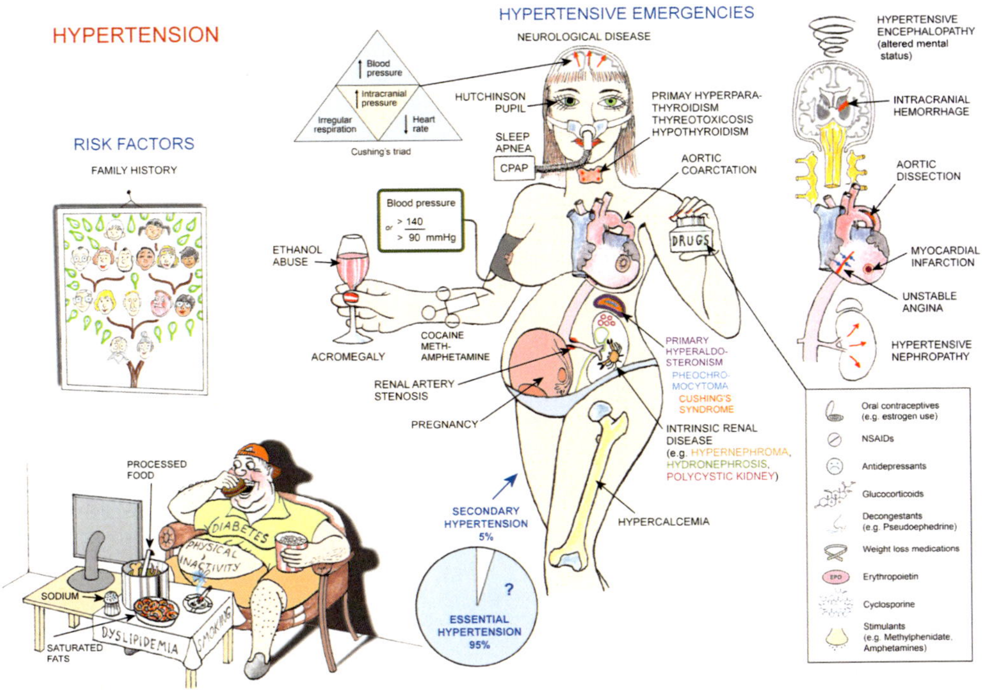
HYPERTENSION
RISK FACTORS
FAMILY HISTORY
PROCESSED FOOD
DIABETES
PHYSICAL INACTIVITY
SODIUM
SATURATED FATS
DYSLIPIDEMIA
SMOKING
HYPERTENSIVE EMERGENCIES
NEUROLOGICAL DISEASE
Blood pressure
Intracranial pressure
Irregular respiration
Heart rate
Cushing's triad
HUTCHINSON PUPIL
SLEEP APNEA
CPAP
PRIMAY HYPERPARA-THYROIDISM
THYREOTOXICOSIS
HYPOTHYROIDISM
AORTIC COARCTATION
Blood pressure
> 140 or > 90 mmHg
ETHANOL ABUSE
DRUGS
ACROMEGALY
COCAINE
METH-AMPHETAMINE
RENAL ARTERY STENOSIS
PREGNANCY
PRIMARY HYPERALDO-STERONISM
PHEOCHRO-MOCYTOMA
CUSHING'S SYNDROME
INTRINSIC RENAL DISEASE
(e.g. HYPERNEPHROMA, HYDRONEPHROSIS, POLYCYSTIC KIDNEY)
HYPERCALCEMIA
SECONDARY HYPERTENSION 5%
?
ESSENTIAL HYPERTENSION 95%
HYPERTENSIVE ENCEPHALOPATHY (altered mental status)
INTRACRANIAL HEMORRHAGE
AORTIC DISSECTION
MYOCARDIAL INFARCTION
UNSTABLE ANGINA
HYPERTENSIVE NEPHROPATHY
Oral contraceptives (e.g. estrogen use)
NSAIDs
Antidepressants
Glucocorticoids
Decongestants (e.g. Pseudoephedrine)
Weight loss medications
EPO
Erythropoietin
Cyclosporine
Stimulants (e.g. Methylphenidate, Amphetamines)

“The visual arts are an important part of a comprehensive education, promoting creativity, critical thinking, problem solving, and innovation.”

National Art Education Association

HYPERTENSION

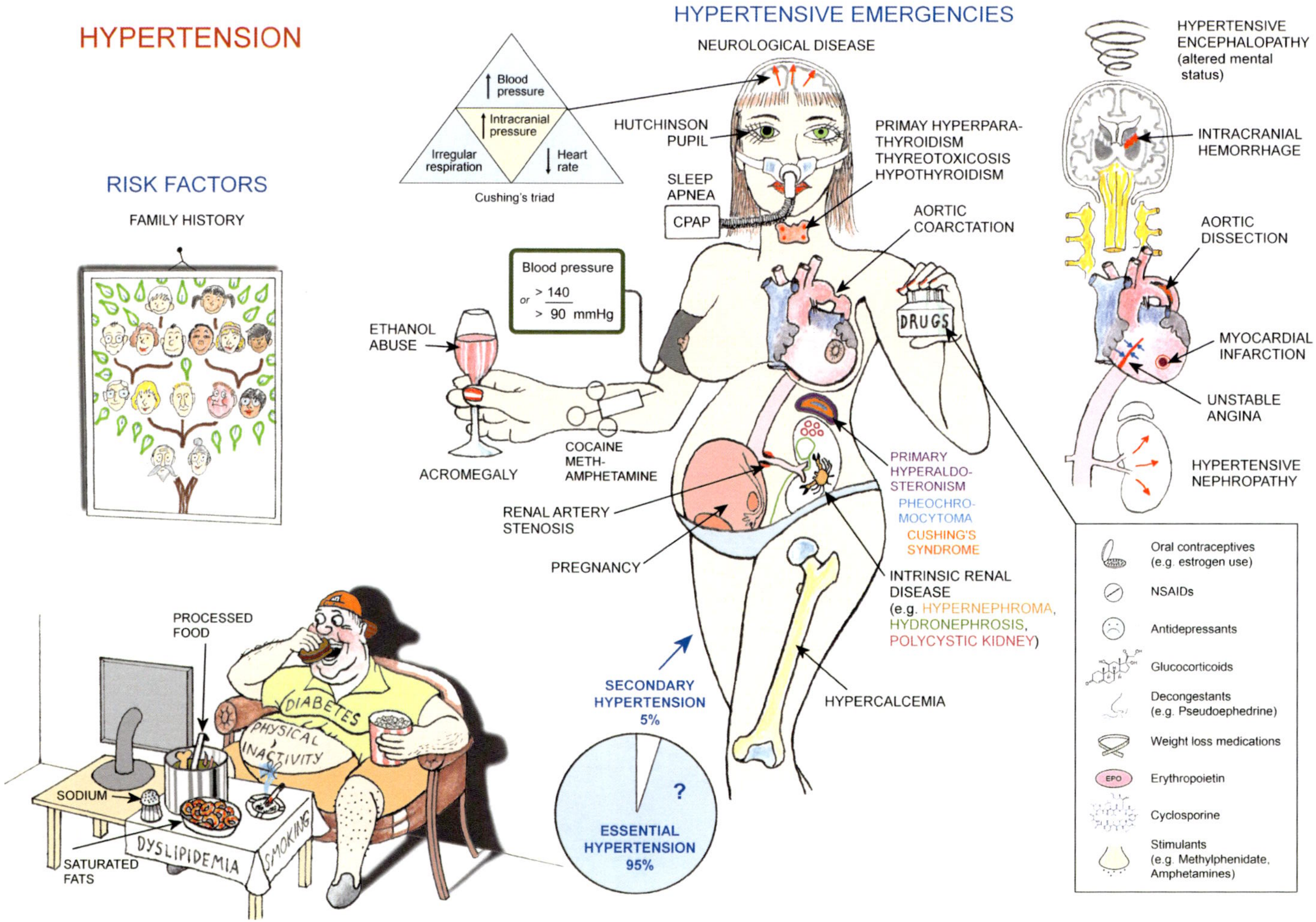

HYPOTENSION

The patient with hypotension should be approached in the **clockwise direction** in the schematic, with the **heart** being the starting point (1), then **hypovolemia** (2), then the **capillary level** (distributive shock, which could be septic and non-septic) (3), and then pulmonary embolus **(PE)** (4). Above the capillaries are **endocrine causes** (5).

An **amniotic fluid embolism** is a very uncommon obstetric emergency in which amniotic fluid enters the circulation of the mother, causing cardiorespiratory collapse and massive coagulopathy.

Fat embolism is caused by the presence of fat globules in the pulmonary circulation. It usually follows the fracture of major bones (like the pelvis or the leg bones).

Beriberi due to thiamine (vitamin B1) deficiency has two clinical presentations: patients with dry beriberi present with neuropathy, while those with wet beriberi present with heart failure, with or without neuropathy.

The red woman ("hot woman") represents sever acidosis which can cause hypotension. (When blue litmus paper is placed in a substance that is acidic, it turns red.) The snowflake in her hand represents the fact that severe hypothermia (body temperature below 30°C [86°F]) is associated with marked depression of the cerebral blood flow and oxygen requirement, reduced cardiac output, and hypotension.

Neurogenic shock is a distributive type of shock resulting in hypotension, often with bradycardia caused by disruption of autonomic nervous system pathways in conditions such as spinal cord injury or traumatic brain injury (TBI). The woman near the patient with the spinal cord injury is calling for help. She holds in her hand a phone, while in the other a snowflake, warning that sometimes patients with hypotension (e.g., drown victims in the cold water) can appear to be clinically dead because of marked depression of brain function, but are still alive, and resuscitation should continue until death is truly confirmed.

Abdominal compartment syndrome occurs when intra-abdominal pressure rises (e.g., in sepsis or severe abdominal trauma) and is sustained at > 20 mmHg. Increasing pressure reduces blood flow to abdominal organs and impairs pulmonary, cardiovascular, renal, and gastrointestinal (GI) function, causing obstructive shock.

The **diver** represents decompression sickness (also called caisson disease). It is caused by dissolved gases emerging from the solution as bubbles inside the body tissues during decompression.

Air trapping is an abnormal retention of air in the lungs where it is difficult to exhale completely. Auto-positive end-expiratory pressure (PEEP) is usually caused by air trapping that results from an inadequate expiratory time, patient-ventilator asynchrony, high respiratory rate, and high minute ventilation. Air trapping can cause overinflation of the lungs, with subsequent compression on the intrathoracic blood vessels and hypotension. [5]

---

5 Abbreviations: SIRS: systemic inflammatory response syndrome.

HYPOTENSION/SHOCK

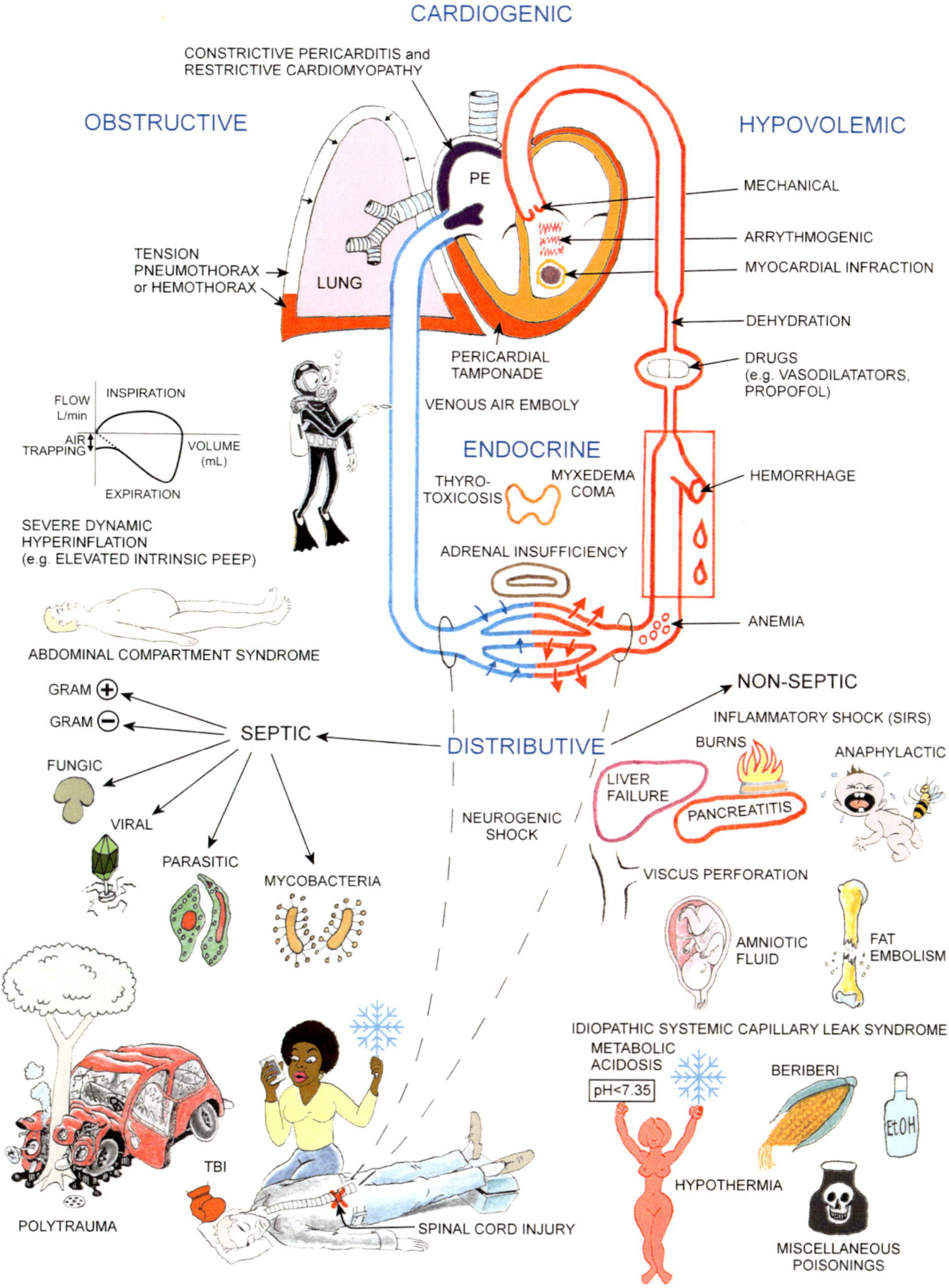

ABDOMINAL PAIN

The most common causes of abdominal pain are not serious, such as gas pains, indigestion or stretched muscles. However, the serious causes should be considered.

1. **Infection**, **obstruction** and **ischemia** may cause abdominal pain in any intra-abdominal organ.
2. **Referred pain** from thorax and pelvis can present as abdominal pain.
3. **Metabolic** and **systemic causes** can cause abdominal pain.

Burning pain is typical of GERD and peptic ulcer disease.

Colicky pain starts and stops abruptly. It occurs due to muscular contractions of a hollow tube (small and large intestine, gall bladder, ureter) to relieve an obstruction. The pain of biliary or renal colic or acute mesenteric ischemia is very strong, while the pain of gastroenteritis is of lesser intensity. (Abrupt onset of midline pain that is out of proportion to the physical exam is suggestive of mesenteric ischemia.)

The pain of chronic mesenteric ischemia usually starts within one hour of eating, while duodenal ulcers may be relieved by eating and recur several hours after a meal. Eating might relieve duodenal ulcer pain because food neutralizes stomach acid; certain foods (such as oatmeal or pears) help protect the ulcer by coating the stomach lining, and the food increases blood flow to the stomach, which can reduce inflammation in the area.

The pain of pancreatitis is typically relieved by sitting up and leaning forward. Peritonitis often causes patients to lie still on their backs because any motion causes pain.

Symptoms such as fevers, chills, fatigue, weight loss, and anorexia would be concerning for infection, malignancy, or systemic illnesses (e.g., inflammatory bowel disease).

Symptoms such as cough, dyspnea, orthopnea, and exertional dyspnea suggest pulmonary or cardiac etiology.

Orthostatic hypotension may indicate early shock or be associated with adrenal insufficiency.

Patients with diabetic ketoacidosis (DKA) will have symptoms of polyuria and thirst.

A patient taking corticosteroids and elderly may have significant masking of pain. [6]

---

6 Abbreviations: RUQ: right upper quadrant; LUQ: left upper quadrant; RLQ: right lower quadrant; LLQ: left lower quadrant.

ABDOMINAL PAIN

1. ABDOMINAL ORGANS

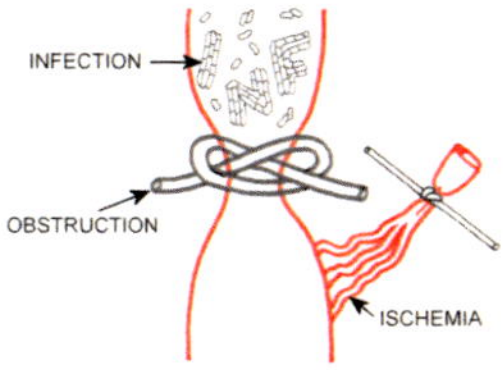

LOCATION

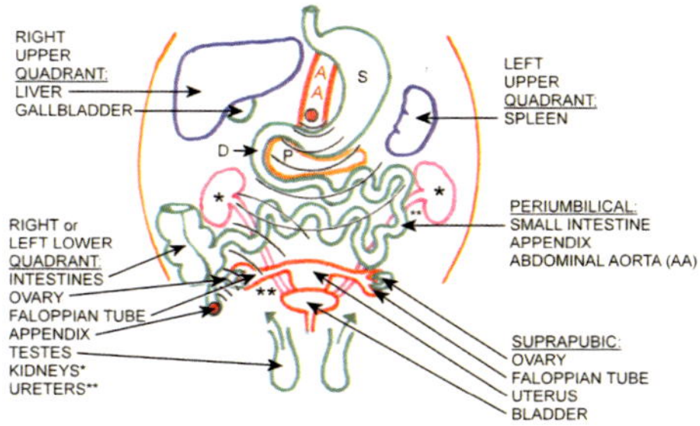

2. REFERRED PAIN FROM THE THORAX AND PELVIS

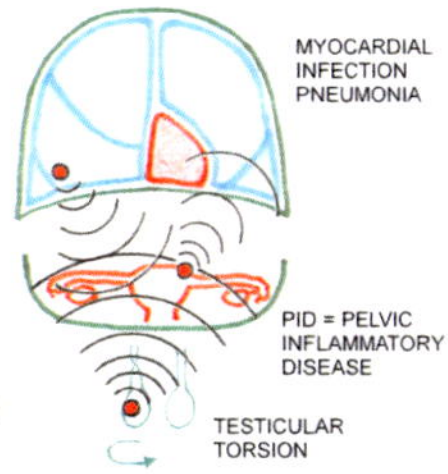

3. METABOLIC AND SYSTEMIC CAUSES

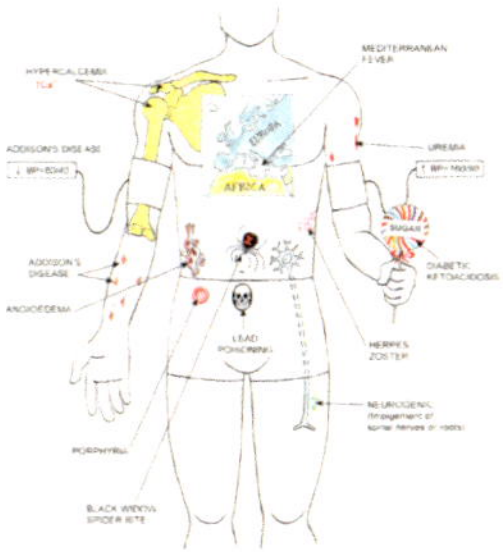

ABDOMINAL QUADRANTS

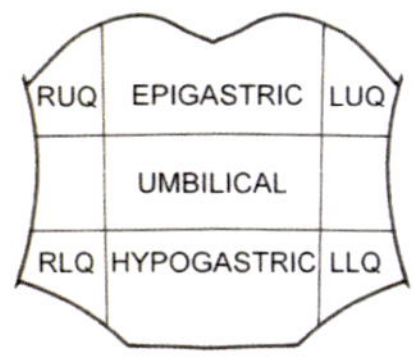

“One day replaces three if one does everything on time.”

Chinese proverb

ABDOMINAL PAIN

1. ABDOMINAL ORGANS

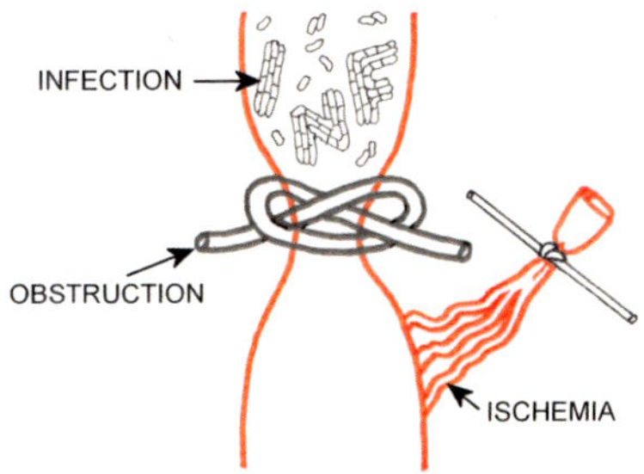

LOCATION

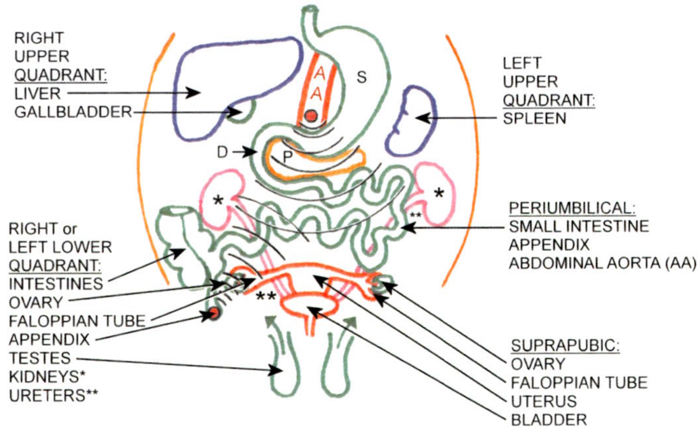

2. REFERRED PAIN FROM THE THORAX AND PELVIS

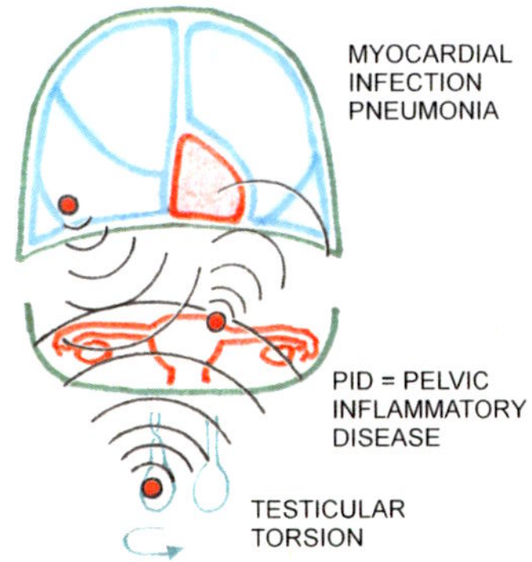

3. METABOLIC AND SYSTEMIC CAUSES

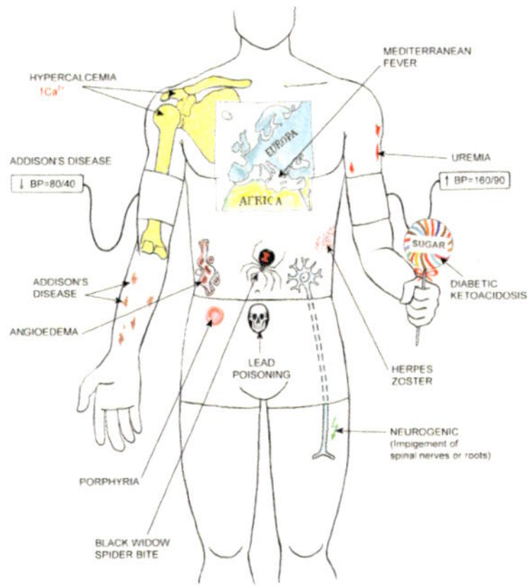

ABDOMINAL QUADRANTS

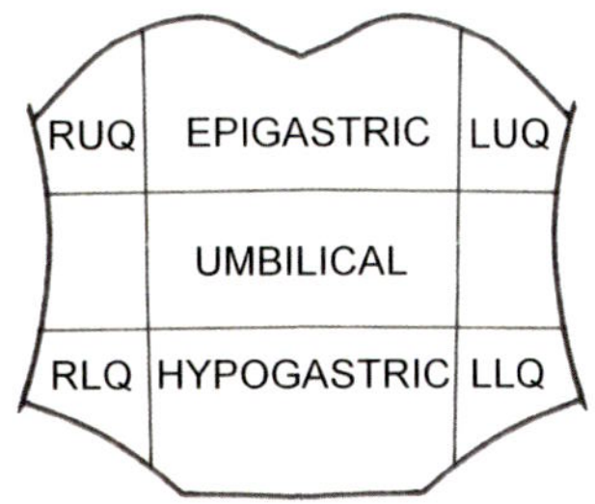

ABDOMINAL PAIN CONTINUED

A tattoo map on the patient's chest in the illustration shows the Mediterranean Sea. Familial **Mediterranean fever** is an inherited autoinflammatory syndrome characterized by recurrent short episodes of high fever associated with abdominal pain, arthritis and skin rash.

The bones rich in calcium represent hypercalcemia. Symptoms of **hypercalcemia** range from nonexistent to severe and can include stomach pain (nausea, vomiting and constipation).

Symptoms of **Addison's disease** usually develop gradually, often over months, but sometimes appear suddenly. Acute adrenal failure can lead to severe pain in the lower back or legs with vomiting and diarrhea. (The latter can be associated with life-threatening dehydration and shock, severe weakness, confusion, altered mental status or delirium, and skin hyperpigmentation.)

The sugar candy which the patient is holding represents diabetic ketoacidosis (**DKA**). Abdominal pain is a frequent DKA manifestation and presents in 40-75% of the cases. Its prevalence increases as arterial pH and serum bicarbonate levels decline.

Angioedema typically causes facial edema, affecting especially the eyes, mouth, lips and tongue, but can also cause digestive problems, including abdominal pain, diarrhea, nausea and vomiting (as well as edema of the hands, feet or genitals).

The most common form of acute **porphyria** (acute intermittent porphyria) may last hours or days and may include severe abdominal pain (and pain in the chest, legs, back, and muscles, as well as red or brown urine mental changes, including anxiety and hallucinations, cardiac arrhythmias, dyspnea, hypertension and seizures).

Common causes of abdominal wall pain include **nerve impingement**, hernia, and surgical or procedural complications. Anterior cutaneous nerve entrapment syndrome is the most common and frequently missed type of abdominal wall pain. It typically presents with acute or chronic localized pain at the lateral edge of the rectus abdominis that worsens with position changes or increased abdominal muscle tension. A positive Carnett test, in which tenderness stays the same or worsens when the patient tenses the abdominal muscles, suggests abdominal wall pain. Abdominal wall pain is often mistaken for intra-abdominal visceral pain, resulting in expensive and unnecessary laboratory tests, imaging studies, consultations, and invasive procedures.

3. METABOLIC AND SYSTEMIC CAUSES

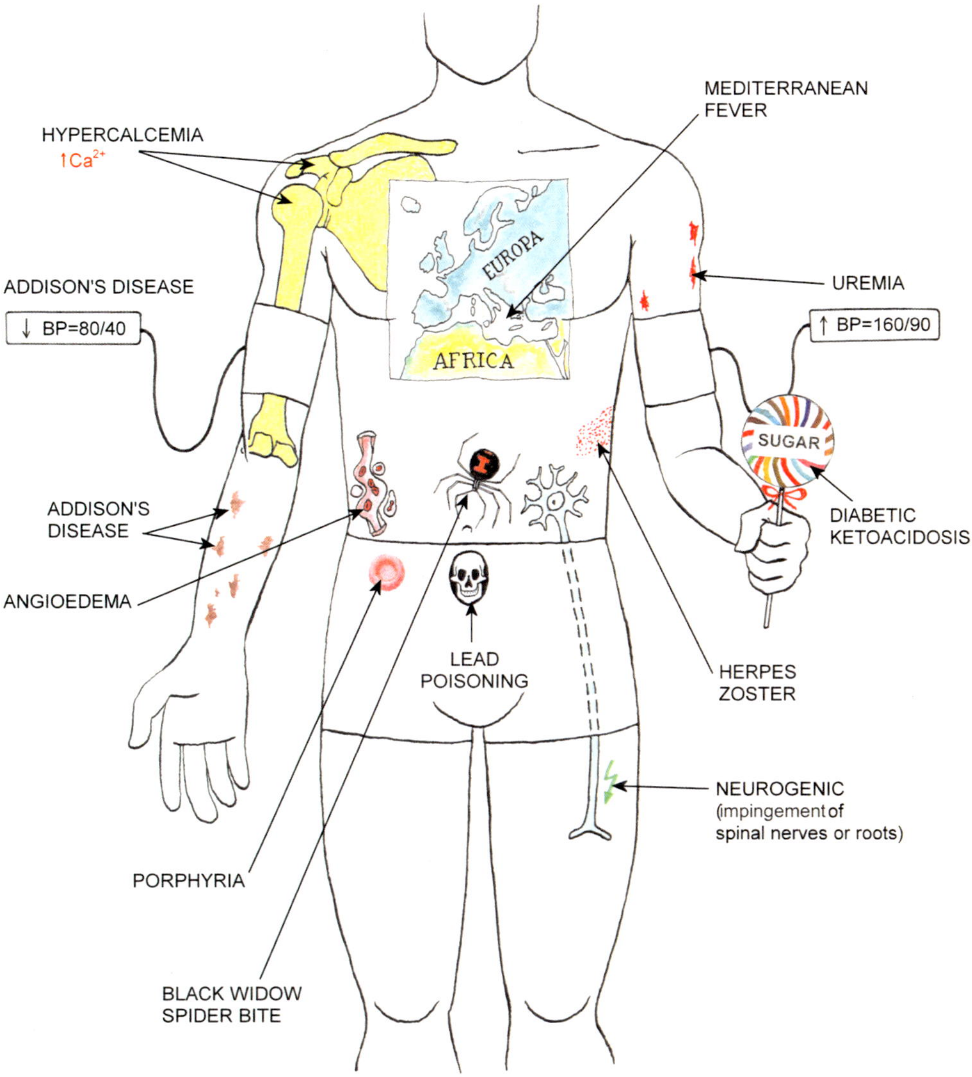

ALTERED MENTAL STATUS

The blister pack of drugs represents the most common drugs which can cause altered mental status.

Hallucinogens such as lysergic acid diethylamide (LSD) and phencyclidine (PCP) are known to significantly alter mental status by affecting perception, mood, and thought patterns.

Arrows pointing down represent withdrawals from the medications such as benzodiazepines and selective serotonin reuptake inhibitors (SSRI), or alcohol. On the other hand, too much serotonin can cause altered mental status through serotonin syndrome.

The patient's eyes are "looking" toward the lesion where a cerebrovascular accident happened.

The antibiotic family of quinolones is represented as the bacterial DNA gyrase (and topoisomerase IV), the enzyme targeted by quinolones. The inhibition of the gyrases normal function by quinolones leads to the formation of a toxic complex that causes lethal DNA fragmentation in the bacteria.

The right lower part of the picture represents the "psychedelic quadrant". The vampire represents porphyria. **In a certain type of porphyria (due to high levels of porphyrins), sun exposure results in painful skin burning, irritation and swelling.** Therefore, the vampire has an umbrella on his head to prevent exposure to the sun. He also holds a muffler in his hand, representing CO poisoning, such as due to car exhaustion, and has a Kaiser-Fleisher ring, a dark ring encircling the cornea of the eye, due to excessive deposits of copper in Wilson's disease.

The tablecloth has blue dots on it, representing lymphocytes, i.e., inflammation, and the legs of the table represent collagen.[7]

---

7 Abbreviations: LSD: Lysergic acid diethylamide; PCP: Phencyclidine; DHT: Dobhoff tube; NGT: Nasogastric tube; SLE: systemic lupus erythematosus.

ALTERED MENTAL STATUS

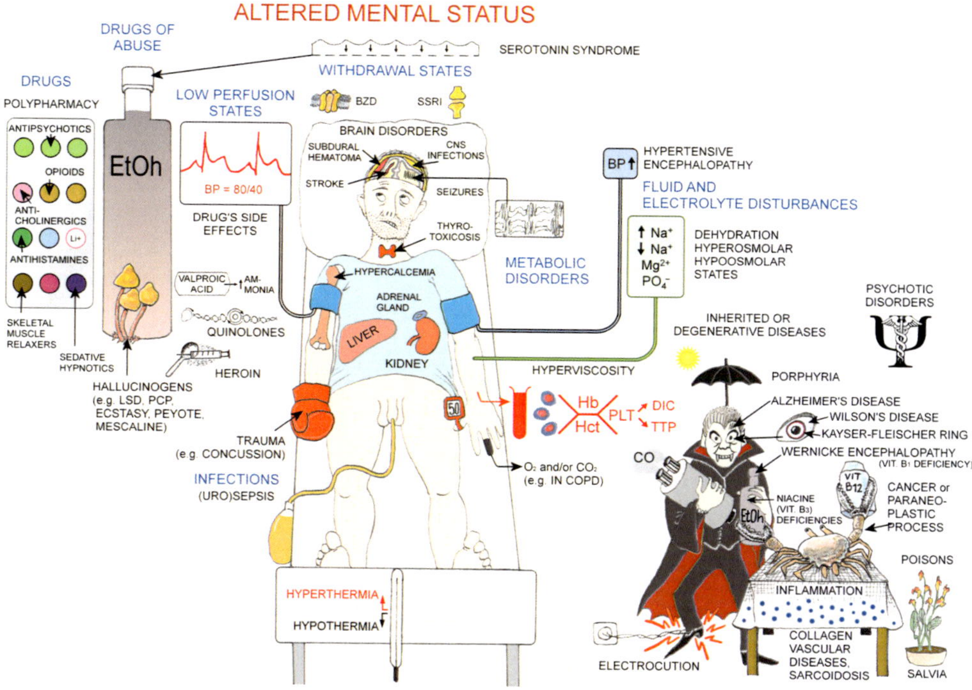

“Speaking is not seeing.”

Arabic wisdom

ALTERED MENTAL STATUS

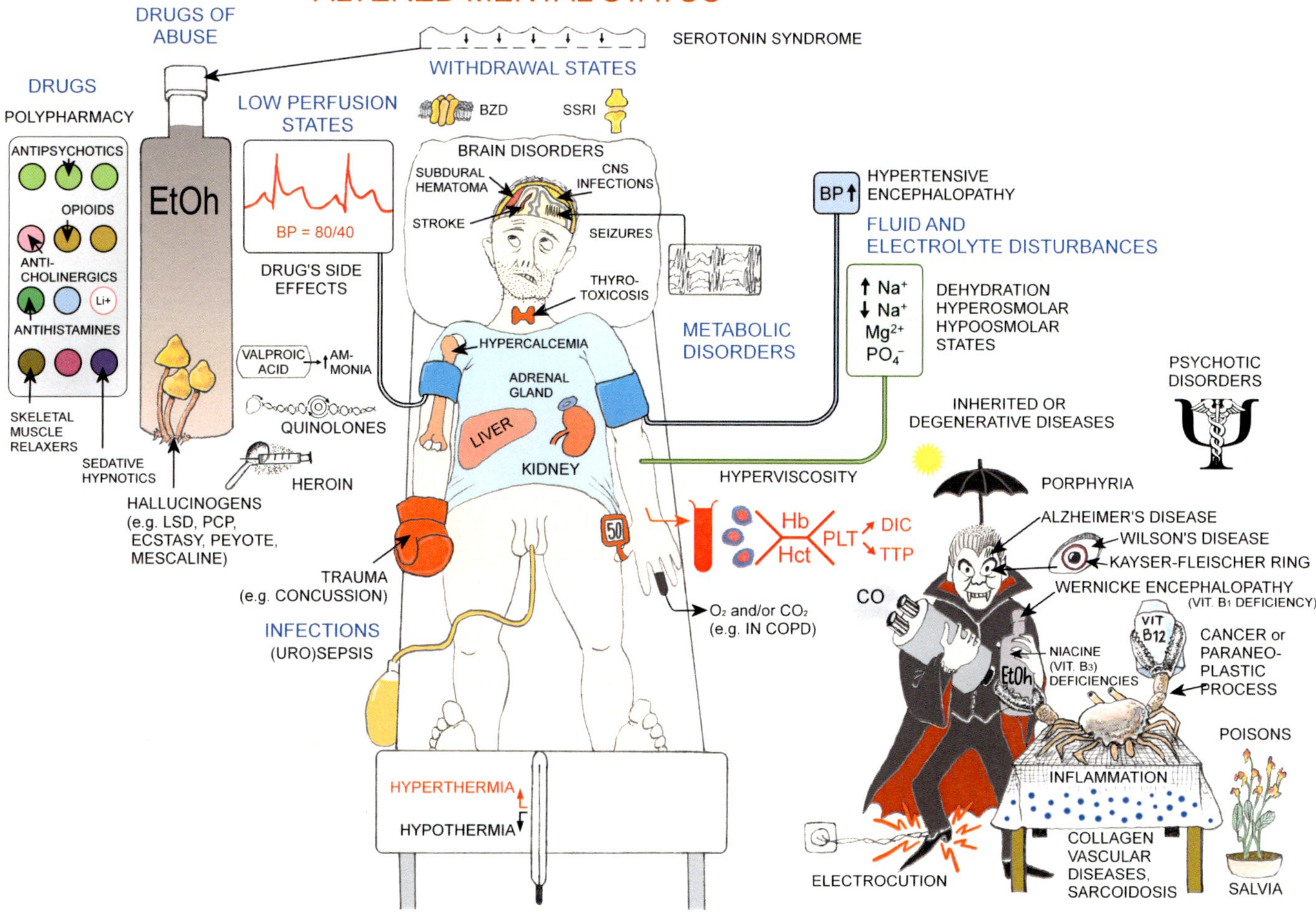

HEADACHE

90% of all headaches are **primary** (not caused by another medical condition) headaches, while **10%** are **secondary** ones (caused by some underlying medical condition). The secondary headaches are more worrisome because they may represent conditions like tumor, stroke or infection.

Cluster headaches are usually associated with severe pain and last 15–180 minutes. They are usually focal around one eye and are associated with autonomic symptoms like red eye, tearing and nasal congestion. This cluster of symptoms usually occurs at the same time every day. The knife represents a stabbing pain. Such headaches are short lasting (1 second to several minutes) and are without autonomic symptoms.

Primary **sex headaches** are dull and bilateral and start during sexual activity. They become much worse during orgasm. (These headaches are assumed to be due to lower pressure in the head during sex). However, such headaches may be due to a subarachnoid hemorrhage, and this needs to be ruled out first.

The witch hitting the head of the patient and watching the time represents a **hypnic headache**. It usually presents in older women, is of moderate-to-severe intensity, and lasts 15–30 minutes. It starts a few hours after falling asleep and may recur several times during the night.

The primary headaches are "framed" with the conditions that might trigger them. The picture representing "crisis" shows a man with empty pockets, indicating financial difficulties.

Temporal arteritis is a medical emergency which could result in blindness. It is an inflammatory disease affecting the large and medium-sized arteries, typically in the head and neck, and classically the temporal arteries. It is common in the elderly (average age 70) and often associated with fever, headache, weight loss, jaw claudication, tender vessels by the temples, and polymyalgia rheumatica.

Increased intraocular pressure (IOP) can sometimes lead to headaches, especially if the pressure rises suddenly. This condition is often associated with glaucoma. When IOP increases acutely, it can cause symptoms like dull or aching headaches, blurred vision, perception of colored halos around lights, and sometimes nausea or vomiting. **Idiopathic intracranial hypertension (IIH)** is caused by an elevation of intracranial pressure (ICP). The condition mainly affects obese young women of childbearing age. The accurate diagnosis of IIH is essential as visual deterioration due to papilledema may be irreversible.

Analgesic rebound headache happens after discontinuation of a pain killer. Headaches due to **hypertension** are usually located in the occipital region of the head. **Lumbar puncture** can be associated with a strong headache.

SNOOP represents a mnemonic for the "red flags" for identifying a dangerous secondary headache. They include:

- Systemic symptoms (fever or weight loss)
- Systemic disease (HIV infection, malignancy)
- Neurologic symptoms or signs
- Onset sudden (thunderclap headache)
- Onset after age 40 years
- Previous headache history (first, worst, or different headache)

HEADACHE

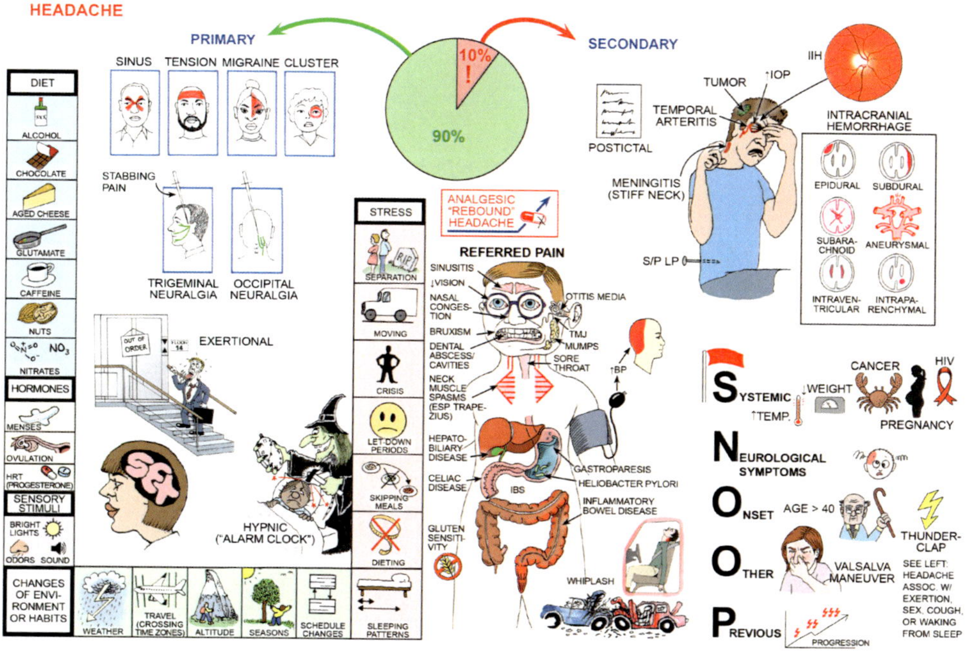

PRIMARY
SECONDARY
10% !
90%
SINUS
TENSION
MIGRAINE
CLUSTER
STABBING PAIN
TRIGEMINAL NEURALGIA
OCCIPITAL NEURALGIA
EXERTIONAL
OUT OF ORDER
HYPNIC ("ALARM CLOCK")
DIET
ALCOHOL
CHOCOLATE
AGED CHEESE
GLUTAMATE
CAFFEINE
NUTS
NO3
NITRATES
HORMONES
MENSES
OVULATION
HRT (PROGESTERONE)
SENSORY STIMULI
BRIGHT LIGHTS
ODORS
SOUND
CHANGES OF ENVIRONMENT OR HABITS
WEATHER
TRAVEL (CROSSING TIME ZONES)
ALTITUDE
SEASONS
SCHEDULE CHANGES
SLEEPING PATTERNS
STRESS
SEPARATION
MOVING
CRISIS
LET-DOWN PERIODS
SKIPPING MEALS
DIETING
ANALGESIC "REBOUND" HEADACHE
REFERRED PAIN
SINUSITIS
↓VISION
NASAL CONGESTION
BRUXISM
DENTAL ABSCESS/ CAVITIES
NECK MUSCLE SPASMS (ESP TRAPEZIUS)
HEPATOBILIARY DISEASE
CELIAC DISEASE
GLUTEN SENSITIVITY
OTITIS MEDIA
TMJ
MUMPS
SORE THROAT
↑BP
GASTROPARESIS
HELIOBACTER PYLORI
IBS
INFLAMMATORY BOWEL DISEASE
WHIPLASH
POSTICTAL
TUMOR
↑IOP
IIH
TEMPORAL ARTERITIS
MENINGITIS (STIFF NECK)
S/P LP
INTRACRANIAL HEMORRHAGE
EPIDURAL
SUBDURAL
SUBARACHNOID
ANEURYSMAL
INTRAVENTRICULAR
INTRAPARENCHYMAL
SYSTEMIC
↓WEIGHT
↑TEMP.
CANCER
HIV
PREGNANCY
NEUROLOGICAL SYMPTOMS
ONSET
AGE > 40
THUNDERCLAP
OTHER
VALSALVA MANEUVER
SEE LEFT: HEADACHE ASSOC. W/ EXERTION, SEX, COUGH, OR WAKING FROM SLEEP
PREVIOUS
PROGRESSION

“There are three classes of people:
those who see,
those who see when they are shown,
those who do not see.”

Leonardo da Vinci

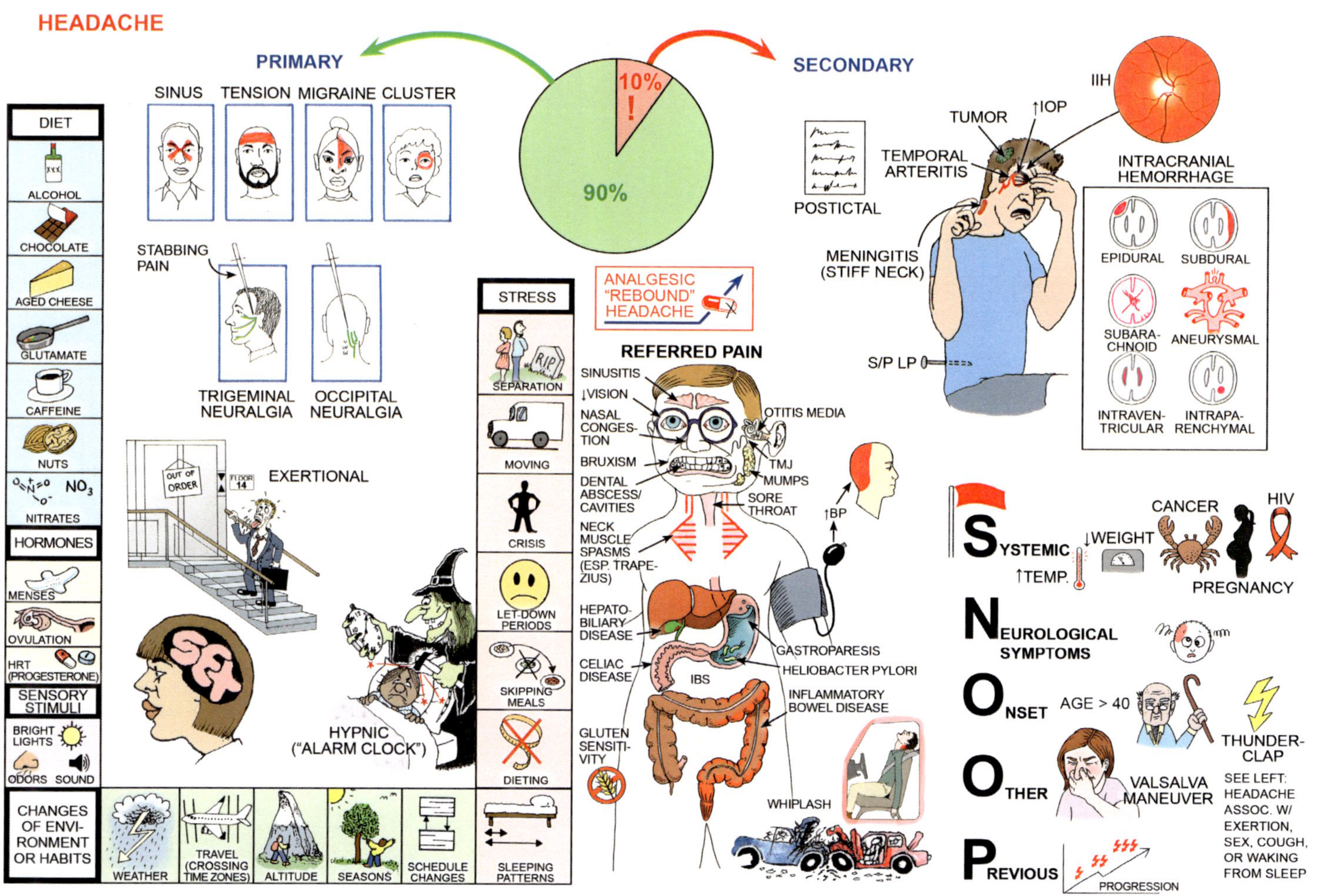
HEADACHE
PRIMARY
SECONDARY
10%
!
90%
SINUS
TENSION
MIGRAINE
CLUSTER
STABBING PAIN
TRIGEMINAL NEURALGIA
OCCIPITAL NEURALGIA
EXERTIONAL
OUT OF ORDER
FLOOR 14
HYPNIC ("ALARM CLOCK")
DIET
ALCOHOL
CHOCOLATE
AGED CHEESE
GLUTAMATE
CAFFEINE
NUTS
NO3
NITRATES
HORMONES
MENSES
OVULATION
HRT (PROGESTERONE)
SENSORY STIMULI
BRIGHT LIGHTS
ODORS
SOUND
CHANGES OF ENVI-RONMENT OR HABITS
WEATHER
TRAVEL (CROSSING TIME ZONES)
ALTITUDE
SEASONS
SCHEDULE CHANGES
SLEEPING PATTERNS
STRESS
SEPARATION
RIP
MOVING
CRISIS
LET-DOWN PERIODS
SKIPPING MEALS
DIETING
ANALGESIC "REBOUND" HEADACHE
REFERRED PAIN
SINUSITIS
↓VISION
NASAL CONGES-TION
BRUXISM
DENTAL ABSCESS/ CAVITIES
NECK MUSCLE SPASMS (ESP. TRAPE-ZIUS)
HEPATO-BILIARY DISEASE
CELIAC DISEASE
GLUTEN SENSITI-VITY
OTITIS MEDIA
TMJ
MUMPS
SORE THROAT
↑BP
GASTROPARESIS
HELIOBACTER PYLORI
IBS
INFLAMMATORY BOWEL DISEASE
WHIPLASH
POSTICTAL
TUMOR
↑IOP
IIH
TEMPORAL ARTERITIS
MENINGITIS (STIFF NECK)
S/P LP
INTRACRANIAL HEMORRHAGE
EPIDURAL
SUBDURAL
SUBARA-CHNOID
ANEURYSMAL
INTRAVEN-TRICULAR
INTRAPA-RENCHYMAL
SYSTEMIC
↑TEMP.
↓WEIGHT
CANCER
HIV
PREGNANCY
NEUROLOGICAL SYMPTOMS
ONSET
AGE > 40
THUNDER-CLAP
OTHER
VALSALVA MANEUVER
SEE LEFT: HEADACHE ASSOC. W/ EXERTION, SEX, COUGH, OR WAKING FROM SLEEP
PREVIOUS
PROGRESSION

FEVER

The picture is self-explanatory.

Fever of unknown origin (FUO) criteria:

- Fever higher than 38.3°C on several occasions
- Duration of fever for at least three weeks
- Uncertain diagnosis after one week of study in the hospital

Certain patients (elderly, immunocompromised, those on steroids, or NSAIDs) may not have a fever, even in the presence of severe infection.

Hypothermia often indicates the presence of an overwhelming infection and should be evaluated systematically as hyperthermia.

The fever should be assumed to be due to infection, unless proven otherwise, because infection causes most of the fevers and can be life-threatening.

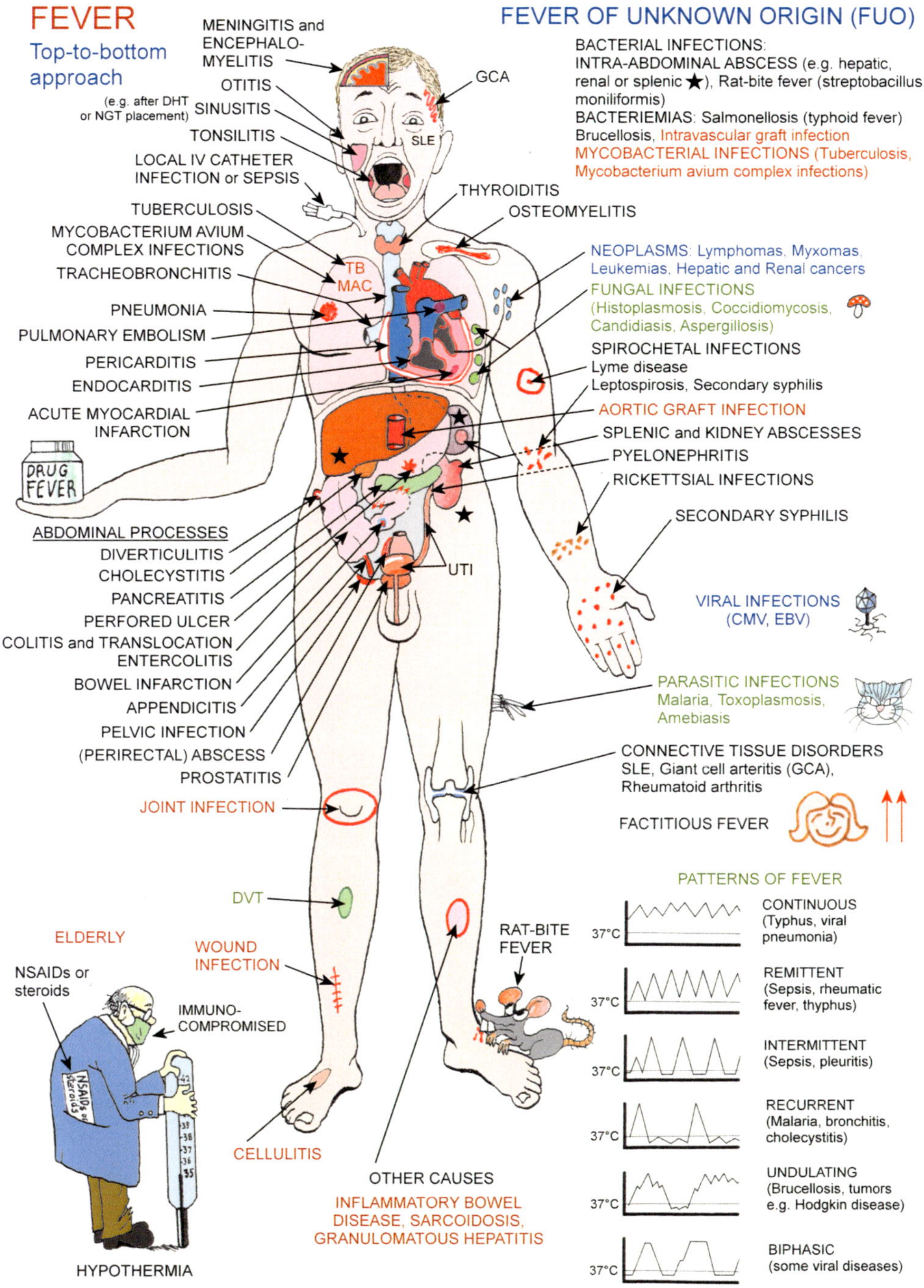
FEVER
Top-to-bottom approach
MENINGITIS and ENCEPHALO-MYELITIS
OTITIS
(e.g. after DHT or NGT placement) SINUSITIS
TONSILITIS
LOCAL IV CATHETER INFECTION or SEPSIS
GCA
SLE
TUBERCULOSIS
MYCOBACTERIUM AVIUM COMPLEX INFECTIONS
TRACHEOBRONCHITIS
TB
MAC
THYROIDITIS
OSTEOMYELITIS
PNEUMONIA
PULMONARY EMBOLISM
PERICARDITIS
ENDOCARDITIS
ACUTE MYOCARDIAL INFARCTION
DRUG FEVER
FEVER OF UNKNOWN ORIGIN (FUO)
BACTERIAL INFECTIONS:
INTRA-ABDOMINAL ABSCESS (e.g. hepatic, renal or splenic ★), Rat-bite fever (streptobacillus moniliformis)
BACTERIEMIAS: Salmonellosis (typhoid fever) Brucellosis, Intravascular graft infection
MYCOBACTERIAL INFECTIONS (Tuberculosis, Mycobacterium avium complex infections)
NEOPLASMS: Lymphomas, Myxomas, Leukemias, Hepatic and Renal cancers
FUNGAL INFECTIONS (Histoplasmosis, Coccidiomycosis, Candidiasis, Aspergillosis)
SPIROCHETAL INFECTIONS
Lyme disease
Leptospirosis, Secondary syphilis
AORTIC GRAFT INFECTION
SPLENIC and KIDNEY ABSCESSES
PYELONEPHRITIS
RICKETTSIAL INFECTIONS
SECONDARY SYPHILIS
ABDOMINAL PROCESSES
DIVERTICULITIS
CHOLECYSTITIS
PANCREATITIS
PERFORED ULCER
COLITIS and TRANSLOCATION ENTERCOLITIS
BOWEL INFARCTION
APPENDICITIS
PELVIC INFECTION
(PERIRECTAL) ABSCESS
PROSTATITIS
UTI
VIRAL INFECTIONS (CMV, EBV)
PARASITIC INFECTIONS Malaria, Toxoplasmosis, Amebiasis
CONNECTIVE TISSUE DISORDERS SLE, Giant cell arteritis (GCA), Rheumatoid arthritis
JOINT INFECTION
FACTITIOUS FEVER
DVT
ELDERLY
NSAIDs or steroids
WOUND INFECTION
IMMUNO-COMPROMISED
RAT-BITE FEVER
NSAIDs or steroids
CELLULITIS
OTHER CAUSES
INFLAMMATORY BOWEL DISEASE, SARCOIDOSIS, GRANULOMATOUS HEPATITIS
HYPOTHERMIA
PATTERNS OF FEVER
37°C
CONTINUOUS (Typhus, viral pneumonia)
REMITTENT (Sepsis, rheumatic fever, thyphus)
INTERMITTENT (Sepsis, pleuritis)
RECURRENT (Malaria, bronchitis, cholecystitis)
UNDULATING (Brucellosis, tumors e.g. Hodgkin disease)
BIPHASIC (some viral diseases)

SYNCOPE

Syncope is a short loss of consciousness and muscle tone due to inadequate cerebral blood flow.

Vasovagal syncope (also known as neurocardiogenic, reflex, situational syncope, or common fainting) is the most common cause of syncope. It is estimated to account for 20%-50% of all syncope. The exact percentage may vary depending on the study population and the diagnostic criteria used.

Precipitating events include standing or stress (physical or emotional), or reflex precipitants (such as micturition, defecation, swallowing, coughing or even hair grooming). The underlying mechanism for the syncopal episode is an exaggeration of reflex-mediated vasomotor tone and heart rate, responsible for maintaining blood pressure.

Carotid sinus sensitivity refers to the overreaction of the carotid sinus to external pressure causing significant bradycardia and/or hypotension.

Approximately 25% of syncope is **cardiac** in origin, including arrhythmias, cardiac ischemia, hypertrophic cardiomyopathy, and orthostatic hypotension. (The edematous legs in the picture emphasize possible cardiac origin.)

Medications that may cause syncope include:

- Beta blockers
- Sodium channel blockers
- Medications that prolong the QT interval
- Antihypertensives
- Peripheral vasodilators
- Diuretics
- Phenothiazines
- Antidepressants
- Nitrates
- Opiates

Neurogenic causes on syncope are rare and include transient ischemic attack (TIA) and autonomic insufficiency (common in the elderly and patients with diabetes.)

SYNCOPE

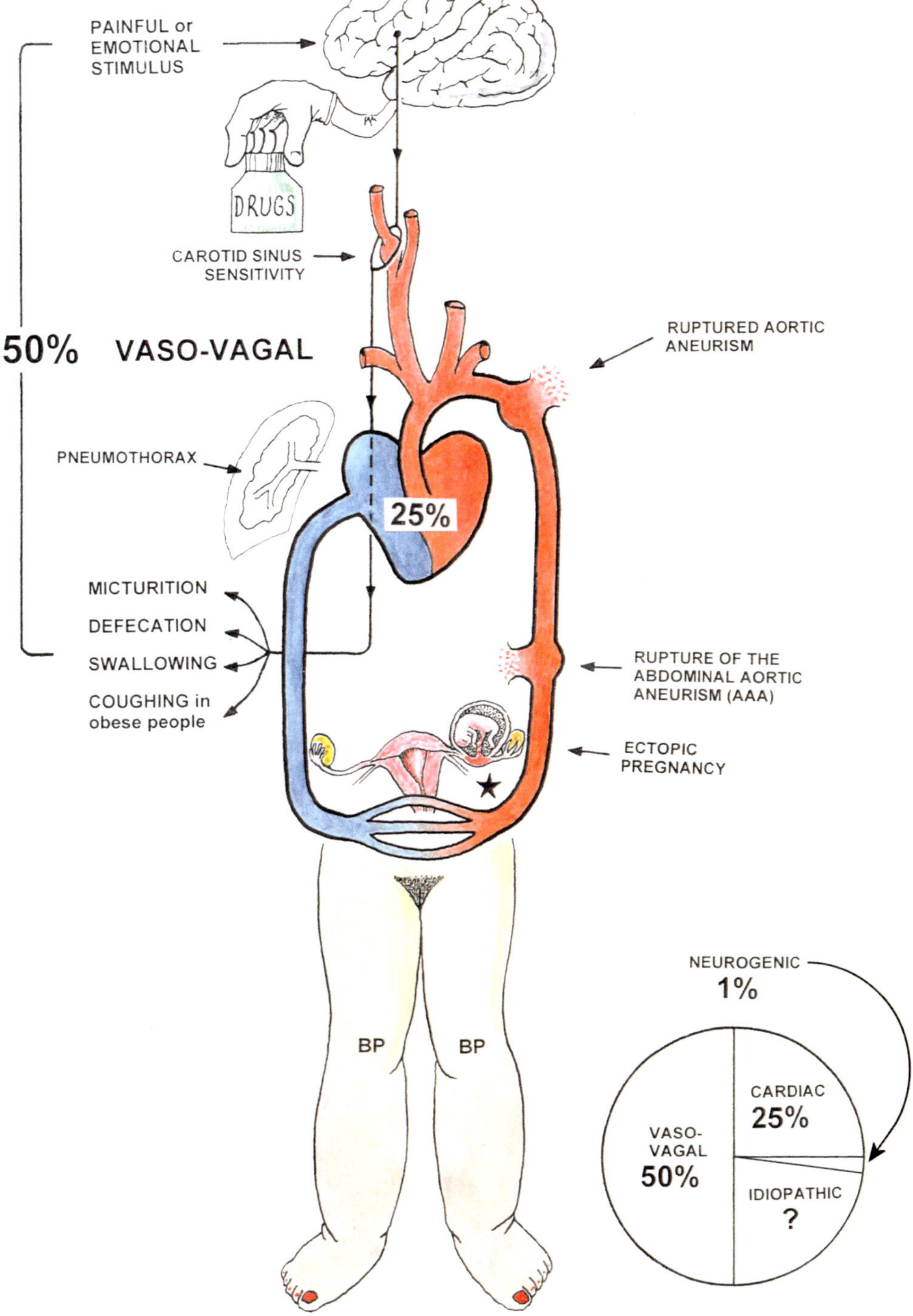
PAINFUL or
EMOTIONAL
STIMULUS
DRUGS
CAROTID SINUS
SENSITIVITY
50%
VASO-VAGAL
RUPTURED AORTIC
ANEURISM
PNEUMOTHORAX
25%
MICTURITION
DEFECATION
SWALLOWING
COUGHING in
obese people
RUPTURE OF THE
ABDOMINAL AORTIC
ANEURISM (AAA)
ECTOPIC
PREGNANCY
BP
BP
NEUROGENIC
1%
CARDIAC
25%
VASO-
VAGAL
50%
IDIOPATHIC
?

FALLS

The picture is self-explanatory.

The nurse is holding the patient with **Parkinson's disease**. They have stooped posture, small shuffling steps, and hypokinesia with the propensity to fall. About 80% of the falls in patients with Parkinson's disease are due to their postural instability.

An **atonic seizure** (drop seizure, akinetic seizure, astatic seizure, or drop attack) consists of partial or complete loss of muscle tone.

Cataplexy is a sudden and transient episode of muscle weakness accompanied by full conscious awareness, typically triggered by emotions such as laughing, crying, or terror. Cataplexy affects approximately 20% of people who have narcolepsy and is caused by an autoimmune destruction of hypothalamic neurons that produce the neuropeptide hypocretin (orexin), which regulates arousal. Cataplexy without narcolepsy is rare.

When patients are **restrained,** they may try to escape by struggling or try to remove the restraint, which can cause them to lose their balance and fall. In addition, restraints can cause patients to become agitated, which can also increase the risk of falls. [8]

8 Abbreviations: ADL: activities of daily living; MI: myocardial infarct; PE: pulmonary embolus; SSRI: selective serotonin reuptake inhibitors.

FALLS

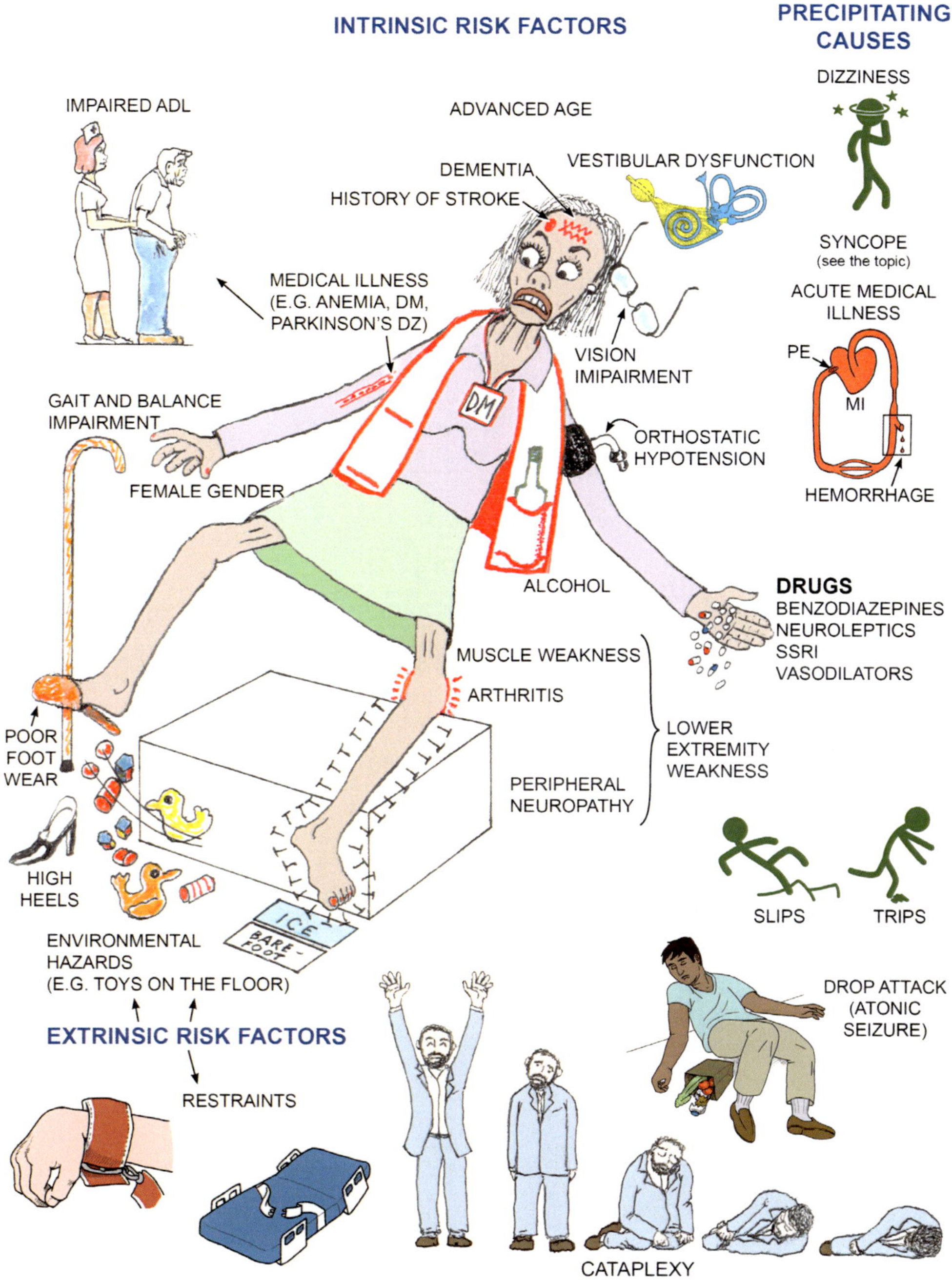
INTRINSIC RISK FACTORS
PRECIPITATING CAUSES
DIZZINESS
IMPAIRED ADL
ADVANCED AGE
DEMENTIA
VESTIBULAR DYSFUNCTION
HISTORY OF STROKE
SYNCOPE
(see the topic)
ACUTE MEDICAL ILLNESS
MEDICAL ILLNESS
(E.G. ANEMIA, DM,
PARKINSON'S DZ)
PE
MI
VISION
IMIPAIRMENT
DM
GAIT AND BALANCE
IMPAIRMENT
ORTHOSTATIC
HYPOTENSION
HEMORRHAGE
FEMALE GENDER
ALCOHOL
DRUGS
BENZODIAZEPINES
NEUROLEPTICS
SSRI
VASODILATORS
MUSCLE WEAKNESS
ARTHRITIS
LOWER
EXTREMITY
WEAKNESS
POOR
FOOT
WEAR
PERIPHERAL
NEUROPATHY
HIGH
HEELS
SLIPS
TRIPS
ICE
BARE-
FOOT
ENVIRONMENTAL
HAZARDS
(E.G. TOYS ON THE FLOOR)
DROP ATTACK
(ATONIC
SEIZURE)
EXTRINSIC RISK FACTORS
RESTRAINTS
CATAPLEXY

COMPLETE BLOOD COUNT (CBC)

1. LEUKOCYTOSIS
2. LEUKOPENIA
3. POLYCYTHEMIA
4. ANEMIA
5. THROMBOCYTOSIS
6. THROMBOCYTOPENIA

COMPLETE BLOOD COUNT (CBC)

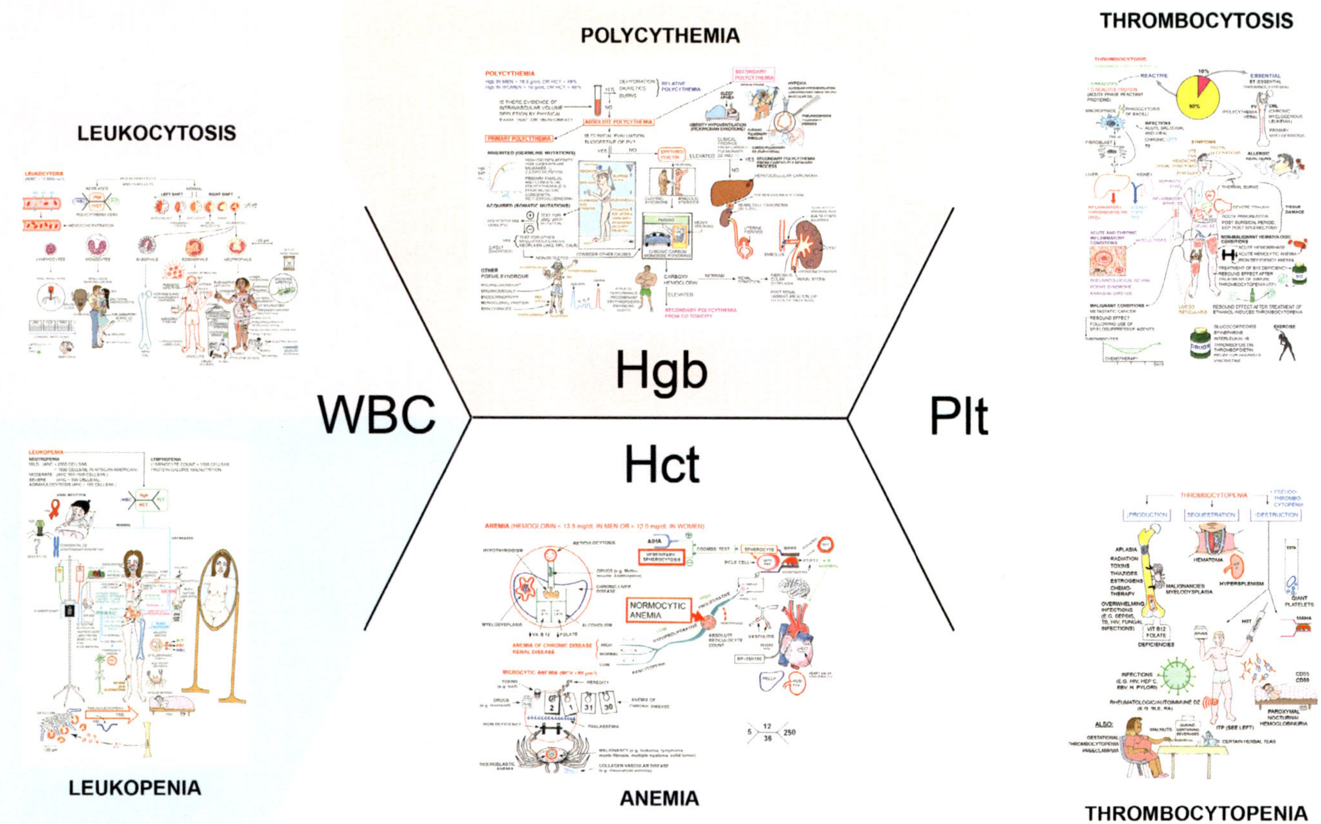

LEUKOCYTOSIS

Leukocytosis could be due to **hemoconcentration**, a part of **polycythemia,** which also has increased red blood cells (RBC) and thrombocytes, or isolated **leukocytosis**.

Hemoconcentration is commonly seen in conditions such as dehydration, burns, shock, and other causes of decreased plasma volume.

Lymphocytosis is associated with chronic and viral infections, while **neutrophilia** is associated with acute and bacterial infections.

Infectious mononucleosis, also known as mono, is sometimes referred to as the "kissing disease" because it is commonly spread through saliva. The Epstein-Barr virus, which causes mono, is present in an infected person's saliva, and it can be passed on through intimate contact, like kissing. However, the virus can also be spread through sharing of utensils, drinking glasses, or other personal items that have been in contact with an infected person's saliva.

Eosinophilia could be a sign of allergic, parasitic or autoimmune disease. However, an increase in the number of eosinophils can also occur during the recovery of bone marrow, known as the "dawn of healing."

Parasitic infection is shown as an ascariasis worm coming out of the nose of the patient. Addison disease represents an autoimmune disease.

Basophilia could be a sign of an underlying bone marrow disorder such as chronic myelogenous leukemia (**CML**) or myeloproliferative neoplasms (**MPNs**).

There are many **drugs** that have been reported to cause eosinophilia as a side effect. Some examples include certain antibiotics like penicillin and cephalosporins, as well as NSAIDs, like ibuprofen and naproxen. Other medications that have been reported to cause eosinophilia include antiepileptic drugs, antidepressants, and antipsychotic medications[9].

---

9 Abbreviations: WBC: white blood cells; Hgb: hemoglobin; HCT: hematocrit; CLL: chronic lymphocytic leukemia; ALL: acute lymphocytic leukemia; CMV: cytomegalovirus; DZ: disease; UC: ulcerative colitis; GI: gastrointestinal.

LEUKOCYTOSIS
(WBC > 11,000/mm³)

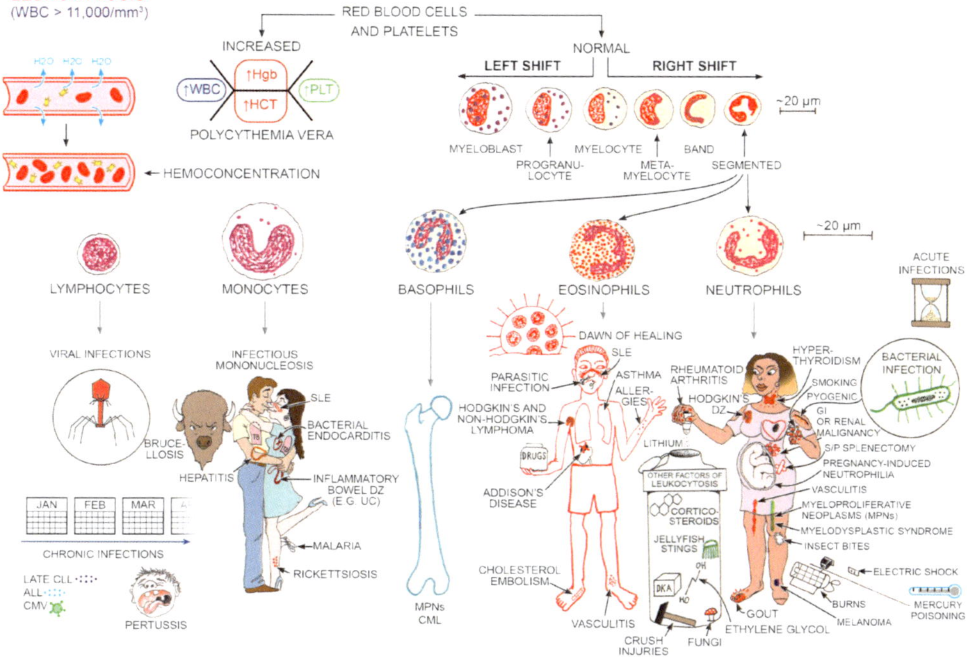

“Silence is a source of great strength.”

Lao Tzu

LEUKOCYTOSIS
(WBC > 11,000/mm³)

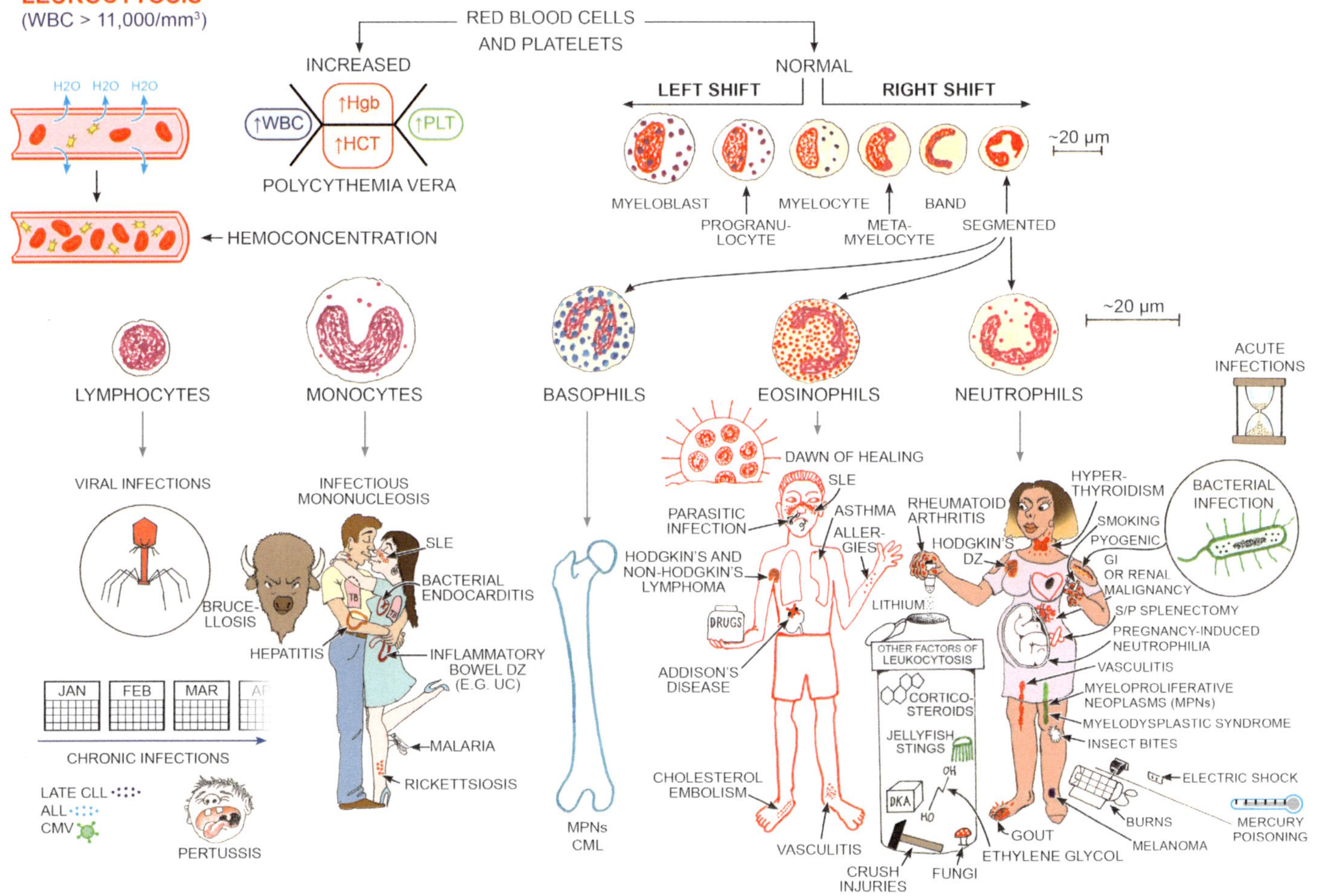

LEUKOPENIA

If only white blood cells (WBC) are reduced, the cause is usually a viral infection, congenital disease, or idiopathic.

If leukopenia is accompanied by reduction of erythrocytes and thrombocytes, the spleen should be evaluated. Splenomegaly suggests hypersplenism. If the spleen is normal in size, the vitamin B12 level should be checked. If the level is reduced, pernicious anemia is the cause. If the vitamin B12 level is normal, bone marrow or PNH is the cause.

Pernicious anemia is an autoimmune disorder affecting intrinsic factor in the stomach, with subsequent diminishment in dietary vitamin B12 absorption, and consequent megaloblastic anemia.

Pernicious anemia can also cause damage to the central nervous system (CNS) leading to paresthesia in extremities, difficulty walking, fatigue and memory loss. (The crossed neuron represents the neurological aspect of vitamin B12 deficiency.)

The red circle with smaller circles inside it (cells in the bone marrow) represents a cross section of a bone, indicating aplastic anemia with impaired production of leukocytes, erythrocytes and thrombocytes.

Paroxysmal nocturnal hemoglobinuria (PNH) is caused by a genetic mutation that causes autoimmune destruction of leukocytes, erythrocytes and thrombocytes, through the hyperactivity of the complement system.

The **pseudo leukopenia** is a laboratory artifact which refers to the false decrease in the WBC count. This can occur during laboratory analysis of blood samples. This happens because the WBCs in the sample aggregate, which can be incorrectly counted as one cell by the machine.

Leukopenia can occur in the beginning of an infection due to the body's immune response to the infection. When infection-causing agents like viruses, bacteria or parasites trigger an activation of WBCs by the bone marrow, their mobilization can lead to their depletion from the blood circulation, leading to temporary leukopenia. In addition, some infections can also directly damage the bone marrow.

The central figure in the picture represents an anorexic patient (with subsequent depletion of nutrients) who sees herself as obese. [10]

10 Abbreviations: SLE: systemic lupus erythematosus; WBC: white blood cell count; PLT: platelets; RBC: red blood cells; DZ: disease

LEUKOPENIA

NEUTROPENIA

MILD (ANC < 2000 CELLS/ML
< 1500 CELLS/ML IN AFRICAN AMERICAN)
MODERATE (ANC 500-1000 CELLS/ML)
SEVERE (ANC < 500 CELLS/ML)
AGRANULOCYTOSIS (ANC < 100 CELLS/ML)

LYMPHOPENIA

LYMPHOCYTE COUNT < 1500 CELLS/ML
PROTEIN-CALORIE MALNUTRITION

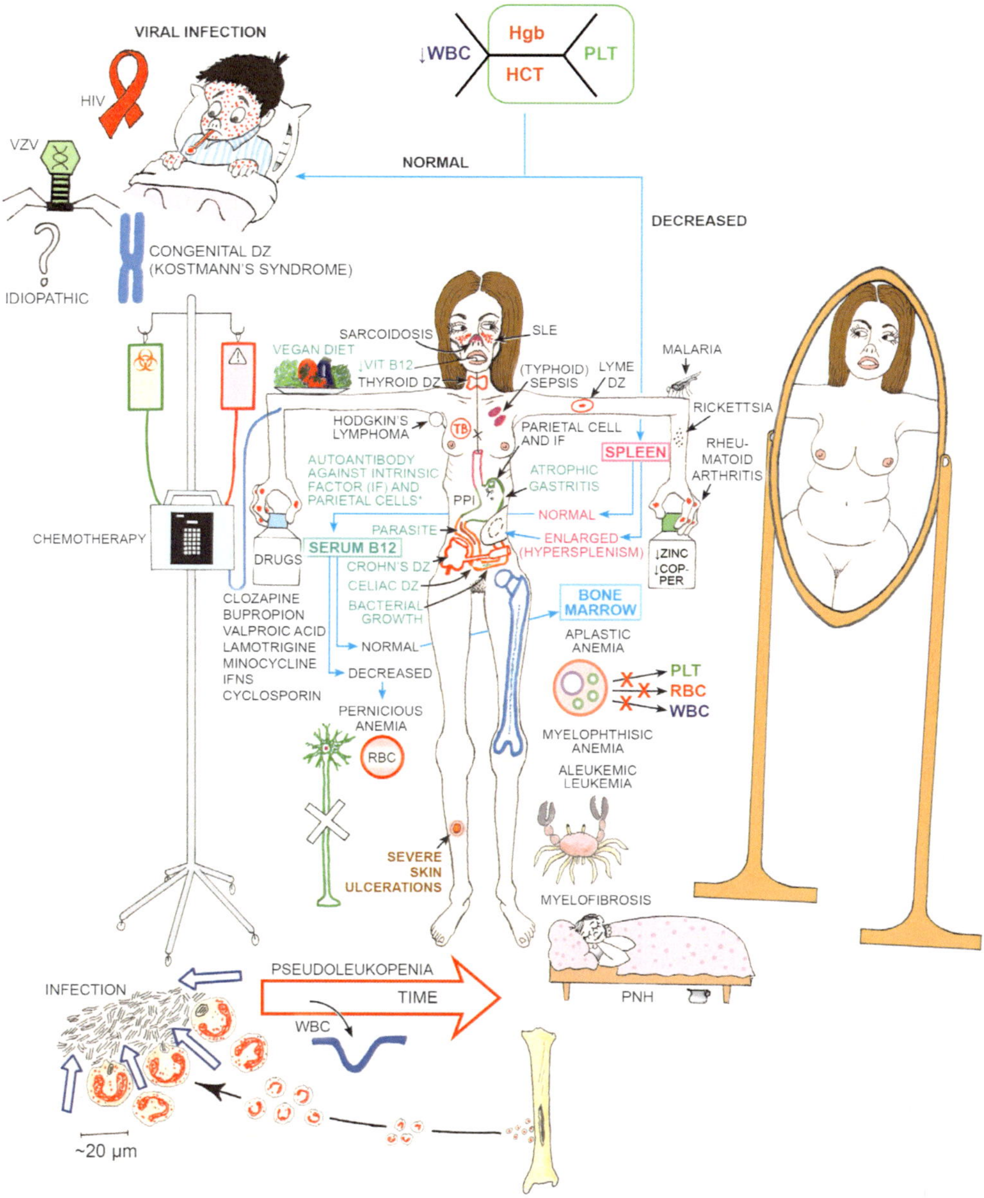

POLYCYTHEMIA

The picture is self-explanatory.

Hypoxia due to sleep apnea, hypoventilation, high altitude or cardio-pulmonary disease stimulates erythropoietin production, which stimulates the production of red blood cells.

The central picture shows symptoms of polycythemia vera, including itchiness after a warm bath.

Some rare mutations of the globin chains can result in a high affinity towards the hemoglobin molecule, changing the affinity to the oxygen with subsequent polycythemia.

A poet holds the book with POEMS.

POEMS syndrome (also known as **osteosclerotic myeloma**, **Crow–Fukase syndrome, Takatsuki disease**, or **PEP syndrome**) is a rare paraneoplastic syndrome caused by a clone of aberrant plasma cells.

A spike of Gamma globulins in electrophoresis can include monoclonal proteins.

A body builder represents the use of recombinant erythropoiesis-enhancing agents which can cause polycythemia.

A garage attendant smokes while inhaling car CO exhaust.

Renal artery stenosis can lead to polycythemia due to reduced blood flow and decrease oxygen delivery to the kidney tissue. This can trigger the release of erythropoietin.

Chronic kidney disease, including long-term obstruction in the urinary tract by a renal stone, can lead to secondary polycythemia.[11]

---

11 Abbreviations: Hgb: hemoglobin; Hct: hematocrit; BUN: blood urea nitrogen; Creat: creatinine; DZ: disease; JAK2 V617F: specific genetic mutation associated with polycythemia vera (PV); MPL, CALR: additional genes implicated in PV pathogenesis.

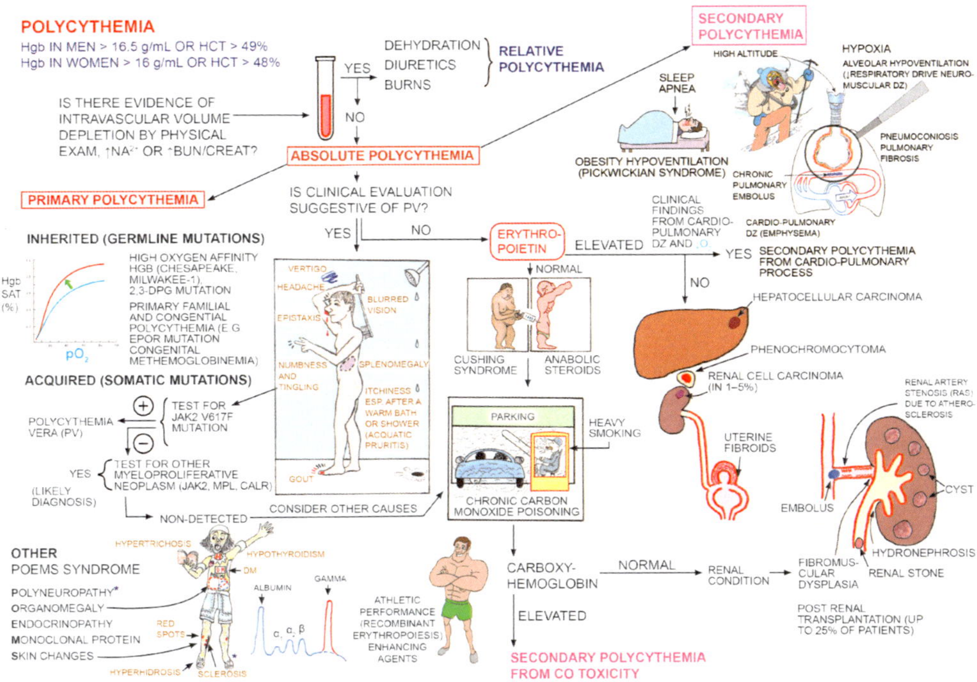
POLYCYTHEMIA
Hgb IN MEN > 16.5 g/mL OR HCT > 49%
Hgb IN WOMEN > 16 g/mL OR HCT > 48%
IS THERE EVIDENCE OF INTRAVASCULAR VOLUME DEPLETION BY PHYSICAL EXAM, ↑NA OR ↑BUN/CREAT?
YES
DEHYDRATION
DIURETICS
BURNS
RELATIVE POLYCYTHEMIA
NO
ABSOLUTE POLYCYTHEMIA
PRIMARY POLYCYTHEMIA
SECONDARY POLYCYTHEMIA
IS CLINICAL EVALUATION SUGGESTIVE OF PV?
YES
NO
INHERITED (GERMLINE MUTATIONS)
HIGH OXYGEN AFFINITY HGB (CHESAPEAKE, MILWAKEE-1), 2,3-DPG MUTATION
PRIMARY FAMILIAL AND CONGENTIAL POLYCYTHEMIA (E.G. EPOR MUTATION CONGENITAL METHEMOGLOBINEMIA)
Hgb SAT (%)
pO2
ACQUIRED (SOMATIC MUTATIONS)
POLYCYTHEMIA VERA (PV)
TEST FOR JAK2 V617F MUTATION
YES
(LIKELY DIAGNOSIS)
TEST FOR OTHER MYELOPROLIFERATIVE NEOPLASM (JAK2, MPL, CALR)
NON-DETECTED
CONSIDER OTHER CAUSES
VERTIGO
HEADACHE
BLURRED VISION
EPISTAXIS
NUMBNESS AND TINGLING
SPLENOMEGALY
ITCHINESS ESP. AFTER A WARM BATH OR SHOWER (ACQUATIC PRURITIS)
GOUT
ERYTHRO-POIETIN
ELEVATED
NORMAL
CUSHING SYNDROME
ANABOLIC STEROIDS
PARKING
HEAVY SMOKING
CHRONIC CARBON MONOXIDE POISONING
CARBOXY-HEMOGLOBIN
NORMAL
ELEVATED
SECONDARY POLYCYTHEMIA FROM CO TOXICITY
RENAL CONDITION
SLEEP APNEA
OBESITY HYPOVENTILATION (PICKWICKIAN SYNDROME)
HIGH ALTITUDE
HYPOXIA
ALVEOLAR HYPOVENTILATION (↓RESPIRATORY DRIVE NEURO-MUSCULAR DZ)
PNEUMOCONIOSIS
PULMONARY FIBROSIS
CHRONIC PULMONARY EMBOLUS
CARDIO-PULMONARY DZ (EMPHYSEMA)
CLINICAL FINDINGS FROM CARDIO-PULMONARY DZ AND ↓O2
YES
SECONDARY POLYCYTHEMIA FROM CARDIO-PULMONARY PROCESS
NO
HEPATOCELLULAR CARCINOMA
PHENOCHROMOCYTOMA
RENAL CELL CARCINOMA (IN 1–5%)
UTERINE FIBROIDS
RENAL ARTERY STENOSIS (RAS) DUE TO ATHERO-SCLEROSIS
CYST
EMBOLUS
HYDRONEPHROSIS
FIBROMUS-CULAR DYSPLASIA
RENAL STONE
POST RENAL TRANSPLANTATION (UP TO 25% OF PATIENTS)
OTHER
POEMS SYNDROME
POLYNEUROPATHY
ORGANOMEGALY
ENDOCRINOPATHY
MONOCLONAL PROTEIN
SKIN CHANGES
HYPERTRICHOSIS
HYPOTHYROIDISM
DM
RED SPOTS
HYPERHIDROSIS
SCLEROSIS
ALBUMIN
GAMMA
α1 α2 β
ATHLETIC PERFORMANCE (RECOMBINANT ERYTHROPOIESIS) ENHANCING AGENTS

"Deep thinking is attainable only to those of deep feelings."

Samuel Taylor Coleridge

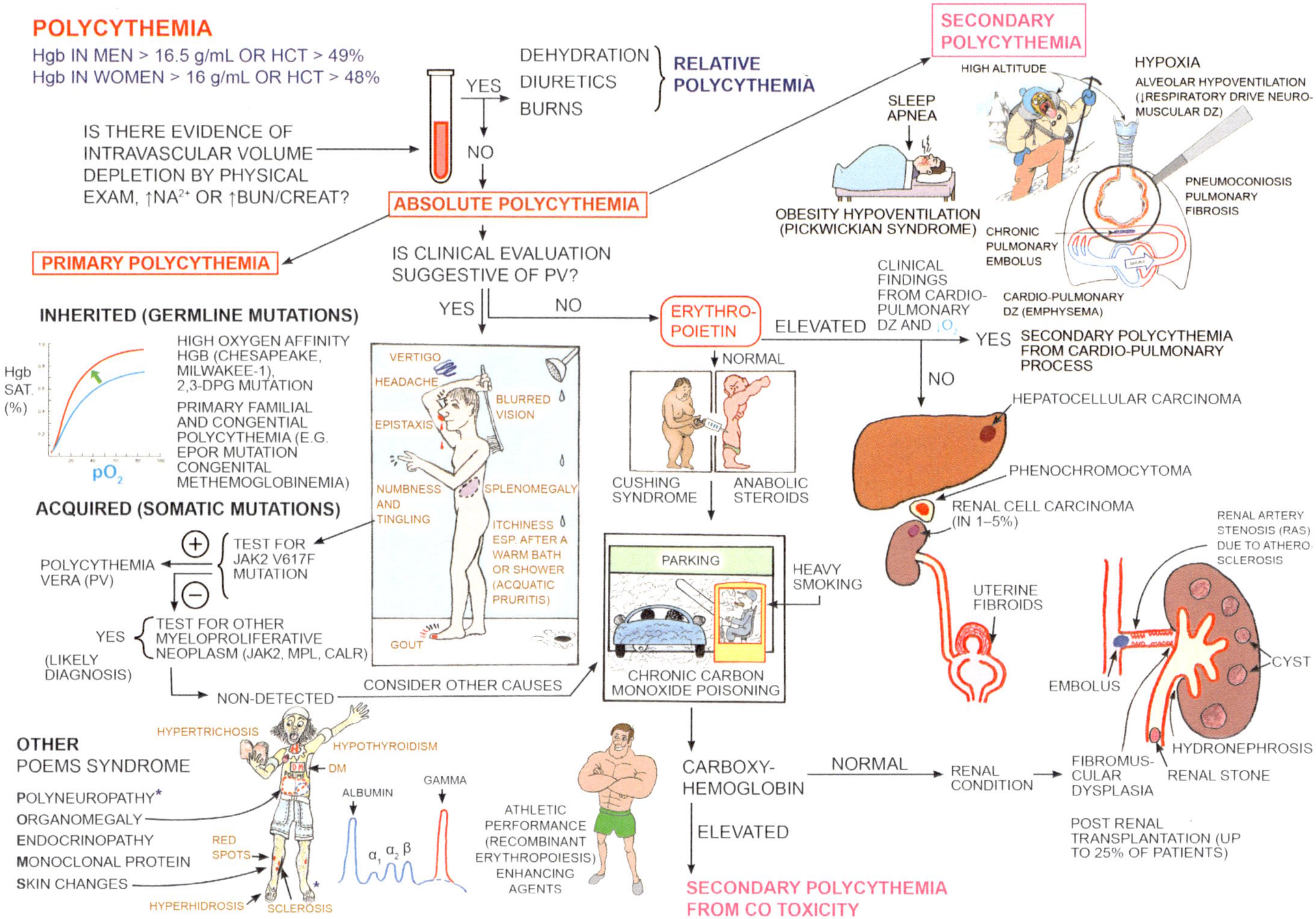
POLYCYTHEMIA
Hgb IN MEN > 16.5 g/mL OR HCT > 49%
Hgb IN WOMEN > 16 g/mL OR HCT > 48%
IS THERE EVIDENCE OF INTRAVASCULAR VOLUME DEPLETION BY PHYSICAL EXAM, ↑NA2+ OR ↑BUN/CREAT?
YES
NO
DEHYDRATION
DIURETICS
BURNS
RELATIVE POLYCYTHEMIA
ABSOLUTE POLYCYTHEMIA
PRIMARY POLYCYTHEMIA
SECONDARY POLYCYTHEMIA
IS CLINICAL EVALUATION SUGGESTIVE OF PV?
YES
NO
INHERITED (GERMLINE MUTATIONS)
Hgb SAT. (%)
pO2
HIGH OXYGEN AFFINITY HGB (CHESAPEAKE, MILWAKEE-1), 2,3-DPG MUTATION
PRIMARY FAMILIAL AND CONGENTIAL POLYCYTHEMIA (E.G. EPOR MUTATION CONGENITAL METHEMOGLOBINEMIA)
ACQUIRED (SOMATIC MUTATIONS)
TEST FOR JAK2 V617F MUTATION
POLYCYTHEMIA VERA (PV)
TEST FOR OTHER MYELOPROLIFERATIVE NEOPLASM (JAK2, MPL, CALR)
YES
(LIKELY DIAGNOSIS)
NON-DETECTED
CONSIDER OTHER CAUSES
VERTIGO
HEADACHE
EPISTAXIS
BLURRED VISION
NUMBNESS AND TINGLING
SPLENOMEGALY
ITCHINESS ESP. AFTER A WARM BATH OR SHOWER (ACQUATIC PRURITIS)
GOUT
ERYTHRO-POIETIN
NORMAL
ELEVATED
CUSHING SYNDROME
ANABOLIC STEROIDS
PARKING
HEAVY SMOKING
CHRONIC CARBON MONOXIDE POISONING
CARBOXY-HEMOGLOBIN
NORMAL
ELEVATED
SECONDARY POLYCYTHEMIA FROM CO TOXICITY
RENAL CONDITION
ATHLETIC PERFORMANCE (RECOMBINANT ERYTHROPOIESIS) ENHANCING AGENTS
OTHER
POEMS SYNDROME
POLYNEUROPATHY*
ORGANOMEGALY
ENDOCRINOPATHY
MONOCLONAL PROTEIN
SKIN CHANGES
HYPERTRICHOSIS
HYPOTHYROIDISM
DM
RED SPOTS
HYPERHIDROSIS
SCLEROSIS
ALBUMIN
GAMMA
α1 α2 β
SLEEP APNEA
OBESITY HYPOVENTILATION (PICKWICKIAN SYNDROME)
HIGH ALTITUDE
HYPOXIA
ALVEOLAR HYPOVENTILATION (↓RESPIRATORY DRIVE NEURO-MUSCULAR DZ)
PNEUMOCONIOSIS
PULMONARY FIBROSIS
CHRONIC PULMONARY EMBOLUS
CARDIO-PULMONARY DZ (EMPHYSEMA)
CLINICAL FINDINGS FROM CARDIO-PULMONARY DZ AND ↓O2
YES
NO
SECONDARY POLYCYTHEMIA FROM CARDIO-PULMONARY PROCESS
HEPATOCELLULAR CARCINOMA
PHENOCHROMOCYTOMA
RENAL CELL CARCINOMA (IN 1–5%)
UTERINE FIBROIDS
RENAL ARTERY STENOSIS (RAS) DUE TO ATHERO-SCLEROSIS
CYST
EMBOLUS
HYDRONEPHROSIS
RENAL STONE
FIBROMUS-CULAR DYSPLASIA
POST RENAL TRANSPLANTATION (UP TO 25% OF PATIENTS)

ANEMIA

The picture was developed in Tony Buzan's Mind Map mnemotechnic style.

For normocytic anemia:

Corrected reticulocyte count = reticulocyte account x patients' hematocrit/expected hematocrit. (The expected range for hematocrit in healthy adults is generally between 39% and 50% for women and between 42% and 54% for men)

If corrected reticulocyte count is < 2%, it suggests decreased RBC production.

If corrected reticulocyte count is > 3%, it indicates hemolysis or blood loss.

If the absolute reticulocyte count is low, it indicates hypoproliferative red blood cells (RBC) condition. Then white blood cells (WBC) and thrombocytes need to be checked; if they are low in number, pancytopenia is the diagnosis. If they are high or normal to high in number, anemia of chronic disease or renal disease is the diagnosis.

The big complete blood count (CBC) grid in the right lower corner of the picture shows that normal hematocrit to hemoglobin ratio is usually 3:1 (in this example 36%:12 g/dL). The number 5 in the CBC grid indicates WBCs in the thousands, while 250 indicates a thrombocyte count in the thousands.

In case of **hemolysis,** a smear (shown in the picture on a glass slide) should be examined. If spherocytes are present, Combs test should be done. If it is positive, it indicates autoimmune hemolytic anemia (**AIHA**) illustrated as an antibody. If the test is negative, the diagnosis is hereditary spherocytosis. The erythrocyte has the left edge in the form of a sickle, suggesting **sickle cell anemia**. Inside the erythrocyte are shown some hereditary conditions which could lead to spontaneous hemolysis, like glucose 6 phosphate dehydrogenase deficiency (**G6PDD**) and paroxysmal nocturnal hemoglobinuria (**PNH**).

The blood vessel on the right side is depicted as narrower, to point microangiopathic hemolytic anemia (**MAHA**) with schistocyte (in the form of a helmet) within. MAHA is a subgroup of hemolytic anemia caused by processes manifest in small blood vessels, like disseminated intravascular coagulation (DIC), hemolytic uremic syndrome/ thrombotic thrombocytopenic purpura (HUS/ TTP), hemolysis, elevated liver enzymes, and low platelet count (HELLP) syndrome or malignant hypertension. If schistocytes are present, PT/PTT should be checked. If they are increased, the diagnosis of **DIC** is established. If PT/PTT are normal, heart valve abnormalities, **HUS/TTP**, vasculitis, severe **hypertension**, or **HELLP** syndrome are possibilities.

HUS = hemolysis, uremia, and thrombocytopenia

TTP = HUS + fever and neurological changes (illustrated as the brain)

A lactose dehydrogenase (LDH) level less than 1000 U/l makes HUS/TTP very unlikely.

In **macrocytic anemia**, the green rectangular bottle shows some of the possible causes. A bottle cap is shown as a reticulocyte.

In **microcytic anemia**, the calendar days indicate anemia of chronic disease.

The rug below the cancer symbolizes collagen vascular disease. The cancer has a sideroblast on its back. (Sideroblasts are immature red blood cells characterized by the presence of iron granules in the cytoplasm. In sideroblastic anemia, the body has iron available but cannot incorporate it into hemoglobin.)

Iron is depicted as a lifting weight made of iron.

Thalassemia is shown as sea waves because the Greek word "thalassa" means "see." The condition is so named because it was first described in people from the Mediterranean region, where the sea was a prominent part of daily life. [12]

---

12 Abbreviations: MCV: mean corpuscular volume

ANEMIA (HEMOGLOBIN ≤ 13.5 mg/dL IN MEN OR < 12.0 mg/dL IN WOMEN)

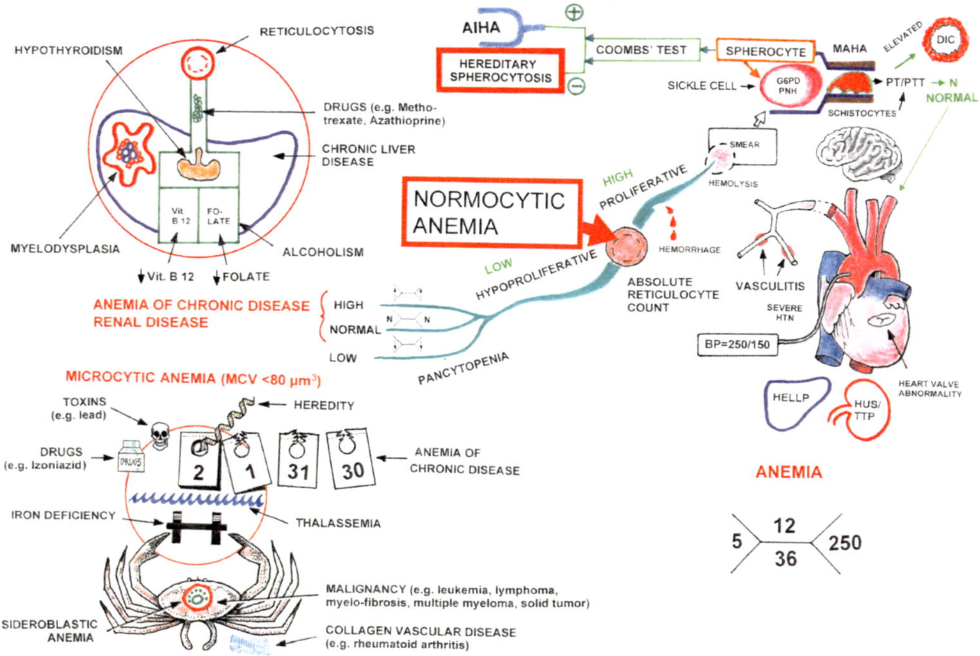

"Diligence is the mother of good fortune."

Miguel de Cervantes

ANEMIA (HEMOGLOBIN < 13.5 mg/dL IN MEN OR < 12.0 mg/dL IN WOMEN)

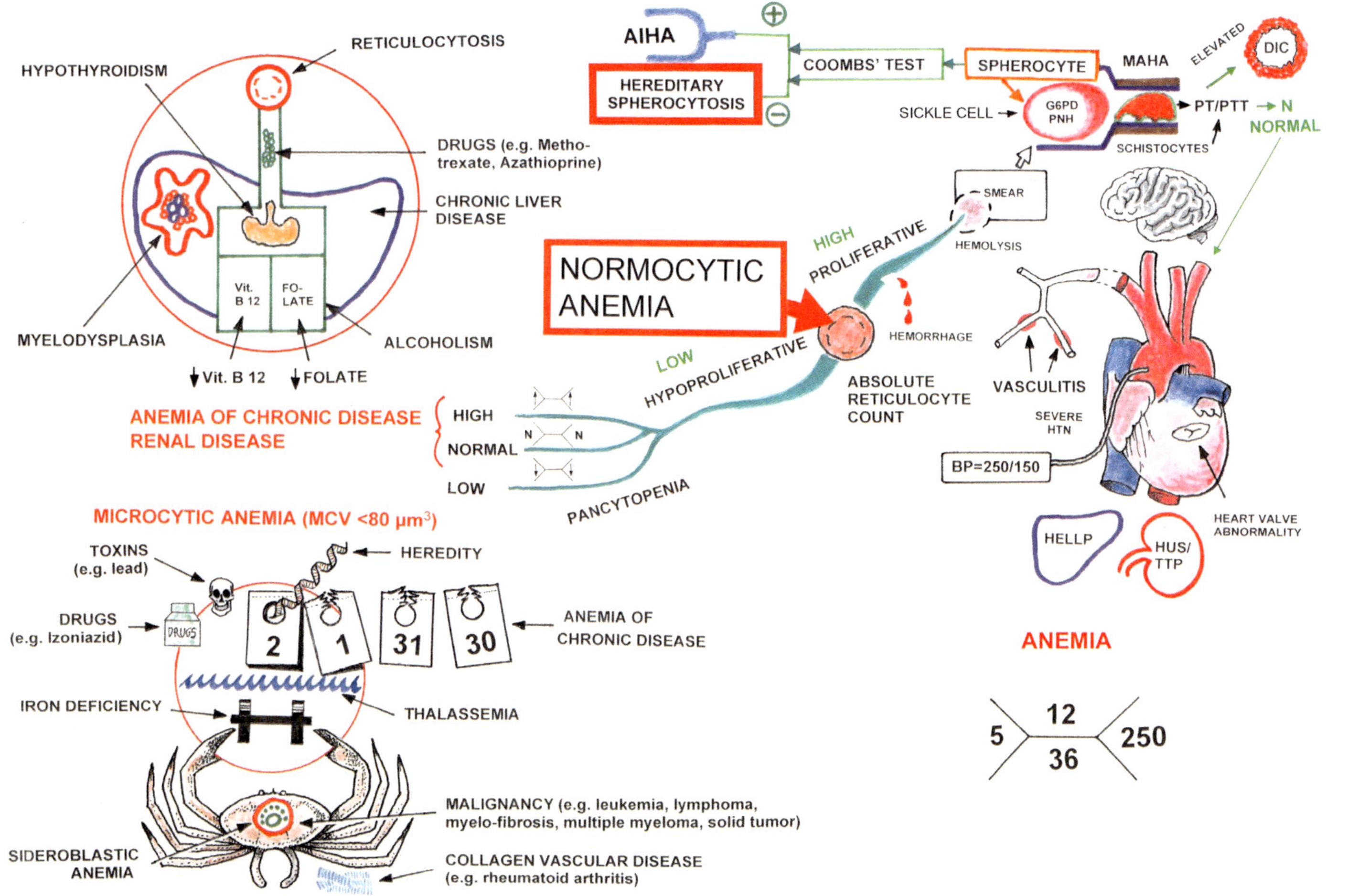

THROMBOCYTOSIS

Normal count is in the range of 150,000 to 450,000 platelets per μL of blood, but investigation is typically considered when the upper limit exceeds 750,000 /μL.

Reactive thrombocytosis develops as a secondary response to another underlying disorder, such as cancer, inflammation or infection.

Essential thrombocytosis, also known as essential thrombocythemia (ET) is one of the myeloproliferative neoplasms. Myeloproliferative neoplasms include polycythemia vera, primary myelofibrosis, and essential polycythemia.

Reactive thrombocytosis relates to reactive processes that are extrinsic to the megakaryocyte, while **primary thrombocytosis** relates to the cell-intrinsic mechanisms (genetic abnormalities) within the megakaryocyte.

Thrombopoietin (TPO), a hormone produced mainly in the liver and kidney, regulates the production of thrombocytes in the bone marrow. The steady state of TPO is achieved by its production, which increases when platelet levels in the blood are low and decreases when platelet levels are high.

Chronic alcohol use can impair the production of thrombocytes in the bone marrow leading to thrombocytopenia. However, stopping alcohol consumption can reverse this process and lead to an increase in platelet production, resulting in the rebound effect. This effect can be observed within a few days after discontinuing alcohol consumption. It is usually self-limiting and resolves on its own within a few weeks.

Vitamin B12 is essential for the production of DNA, RNA and proteins, including those involved in the production of red blood cells and thrombocytes. When vitamin B12 deficiency is treated there is an increase in DNA synthesis and production of new cells including thrombocytes, which can lead to thrombocytosis.

Acute hemolytic anemia can lead to an increase in the production of thrombopoietin.

Iron deficiency can cause a reduction in the size of red blood cells, which in turn can activate platelets and lead to thrombocytosis. Iron deficiency can also stimulate the production of TPO. [13]

---

13 Abbreviations: TB: tuberculosis; DZ: disease; RA; rheumatoid arthritis; VTE: Venous thromboembolism; CVA: cerebrovascular accident.

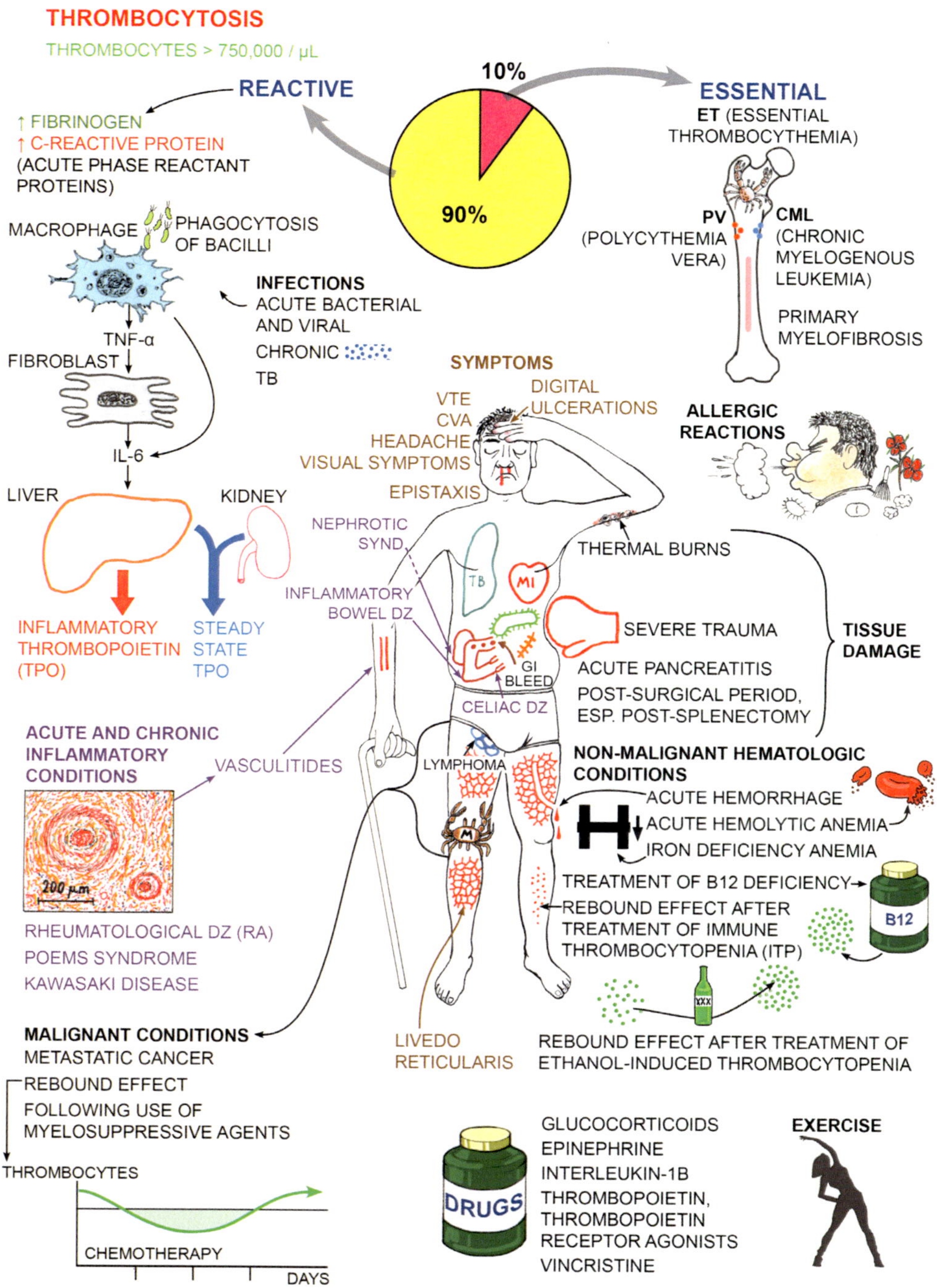

THROMBOCYTOSIS
THROMBOCYTES > 750,000 / μL
REACTIVE
10%
90%
ESSENTIAL
ET (ESSENTIAL THROMBOCYTHEMIA)
PV (POLYCYTHEMIA VERA)
CML (CHRONIC MYELOGENOUS LEUKEMIA)
PRIMARY MYELOFIBROSIS
↑ FIBRINOGEN
↑ C-REACTIVE PROTEIN
(ACUTE PHASE REACTANT PROTEINS)
MACROPHAGE
PHAGOCYTOSIS OF BACILLI
INFECTIONS
ACUTE BACTERIAL AND VIRAL
CHRONIC
TB
TNF-α
FIBROBLAST
IL-6
LIVER
KIDNEY
INFLAMMATORY THROMBOPOIETIN (TPO)
STEADY STATE TPO
SYMPTOMS
VTE
CVA
HEADACHE
VISUAL SYMPTOMS
EPISTAXIS
DIGITAL ULCERATIONS
ALLERGIC REACTIONS
NEPHROTIC SYND
INFLAMMATORY BOWEL DZ
TB
MI
GI BLEED
CELIAC DZ
THERMAL BURNS
SEVERE TRAUMA
ACUTE PANCREATITIS
POST-SURGICAL PERIOD, ESP. POST-SPLENECTOMY
TISSUE DAMAGE
ACUTE AND CHRONIC INFLAMMATORY CONDITIONS
VASCULITIDES
200 μm
RHEUMATOLOGICAL DZ (RA)
POEMS SYNDROME
KAWASAKI DISEASE
LYMPHOMA
M
NON-MALIGNANT HEMATOLOGIC CONDITIONS
ACUTE HEMORRHAGE
ACUTE HEMOLYTIC ANEMIA
IRON DEFICIENCY ANEMIA
TREATMENT OF B12 DEFICIENCY
B12
REBOUND EFFECT AFTER TREATMENT OF IMMUNE THROMBOCYTOPENIA (ITP)
XXX
LIVEDO RETICULARIS
REBOUND EFFECT AFTER TREATMENT OF ETHANOL-INDUCED THROMBOCYTOPENIA
MALIGNANT CONDITIONS
METASTATIC CANCER
REBOUND EFFECT FOLLOWING USE OF MYELOSUPPRESSIVE AGENTS
THROMBOCYTES
CHEMOTHERAPY
DAYS
DRUGS
GLUCOCORTICOIDS
EPINEPHRINE
INTERLEUKIN-1B
THROMBOPOIETIN, THROMBOPOIETIN RECEPTOR AGONISTS
VINCRISTINE
EXERCISE

THROMBOCYTOPENIA

Pseudothrombocytopenia or **spurious thrombocytopenia** is an in-vitro sampling problem, reported in association with the use of Ethylenediaminetetraacetic acid (EDTA) as an anticoagulant.

Other risk factors associated with pseudothrombocytopenia are autoimmune diseases, infections, pregnancy and the treatment with some medications such as low-molecular-weight heparin, valproic acid, insulin, antibiotics and chemotherapy medications.

Giant platelet disorders, also known as **macrothrombocytopenia**, are rare disorders featuring abnormally large platelets, thrombocytopenia and a tendency for bleeding. Giant platelets cannot adhere adequately to injured blood vessel walls, resulting in abnormal bleeding when injured. Giant platelet disorder occurs for inherited diseases such as Bernard–Soulier syndrome.

Heparin-induced thrombocytopenia (HIT) is a serious condition that can occur in patients treated with heparin. A fall in platelet counts and a hypercoagulable state characterize HIT.

Type I HIT, also known as heparin-associated thrombocytopenia (HAT), is a non-immune mediated reaction. Type I HIT is much more common than type II and can occur as early as day 1 of therapy. This is a mild reaction, it is not associated with any complications, and platelet counts will spontaneously normalize even if heparin is continued.

Type II HIT is an immune, antibody-mediated reaction. Because it takes time for the antibodies to form, this reaction usually occurs **after 5 to 14 days** of receiving heparin. However, if a patient has been exposed to heparin within the last 100 days, antibodies may remain in the system, causing this reaction to manifest as soon as **day one of re-exposure** to heparin. This is a very serious reaction that causes a hypercoagulable state and can lead to life-threatening complications such are cerebrovascular accident (CVA), myocardial infarct (MI), deep vein thrombosis (DVT) or pulmonary embolus (PE).

Besides heparin, **drug-induced** nonimmune thrombocytopenia can be caused by chemotherapy, valproic acid, furosemide, gold, used to treat arthritis, NSAIDs, penicillin, quinidine, quinine, ranitidine, sulfonamides, linezolid and other antibiotics and statins.

MAHA, often caused by underlying medical conditions, such as systemic lupus erythematosus (SLE), hemolytic uremic syndrome (HUS), or thrombotic thrombocytopenic purpura (TTP), is characterized by hemolysis, thrombocyte activation and the formation of small thrombi, which can lead to thrombocytopenia.

Paroxysmal nocturnal hemoglobinuria (**PNH**) is a rare clonal disorder caused by an acquired mutation in the *PIGA* gene in hematopoietic stem cells, which results in the abnormal expression of proteins on the surface of blood cells. This can trigger an immune response with subsequent thrombocytopenia. [14]

---

14 Abbreviations: TB: tuberculosis; HIV: human immunodeficiency virus. DZ: disease.

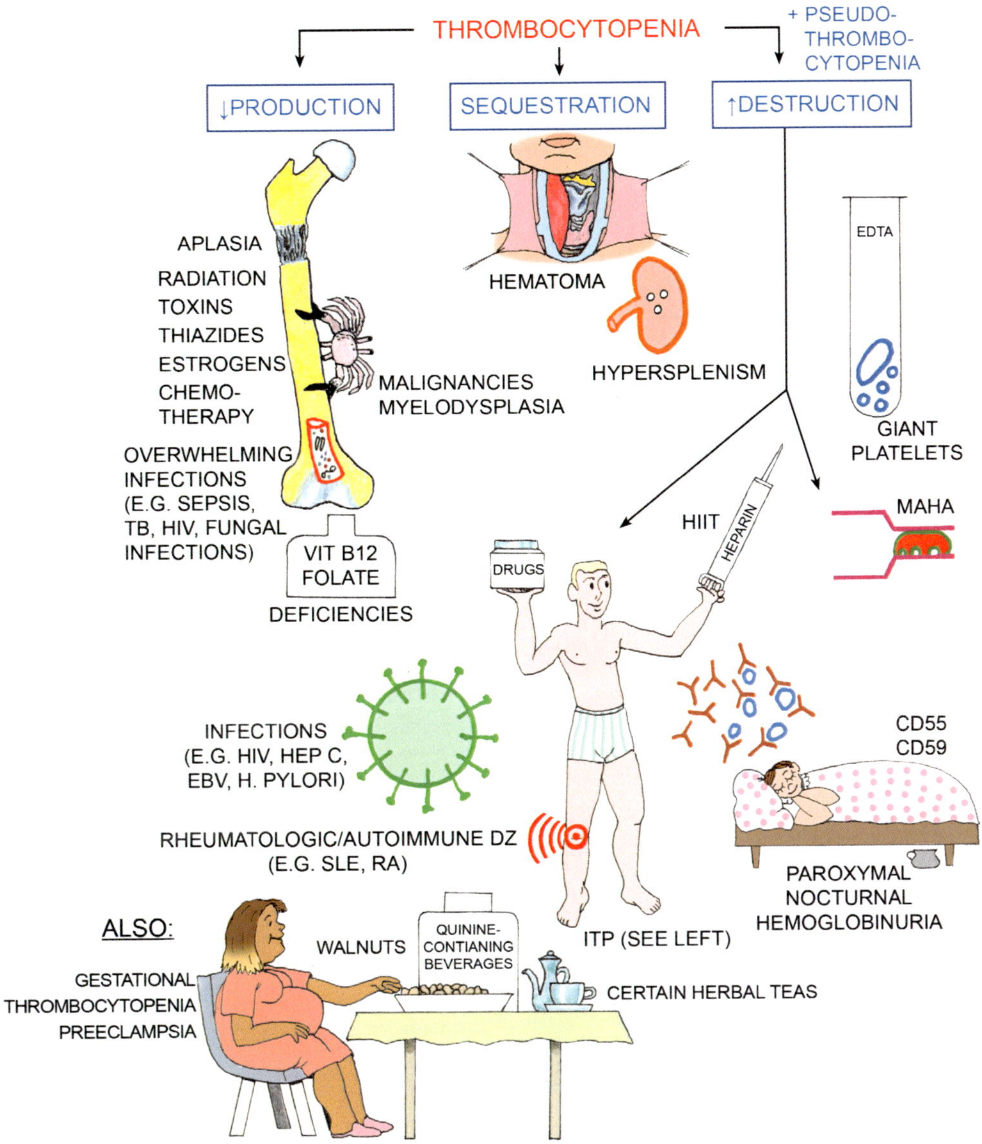
THROMBOCYTOPENIA
+ PSEUDO-THROMBO-CYTOPENIA
↓PRODUCTION
SEQUESTRATION
↑DESTRUCTION
APLASIA
RADIATION
TOXINS
THIAZIDES
ESTROGENS
CHEMO-THERAPY
MALIGNANCIES
MYELODYSPLASIA
OVERWHELMING INFECTIONS (E.G. SEPSIS, TB, HIV, FUNGAL INFECTIONS)
VIT B12
FOLATE
DEFICIENCIES
HEMATOMA
HYPERSPLENISM
EDTA
GIANT PLATELETS
MAHA
HIIT
HEPARIN
DRUGS
CD55
CD59
INFECTIONS (E.G. HIV, HEP C, EBV, H. PYLORI)
RHEUMATOLOGIC/AUTOIMMUNE DZ (E.G. SLE, RA)
PAROXYMAL NOCTURNAL HEMOGLOBINURIA
ITP (SEE LEFT)
ALSO:
GESTATIONAL THROMBOCYTOPENIA
PREECLAMPSIA
WALNUTS
QUININE-CONTIANING BEVERAGES
CERTAIN HERBAL TEAS

BASIC METABOLIC PANEL (BMP)

1. HYPERNATREMIA
2. HYPONATREMIA
3. HYPERKALEMIA
4. HYPOKALEMIA
5. HYPER AND HYPOCHLOREMIA
6. BICARBONATE (ACID-BASE BALANCE) Respiratory Acidosis, Metabolic acidosis, Metabolic alkalosis, Respiratory alkalosis
7. INCREASED and REDUCED BUN AND CREATININE
8. HYPER AND HYPOGLYCEMIA

BASIC METABOLIC PANEL (BMP)

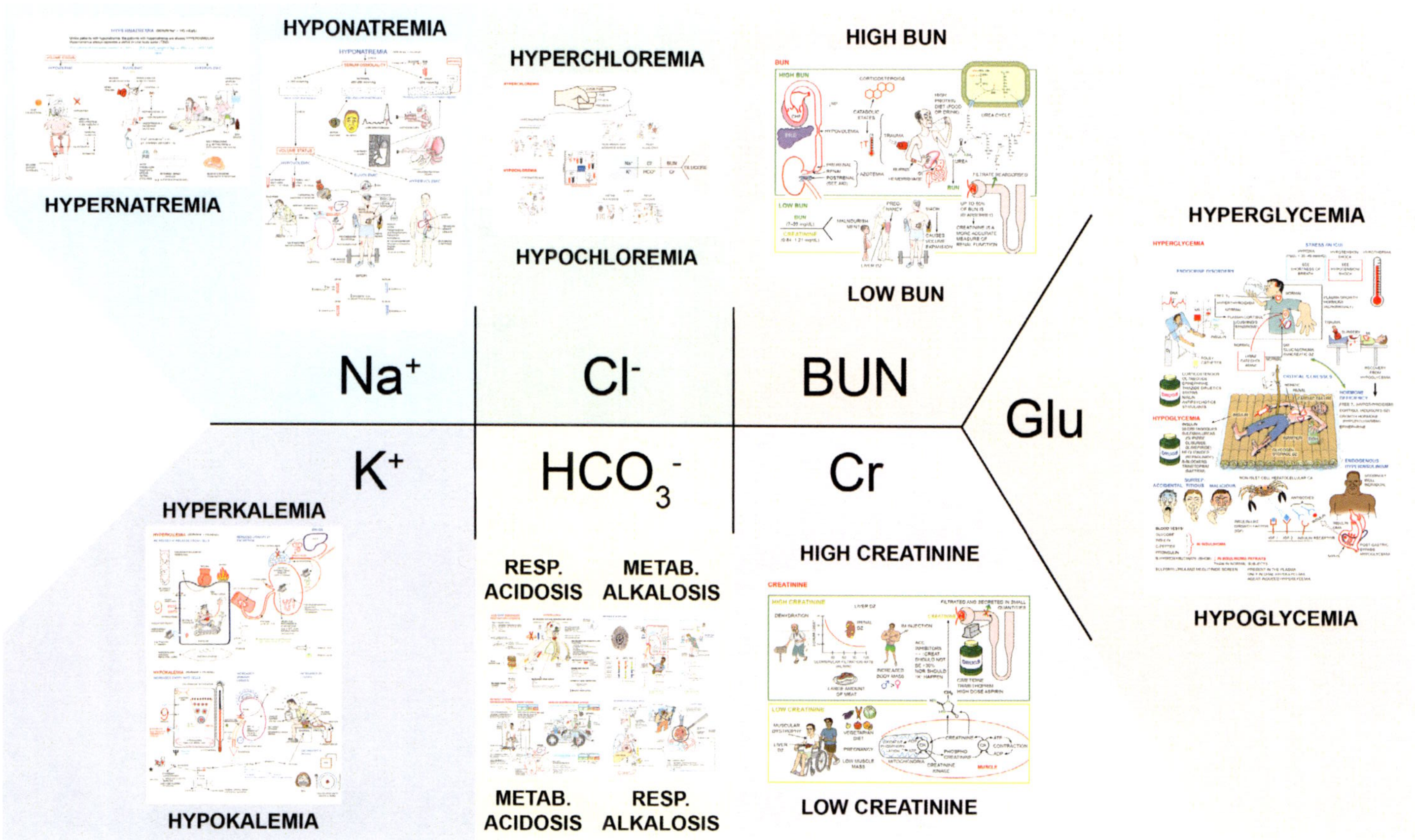

HYPERNATREMIA

Patients with hypernatremia have increased osmolarity, which is a measure of the concentration of solutes in the blood. This is because sodium is one of the primary osmotically active substances in the blood, and an increase in sodium concentration can lead to an increase in the osmolarity of the blood.

Additionally, hypernatremia often occurs when there is a relative deficit of water in the body, leading to dehydration and a decrease in total body water. This can further increase the osmolarity of the blood, as there is a higher concentration of solutes in a smaller volume of water.

As a compensatory mechanism to hypernatremia in **hypovolemic** and **euvolemic conditions**, the body may **increase the amount of chloride** in the blood to maintain a balance of electrical charges in the body's fluids.

In hypervolemic hypernatremia, the concentration of chloride in the blood may also increase. However, the association between hypervolemic hypernatremia and chloride levels is complex and may be influenced by other factors as well.

In **Cushing syndrome** there is an excessive production of cortisol by the adrenal glands. This can lead to hypernatremia. As a compensatory mechanism, the body may excrete excess sodium in the urine and retain chlorides to maintain a balance of electrical charges in the body fluids, therefore leading to **hypochloremia** in the blood.

Elderly people are prone to hypernatremia because their thirst sensation may decrease. Additionally, older adults are more likely to have chronic medical conditions such as diabetes insipidus (DI), kidney disease or heart failure. Furthermore, some medications commonly used in older adults can increase hypernatremia such as diuretics, laxatives and anticholinergics.

Particular types of **brain tumors**, such as craniopharyngioma, meningioma and glioma can cause lesions in the parts of the brain that control thirst and fluid balance. This can result in a decreased sense of thirst and reduce fluid intake, leading to dehydration and hypernatremia. Additionally, the tumor can release Antidiuretic hormone (ADH).

Head trauma can cause disruption of the hypothalamic-pituitary-adrenal axis which controls the release of ADH.

In **nephrogenic diabetes insipidus,** when kidneys are unable to respond to ADH (vasopressin), hypernatremia occurs because of increased water loss due to excessive urine production.

Hypercalcemia may lead to dehydration, which can then lead to an increase in the concentration of sodium in the blood. Additionally, certain medications used to treat hypercalcemia, such as some diuretics can cause increased secretion of sodium in water which can also lead to hypernatremia.

Loss of potassium from the body can cause an imbalance in the electrical charges of the body fluids. To compensate for it, the body will retain sodium.[15]

15 Abbreviations: HCTZ: hydrochlorothiazide

HYPERNATREMIA (SERUM Na^+ > 145 mEq/L)

Unlike patients with hyponatremia, the patients with hypernatremia are always HYPEROSMOLAR.
Hypernatremia always reprensts a deficit in total body water (TBW)

The volume of free water needed is: $Vol_{H_2O} = \underbrace{(0.6 \times \text{body weight in kg})}_{TBW} \times ([Na^+_{serum} - 140] / 140)$

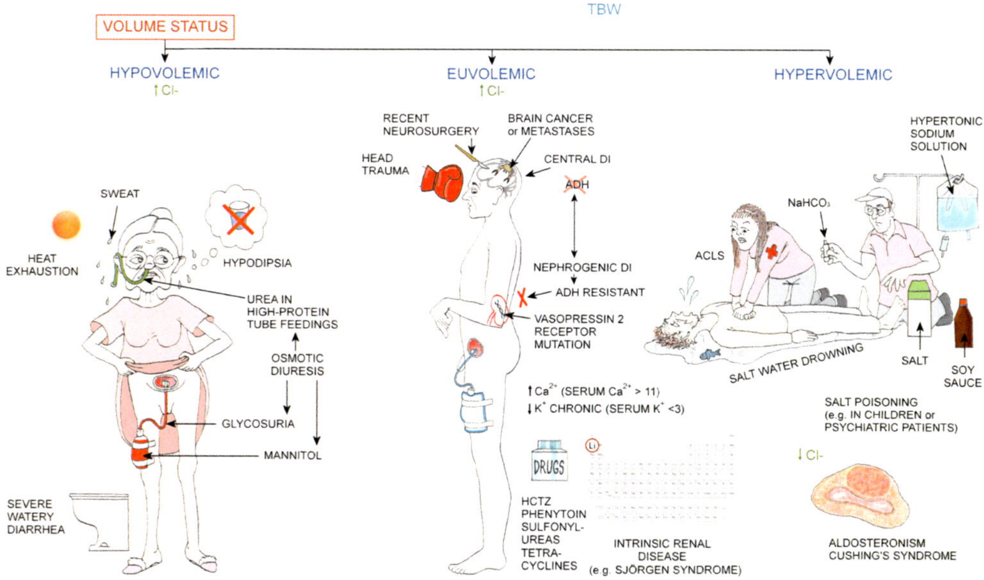

“Showing once is worth more than saying a hundred times.”

Chinese proverb

HYPERNATREMIA (SERUM $Na^+ > 145$ mEq/L)

Unlike patients with hyponatremia, the patients with hypernatremia are always HYPEROSMOLAR. Hypernatremia always reprensts a deficit in total body water (TBW)

The volume of free water needed is: $Vol_{H_2O} = \underbrace{(0.6 \times \text{body weight in kg})}_{TBW} \times ([Na^+_{serum} - 140] / 140)$

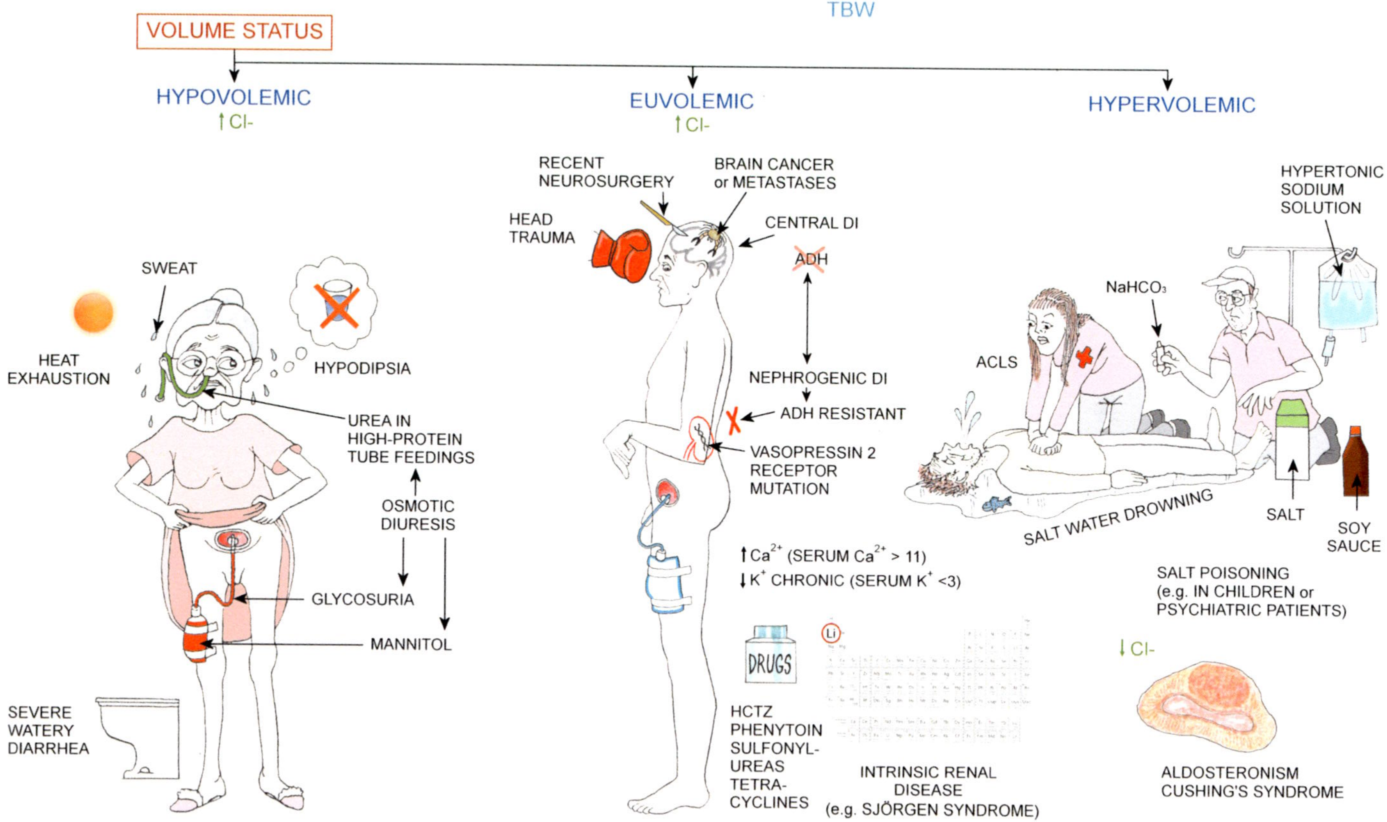

HYPONATREMIA

Patients with hyponatremia often look "truly sick."

Hypotonic hyponatremia is usually caused by primary water gain or sodium loss. Sodium loss may be the result of renal or external causes. (Polydipsia as the cause of hyponatremia is extremely rare, except in rare psychiatric patients who drink water excessively. An individual with normal kidney function would have to drink more than 20 liters of water per day before developing hyponatremia.)

Isotonic hyponatremia (pseudohyponatremia) occurs because of a decrease in the aqueous phase of plasma (hyperproteinemia, hyperlipidemia). High levels of protein and lipids in the blood can increase the concentration of other solutes, such as sodium, making the blood more concentrated. As the body tries to dilute the blood to maintain a normal balance of solutes, excess water is taken up by cells, leading to hyponatremia. Liver disease can cause jaundice and hyponatremia at the same time.

Hypertonic hyponatremia is caused by an increase in extravascular solute concentration, e.g., hyperglycemia or intravenous (IV) mannitol or intravenous immunoglobulin (IVIG) administration.

Translocational hyponatremia is a rare type of hyponatremia that occurs when water moves from the intracellular space to the extracellular space, causing a diluted concentration of sodium in the blood (in procedures such as hysteroscopy, transurethral resection of prostate [TURP], or administration of contrast agents).

In hyponatremia, an **increased chloride** level suggests diabetic ketoacidosis (DKA), Addison disease, renal tubular acidosis (RTA), nephritis and use of certain diuretics as the cause.

A decreased chloride level suggests congestive heart failure (CHF), syndrome of inappropriate ADB secretion (SIADH), pyloric obstruction, vomiting, malabsorption syndrome and diuretics as possible causes.

A **low plasma cortisol** level coupled with a low sodium level and elevated chloride level suggest Addison disease.

A low sodium and elevated chloride but **normal plasma cortisol** should suggest RTA, nephritis, and use of certain diuretics.

The mechanism by which hypothyroidism causes hyponatremia is not completely understood, but it is thought to be related to the changes in the activity of the renin-angiotensin-aldosterone system (RAAS).

SIADH typically reflects pathology in the lungs (such as lung cancer or a pulmonary process) or the brain (such as brain trauma or some medications affecting the central nervous system [CNS]).

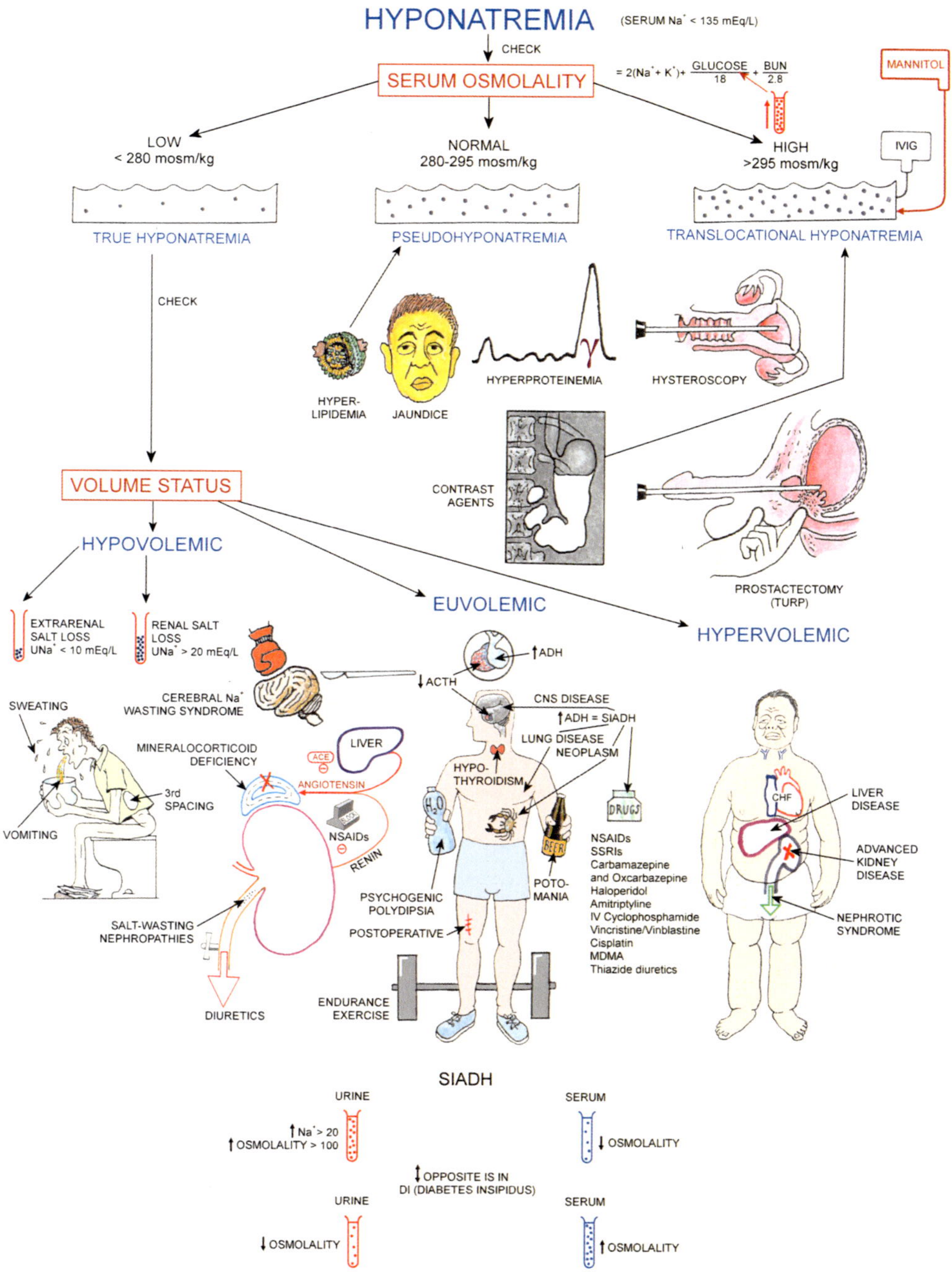
HYPONATREMIA
(SERUM Na+ < 135 mEq/L)
CHECK
SERUM OSMOLALITY
= 2(Na+ + K+)+ GLUCOSE/18 + BUN/2.8
MANNITOL
LOW
< 280 mosm/kg
NORMAL
280-295 mosm/kg
HIGH
>295 mosm/kg
IVIG
TRUE HYPONATREMIA
PSEUDOHYPONATREMIA
TRANSLOCATIONAL HYPONATREMIA
CHECK
HYPER-
LIPIDEMIA
JAUNDICE
HYPERPROTEINEMIA
HYSTEROSCOPY
CONTRAST
AGENTS
PROSTACTECTOMY
(TURP)
VOLUME STATUS
HYPOVOLEMIC
EUVOLEMIC
HYPERVOLEMIC
EXTRARENAL
SALT LOSS
UNa+ < 10 mEq/L
RENAL SALT
LOSS
UNa+ > 20 mEq/L
CEREBRAL Na+
WASTING SYNDROME
SWEATING
VOMITING
3rd
SPACING
MINERALOCORTICOID
DEFICIENCY
LIVER
ACE
ANGIOTENSIN
NSAIDs
RENIN
SALT-WASTING
NEPHROPATHIES
DIURETICS
↑ADH
↓ACTH
CNS DISEASE
↑ADH = SIADH
LUNG DISEASE
NEOPLASM
HYPO-
THYROIDISM
DRUGS
NSAIDs
SSRIs
Carbamazepine
and Oxcarbazepine
Haloperidol
Amitriptyline
IV Cyclophosphamide
Vincristine/Vinblastine
Cisplatin
MDMA
Thiazide diuretics
BEER
POTO-
MANIA
PSYCHOGENIC
POLYDIPSIA
POSTOPERATIVE
ENDURANCE
EXERCISE
CHF
LIVER
DISEASE
ADVANCED
KIDNEY
DISEASE
NEPHROTIC
SYNDROME
SIADH
URINE
↑Na+ > 20
↑OSMOLALITY > 100
SERUM
↓OSMOLALITY
↕OPPOSITE IS IN
DI (DIABETES INSIPIDUS)
URINE
↓OSMOLALITY
SERUM
↑OSMOLALITY

HYPERKALEMIA

Pseudohyperkalemia is a laboratory finding in which a blood test indicates a high level of potassium in the blood, but the actual potassium level in the body is within normal range. It occurs due to leakage of potassium from the cells during or after blood collection. It could happen due to prolonged tourniquet application, excessive exercise, any other form of muscle injury, or hemolysis.

In **metabolic acidosis** the potassium ions move out of the cell due to a change in the pH balance of the body.

Exercising can cause a brief increase in potassium levels in the blood. So, the patients with hyperkalemia should be cautious about it. However, regular exercise can also help manage the underlying conditions that may be contributing to hyperkalemia such as renal disease or hypertension.

The **increase in plasma osmolality** results in osmotic water movement from the cells into the extracellular fluid. The loss of cell water raises the cell potassium concentration, thereby creating a favorable gradient for passive potassium to exit through potassium channels in the cell membrane.

Insulin promotes potassium entry **into** cells. Therefore, **insulin deficiency** leads to hyperkalemia.

Some **beta blockers** can directly affect the renal excretion of potassium from the body, which can contribute to hyperkalemia.

Any cause of **increased tissue catabolism** (like in trauma or burns) leads to the release of intracellular potassium into the extracellular fluid.

If a large number of older red blood cells (**RBC) are transfused** quickly this can lead to hyperkalemia.

The muscle relaxant **succinylcholine** (used for temporary paralysis of skeletal muscles, allowing for easier intubation and surgery) causes muscle cell depolarization, to prevent muscle contraction. As a result of this depolarization, intracellular potassium can leak out into the bloodstream, leading to hyperkalemia.

L-arginine is an amino acid commonly used as a dietary supplement. It helps the body produce nitric oxide (NO) which can improve blood flow and cardiovascular health. However, excessive intake of L-arginine may lead to certain side effects including hyperkalemia. L-arginine is converted to NO which can interact with certain potassium channels.

Ureterojejunostomy is the surgical procedure performed in people who have their bladder removed due to cancer or other conditions. [16]

16 Abbreviations: RTA: renal tubular acidosis.

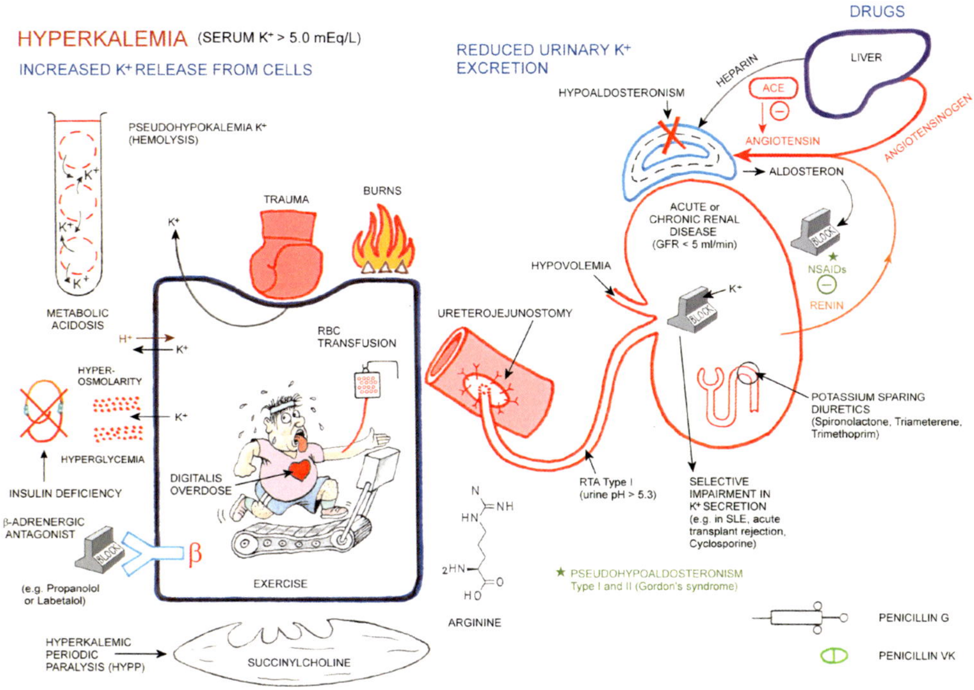

HYPERKALEMIA (SERUM K+ > 5.0 mEq/L)
INCREASED K+ RELEASE FROM CELLS
PSEUDOHYPOKALEMIA K+
(HEMOLYSIS)
K+
METABOLIC
ACIDOSIS
H+
HYPER-
OSMOLARITY
HYPERGLYCEMIA
INSULIN DEFICIENCY
β-ADRENERGIC
ANTAGONIST
BLOCK
(e.g. Propanolol
or Labetalol)
β
TRAUMA
BURNS
RBC
TRANSFUSION
DIGITALIS
OVERDOSE
EXERCISE
HYPERKALEMIC
PERIODIC
PARALYSIS (HYPP)
SUCCINYLCHOLINE
ARGININE
REDUCED URINARY K+
EXCRETION
DRUGS
LIVER
HEPARIN
ACE
ANGIOTENSIN
ANGIOTENSINOGEN
HYPOALDOSTERONISM
ALDOSTERON
ACUTE or
CHRONIC RENAL
DISEASE
(GFR < 5 ml/min)
NSAIDs
RENIN
HYPOVOLEMIA
URETEROJEJUNOSTOMY
POTASSIUM SPARING
DIURETICS
(Spironolactone, Triameterene,
Trimethoprim)
RTA Type I
(urine pH > 5.3)
SELECTIVE
IMPAIRMENT IN
K+ SECRETION
(e.g. in SLE, acute
transplant rejection,
Cyclosporine)
★ PSEUDOHYPOALDOSTERONISM
Type I and II (Gordon's syndrome)
PENICILLIN G
PENICILLIN VK

"Drawing is vision on paper."

Andrew Loomis

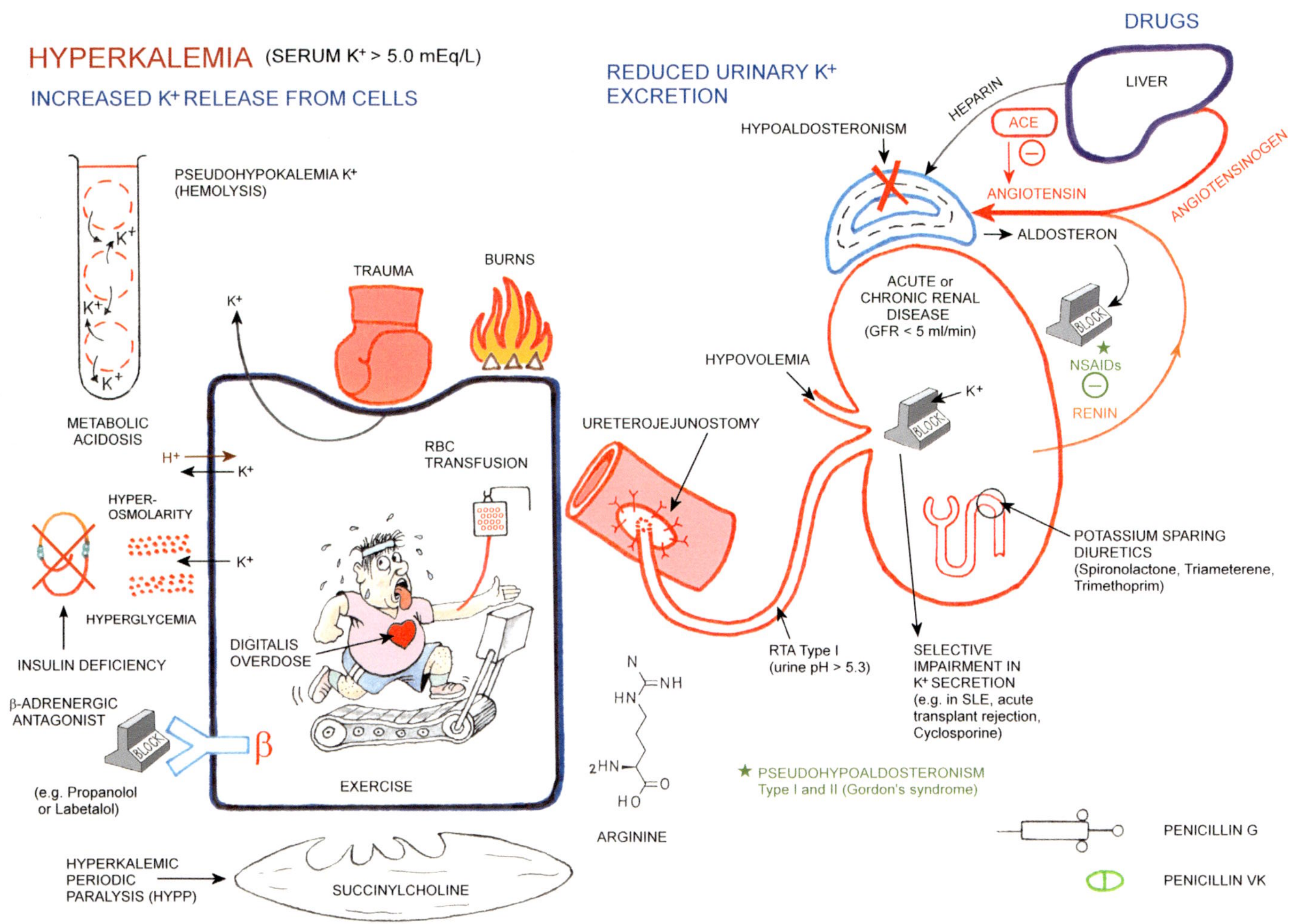
HYPERKALEMIA (SERUM K+ > 5.0 mEq/L)
INCREASED K+ RELEASE FROM CELLS
PSEUDOHYPOKALEMIA K+ (HEMOLYSIS)
K+
METABOLIC ACIDOSIS
H+
K+
HYPER-OSMOLARITY
HYPERGLYCEMIA
INSULIN DEFICIENCY
β-ADRENERGIC ANTAGONIST
BLOCK
(e.g. Propanolol or Labetalol)
β
TRAUMA
BURNS
RBC TRANSFUSION
DIGITALIS OVERDOSE
EXERCISE
HYPERKALEMIC PERIODIC PARALYSIS (HYPP)
SUCCINYLCHOLINE
REDUCED URINARY K+ EXCRETION
DRUGS
LIVER
HEPARIN
ACE
ANGIOTENSINOGEN
HYPOALDOSTERONISM
ANGIOTENSIN
ALDOSTERON
ACUTE or CHRONIC RENAL DISEASE (GFR < 5 ml/min)
NSAIDs
RENIN
HYPOVOLEMIA
URETEROJEJUNOSTOMY
POTASSIUM SPARING DIURETICS (Spironolactone, Triameterene, Trimethoprim)
RTA Type I (urine pH > 5.3)
SELECTIVE IMPAIRMENT IN K+ SECRETION (e.g. in SLE, acute transplant rejection, Cyclosporine)
ARGININE
★ PSEUDOHYPOALDOSTERONISM Type I and II (Gordon's syndrome)
PENICILLIN G
PENICILLIN VK

HYPOKALEMIA

In **alkalosis** in response to decreased concentration of hydrogen ions, the body may try to excrete more potassium ions in the urine. This can lead to a decrease in the level of potassium in the blood.

In diabetic keto acidosis (DKA) or a hyperosmolar hyperglycemic state (nonketotic hyperglycemia), hyperosmolality and insulin deficiency favor the movement of potassium out of cells. As a result, the serum potassium concentration at presentation may be normal or even elevated despite a marked potassium deficit due to urinary and, in some patients, gastrointestinal losses. The initiation of **insulin** therapy and fluid replacement will lower the serum potassium.

Beta agonists cause the movement of potassium out of the blood and into the cells.

Activation of the renin-angiotensin-aldosterone system (RAAS) by paraneoplastic production of renin-like activity in **AML** blast cells might contribute to hypokalemia.

Granulocyte-macrophage colony-stimulating factor (**GM-CSF**) can lead to hypokalemia by increasing the production and release of certain hormones, particularly cortisol, which can increase potassium to move from the bloodstream into cells. In addition, GM-CSF can also increase the number of white blood cells in the circulation, which can lead to an increased demand for nutrients such as potassium.

Vitamin B12 deficiency can cause hypokalemia because vitamin B12 is essential for the proper functioning of the nervous system, and it plays an important role in the regulation of the potassium level in the body. In addition, pernicious anemia itself can lead to an increase in the excretion of potassium in the urine.

Periodic paralysis (PP) is a rare neuromuscular disorder related to a defect in muscle ion channels, characterized by episodes of painless muscle weakness, which may be precipitated by heavy exercise, fasting, or high-carbohydrate meals.

PP is classified as hypokalemic when episodes occur in association with low potassium blood levels or as hyperkalemic when episodes can be induced by elevated potassium. Most cases of PP are hereditary, usually with an autosomal dominant inheritance pattern. Acquired cases of hypokalemic PP have been described in association with hyperthyroidism.

Patients with hypokalemia may also have **hypomagnesemia** due to concurrent loss with diarrhea or diuretic therapy or, in patients with hypomagnesemia as the primary abnormality, renal potassium wasting. Such patients can be refractory to potassium replacement alone. Thus, measurement of serum magnesium should be considered in patients with hypokalemia.

Hypothermia can cause hypokalemia by its effect on the movement of the potassium ions across cell membranes. Also, hypothermia can decrease the rate at which the kidneys excrete potassium. [17]

---

17 Abbreviations: PCA/PRA: plasma aldosterone concentration (PAC) to plasma renin activity (PRA) ratio; RTA: renal tubular acidosis.

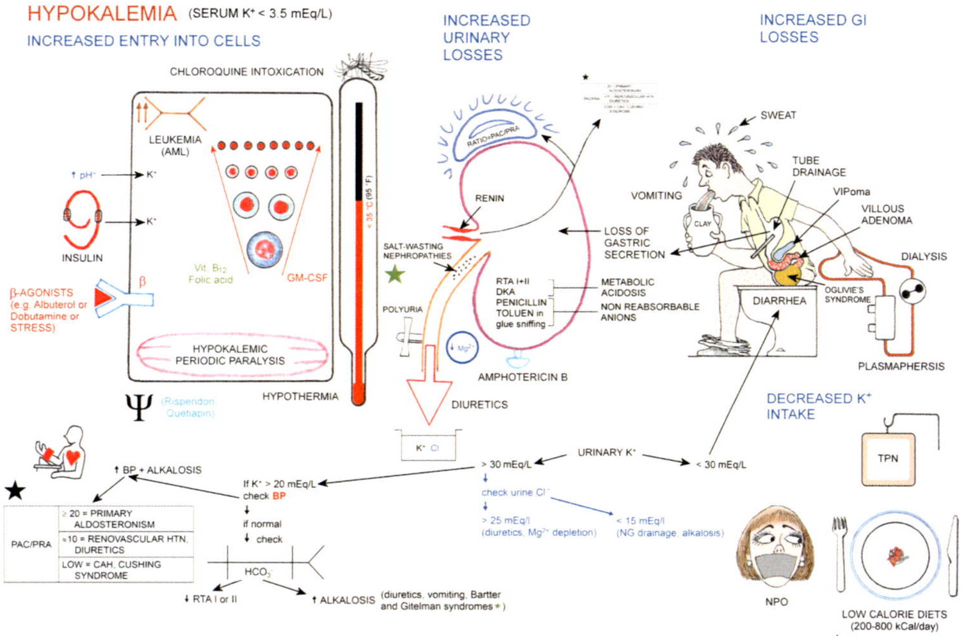
HYPOKALEMIA (SERUM K+ < 3.5 mEq/L)
INCREASED ENTRY INTO CELLS
CHLOROQUINE INTOXICATION
LEUKEMIA (AML)
↑ pH → K+
K+
INSULIN
Vit. B12 Folic acid
GM-CSF
β
β-AGONISTS (e.g. Albuterol or Dobutamine or STRESS)
HYPOKALEMIC PERIODIC PARALYSIS
< 35 °C (95 °F)
HYPOTHERMIA
Ψ (Rispendon Quetiapin)
INCREASED URINARY LOSSES
RATIO=PAC/PRA
RENIN
SALT-WASTING NEPHROPATHIES
POLYURIA
↓ Mg2+
RTA I+II
DKA
PENICILLIN
TOLUEN in glue sniffing
METABOLIC ACIDOSIS
NON REABSORBABLE ANIONS
LOSS OF GASTRIC SECRETION
AMPHOTERICIN B
DIURETICS
K+ Cl
INCREASED GI LOSSES
SWEAT
TUBE DRAINAGE
VOMITING
CLAY
VIPoma
VILLOUS ADENOMA
DIALYSIS
OGLIVIE'S SYNDROME
DIARRHEA
PLASMAPHERSIS
DECREASED K+ INTAKE
TPN
URINARY K+
> 30 mEq/L
< 30 mEq/L
check urine Cl−
> 25 mEq/l (diuretics, Mg2+ depletion)
< 15 mEq/l (NG drainage, alkalosis)
If K+ > 20 mEq/L check BP
↑ BP + ALKALOSIS
if normal
check
HCO3−
↓ RTA I or II
↑ ALKALOSIS (diuretics, vomiting, Bartter and Gitelman syndromes)
PAC/PRA
≥ 20 = PRIMARY ALDOSTERONISM
≈10 = RENOVASCULAR HTN, DIURETICS
LOW = CAH, CUSHING SYNDROME
NPO
LOW CALORIE DIETS (200-800 kCal/day)

"Be slow on the tongue and quick on the eyes."

Miguel de Cervantes

HYPOKALEMIA (SERUM K⁺ < 3.5 mEq/L)

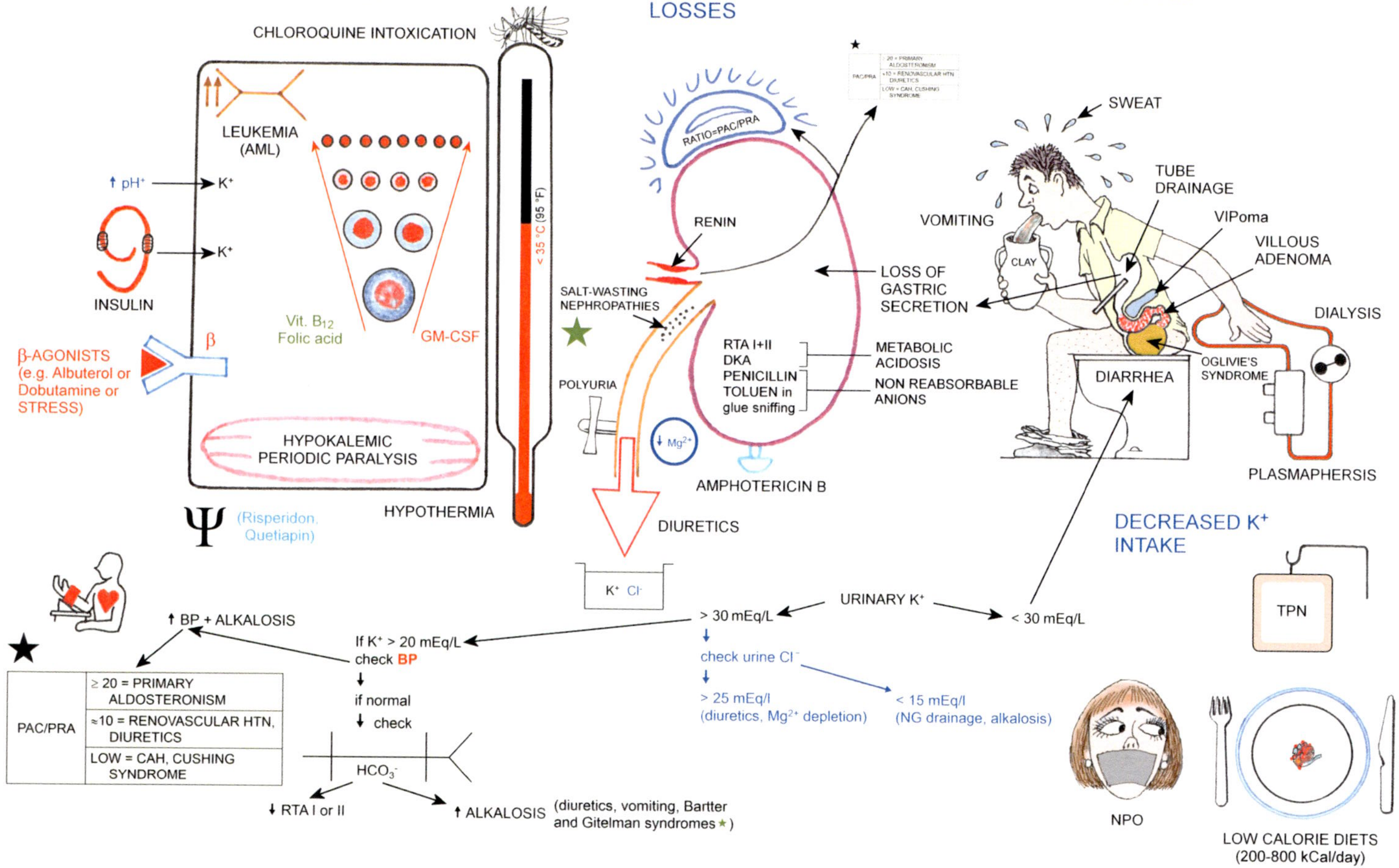

PAC/PRA	≥ 20 = PRIMARY ALDOSTERONISM
	≈10 = RENOVASCULAR HTN, DIURETICS
	LOW = CAH, CUSHING SYNDROME

"Vision is the art of seeing what is invisible to others."

Jonathan Swift

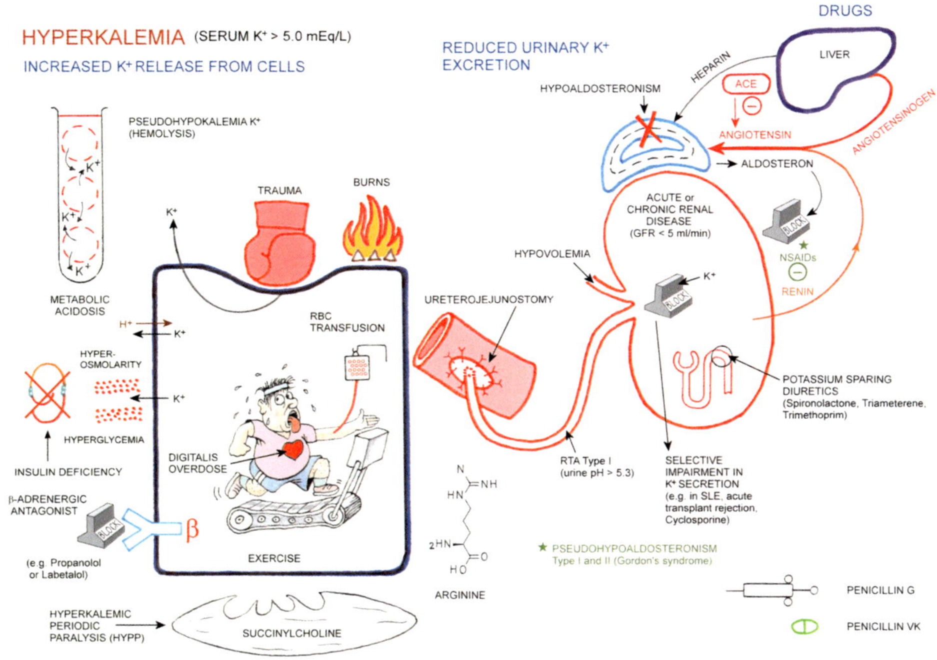
HYPERKALEMIA (SERUM K+ > 5.0 mEq/L)
INCREASED K+ RELEASE FROM CELLS
PSEUDOHYPOKALEMIA K+ (HEMOLYSIS)
METABOLIC ACIDOSIS
H+
K+
HYPER-OSMOLARITY
HYPERGLYCEMIA
INSULIN DEFICIENCY
β-ADRENERGIC ANTAGONIST
BLOCK
β
(e.g. Propanolol or Labetalol)
TRAUMA
BURNS
RBC TRANSFUSION
DIGITALIS OVERDOSE
EXERCISE
HYPERKALEMIC PERIODIC PARALYSIS (HYPP)
SUCCINYLCHOLINE
ARGININE
REDUCED URINARY K+ EXCRETION
DRUGS
LIVER
HEPARIN
ACE
ANGIOTENSIN
ANGIOTENSINOGEN
HYPOALDOSTERONISM
ALDOSTERON
ACUTE or CHRONIC RENAL DISEASE (GFR < 5 ml/min)
NSAIDs
RENIN
HYPOVOLEMIA
URETEROJEJUNOSTOMY
POTASSIUM SPARING DIURETICS (Spironolactone, Triameterene, Trimethoprim)
RTA Type I (urine pH > 5.3)
SELECTIVE IMPAIRMENT IN K+ SECRETION (e.g. in SLE, acute transplant rejection, Cyclosporine)
★ PSEUDOHYPOALDOSTERONISM Type I and II (Gordon's syndrome)
PENICILLIN G
PENICILLIN VK

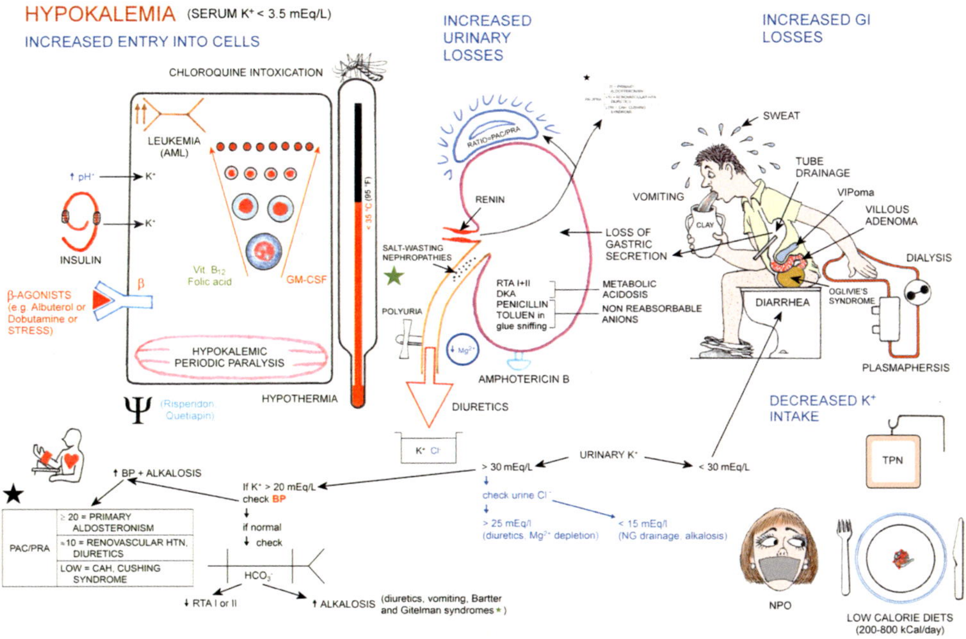
HYPOKALEMIA (SERUM K+ < 3.5 mEq/L)
INCREASED ENTRY INTO CELLS
CHLOROQUINE INTOXICATION
LEUKEMIA (AML)
↑ pH
K+
INSULIN
Vit. B12 Folic acid
GM-CSF
β-AGONISTS (e.g. Albuterol or Dobutamine or STRESS)
HYPOKALEMIC PERIODIC PARALYSIS
< 35 °C (95 °F)
HYPOTHERMIA
(Rispendon Quetiapin)
INCREASED URINARY LOSSES
RATIO=PAC/PRA
RENIN
SALT-WASTING NEPHROPATHIES
POLYURIA
Mg2+
LOSS OF GASTRIC SECRETION
RTA I+II
DKA
PENICILLIN
TOLUEN in glue sniffing
METABOLIC ACIDOSIS
NON REABSORBABLE ANIONS
AMPHOTERICIN B
DIURETICS
K+ Cl-
URINARY K+
> 30 mEq/L
< 30 mEq/L
check urine Cl-
> 25 mEq/l (diuretics, Mg2+ depletion)
< 15 mEq/l (NG drainage, alkalosis)
If K+ > 20 mEq/L check BP
↑ BP + ALKALOSIS
if normal
check
HCO3-
↓ RTA I or II
↑ ALKALOSIS (diuretics, vomiting, Bartter and Gitelman syndromes ★)
PAC/PRA
≥ 20 = PRIMARY ALDOSTERONISM
≈10 = RENOVASCULAR HTN, DIURETICS
LOW = CAH, CUSHING SYNDROME
INCREASED GI LOSSES
SWEAT
TUBE DRAINAGE
VOMITING
CLAY
VIPoma
VILLOUS ADENOMA
DIALYSIS
DIARRHEA
OGLIVIE'S SYNDROME
PLASMAPHERSIS
DECREASED K+ INTAKE
TPN
NPO
LOW CALORIE DIETS (200-800 kCal/day)

HYPER AND HYPOCHLOREMIA

Hyperchloremia is often a secondary condition caused by an underlying medical condition. The most common cause of hyperchloremia is **dehydration**. Other medical causes may include:

kidney disease, such as renal tubular acidosis (RTA)

medications such as diuretics or corticosteroids

diabetic keto acidosis (**DKA**)

non anion gap metabolic acidosis (Decrease in pH triggers the kidneys to excrete more acids. Chloride ions and negatively charged anions and their concentration in the blood can increase to compensate for the decrease in bicarbonate ions.)

respiratory alkalosis (When there is too little carbon dioxide in the blood, the kidneys excrete bicarbonate ions to help rebalance the increased pH level. The kidneys then absorb more chloride ions to help compensate for the loss of bicarbonate ions.)

severe infection (The body's immune response to the infection can cause an increase in the production of inflammatory cytokines. These cytokines can cause a decrease in the secretion of bicarbonate ions from the kidneys and increase in the secretion of chloride ions. Severe infection can also cause vomiting and diarrhea with subsequent dehydration and increased concentration of chlorides in the blood).

Adrenal gland disorders such as Addison disease. (The lack of aldosterone causes a decrease in reabsorption of sodium or chloride from the kidneys, leading to an excess loss of these ions in the urine. However, over time the kidneys may increase the reabsorption of chloride ions to compensate, leading to hyperchloremia.).

The most common cause of **hypochloremia** is **overhydration**. Other medical causes include:

- **diuretic use**
- **vomiting and diarrhea**
- **kidney disease,** such as chronic renal failure

metabolic alkalosis (When there is too much bicarbonate in the blood, the kidneys excrete more bicarbonate ions to achieve acid-base balance. As the kidneys excrete more bicarbonate ions, more chloride ions are also excreted in the urine.)

respiratory acidosis (The exact mechanism linking respiratory acidosis to hypochloremia is not fully understood, but it likely involves kidney function and electrolyte regulation.)

Primary hyperparathyroidism disrupts calcium regulation (through increased renal bicarbonate loss and resulting normal anion gap metabolic acidosis), which indirectly impacts chloride levels and can contribute to hyperchloremia.

Chemotherapy drugs may cause electrolyte imbalances, including hypochloremia.

HYPERCHLOREMIA

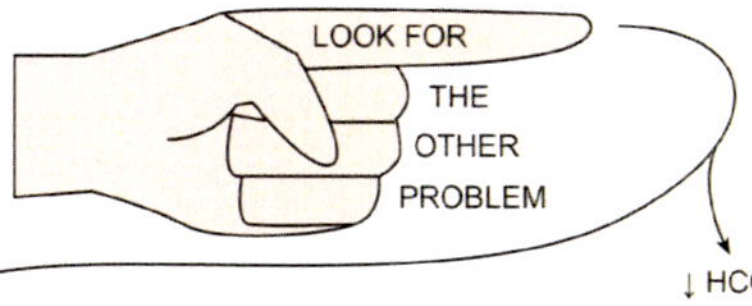

↓ HCO_3^-

HYPERNATREMIA

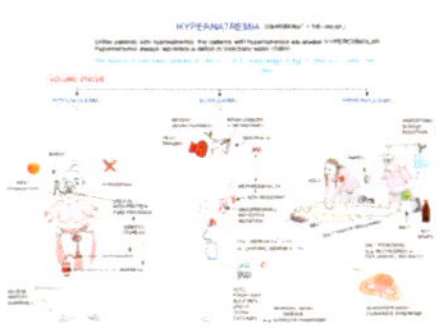

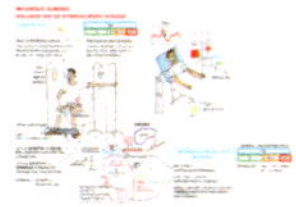

NON-ANION GAP ACIDOSIS W/DKA

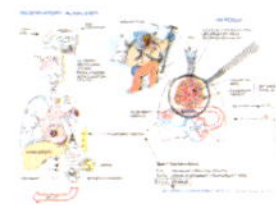

RESP. ALKALOSIS

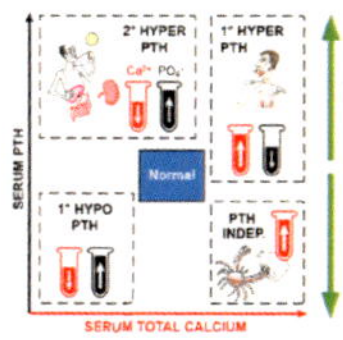

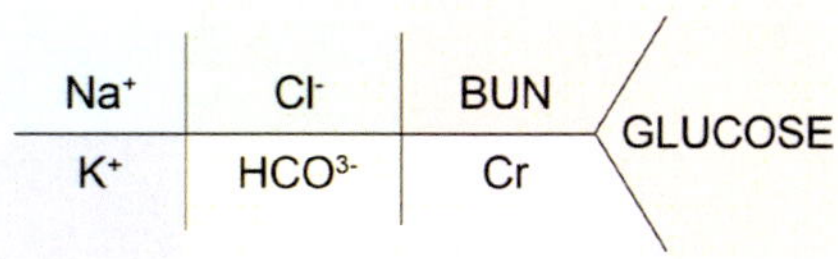

HYPOCHLOREMIA

HYPONATREMIA

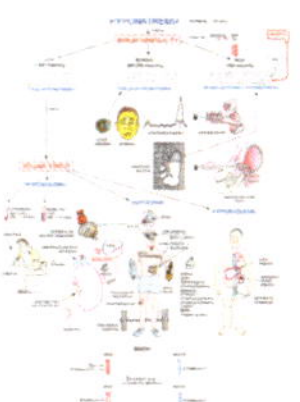

↑ HCO_3^-

METAB. ALKALOSIS

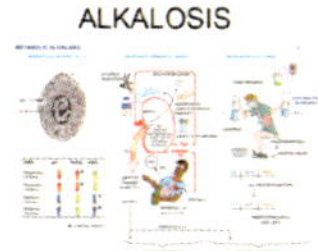

RESP. ACIDOSIS

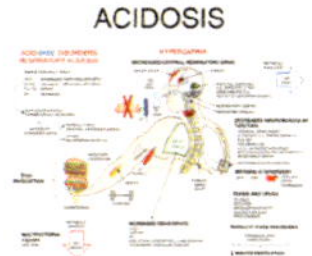

“Art is the lesser sister to medicine. It aims to heal.”

Andrew Lam

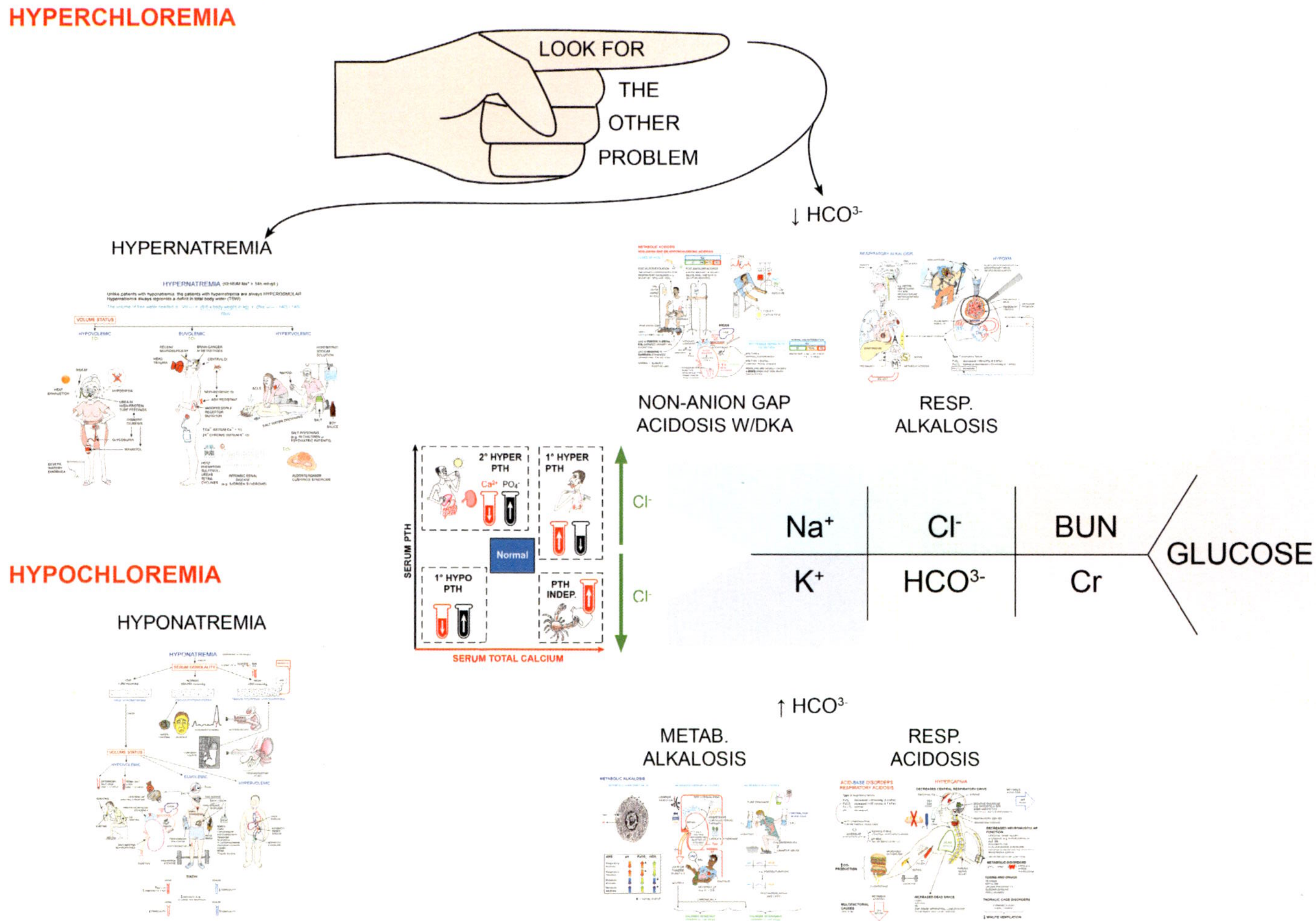
HYPERCHLOREMIA
LOOK FOR
THE
OTHER
PROBLEM
↓ HCO3-
HYPERNATREMIA
NON-ANION GAP ACIDOSIS W/DKA
RESP. ALKALOSIS
2° HYPER PTH
1° HYPER PTH
1° HYPO PTH
PTH INDEP.
Normal
SERUM PTH
SERUM TOTAL CALCIUM
Cl-
Cl-
Na+
Cl-
BUN
K+
HCO3-
Cr
GLUCOSE
HYPOCHLOREMIA
HYPONATREMIA
↑ HCO3-
METAB. ALKALOSIS
RESP. ACIDOSIS

ACID-BASE BALANCE NOMOGRAM

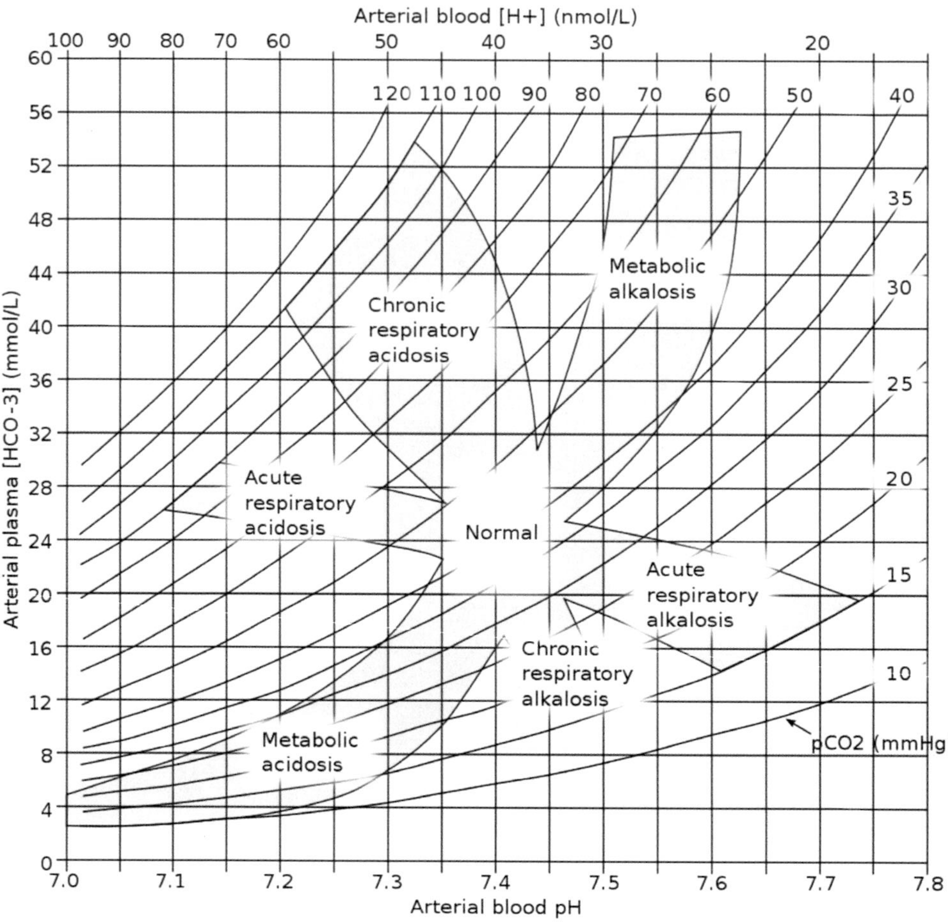

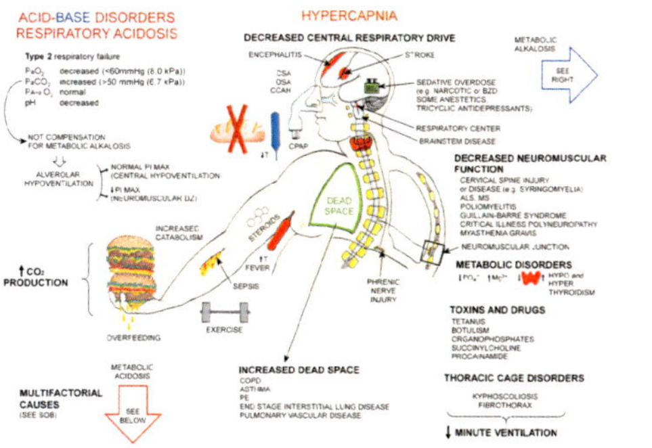
ACID-BASE DISORDERS
RESPIRATORY ACIDOSIS
Type 2 respiratory failure
P_aO_2 decreased (<60mmHg (8.0 kPa))
P_aCO_2 increased (>50 mmHg (6.7 kPa))
$P_{A-a}O_2$ normal
pH decreased
NOT COMPENSATION FOR METABOLIC ALKALOSIS
ALVEROLAR HYPOVENTILATION
NORMAL PI MAX (CENTRAL HYPOVENTILATION
↓PI MAX (NEUROMUSCULAR DZ)
HYPERCAPNIA
DECREASED CENTRAL RESPIRATORY DRIVE
ENCEPHALITIS
STROKE
CSA
OSA
CCAH
SEDATIVE OVERDOSE (e.g. NARCOTIC or BZD SOME ANESTETICS TRICYCLIC ANTIDEPRESSANTS)
RESPIRATORY CENTER
BRAINSTEM DISEASE
↓T
CPAP
METABOLIC ALKALOSIS
SEE RIGHT
DECREASED NEUROMUSCULAR FUNCTION
CERVICAL SPINE INJURY or DISEASE (e.g. SYRINGOMYELIA)
ALS, MS
POLIOMYELITIS
GUILLAIN-BARRE SYNDROME
CRITICAL ILLNESS POLYNEUROPATHY
MYASTHENIA GRAVIS
NEUROMUSCULAR JUNCTION
DEAD SPACE
STEROIDS
INCREASED CATABOLISM
↑T FEVER
SEPSIS
↑CO₂ PRODUCTION
OVERFEEDING
EXERCISE
PHRENIC NERVE INJURY
METABOLIC DISORDERS
HYPO and HYPER THYROIDISM
TOXINS AND DRUGS
TETANUS
BOTULISM
ORGANOPHOSPHATES
SUCCINYLCHOLINE
PROCAINAMIDE
METABOLIC ACIDOSIS
MULTIFACTORIAL CAUSES (SEE SOB)
SEE BELOW
INCREASED DEAD SPACE
COPD
ASTHMA
PE
END STAGE INTERSTITIAL LUNG DISEASE
PULMONARY VASCULAR DISEASE
THORACIC CAGE DISORDERS
KYPHOSCOLIOSIS
FIBROTHORAX
↓ MINUTE VENTILATION

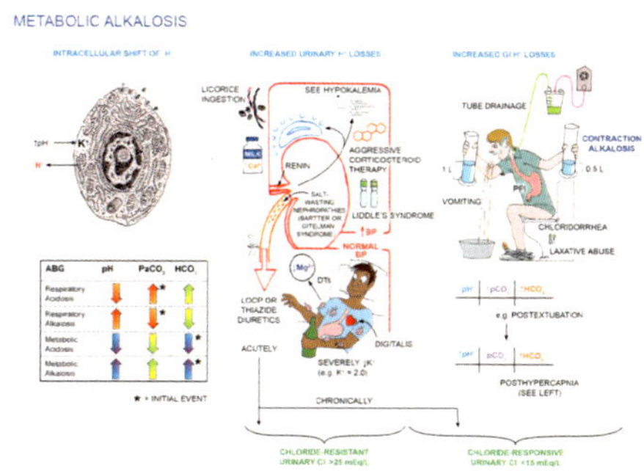
METABOLIC ALKALOSIS
INTRACELLULAR SHIFT OF H⁺
INCREASED URINARY H⁺ LOSSES
INCREASED GI H⁺ LOSSES
↑pH
K⁺
H⁺
LICORICE INGESTION
SEE HYPOKALEMIA
RENIN
AGGRESSIVE CORTICOSTEROID THERAPY
SALT-WASTING NEPHROPATHIES (BARTTER OR GITELMAN SYNDROME)
LIDDLE'S SYNDROME
↑BP
NORMAL BP
Mg²⁺
DTs
LOOP OR THIAZIDE DIURETICS
DIGITALIS
ACUTELY
SEVERELY ↓K⁺ (e.g. K⁺ = 2.0)
TUBE DRAINAGE
CONTRACTION ALKALOSIS
1 L
0.5 L
VOMITING
PPI
CHLORIDORRHEA
LAXATIVE ABUSE
e.g. POSTEXTUBATION
POSTHYPERCAPNIA (SEE LEFT)
CHRONICALLY
CHLORIDE-RESISTANT URINARY Cl⁻ >25 mEq/L
CHLORIDE-RESPONSIVE URINARY Cl⁻ <15 mEq/L
ABG
pH
$PaCO_2$
HCO_3^-
Respiratory Acidosis
Respiratory Alkalosis
Metabolic Acidosis
Metabolic Alkalosis
★ = INITIAL EVENT

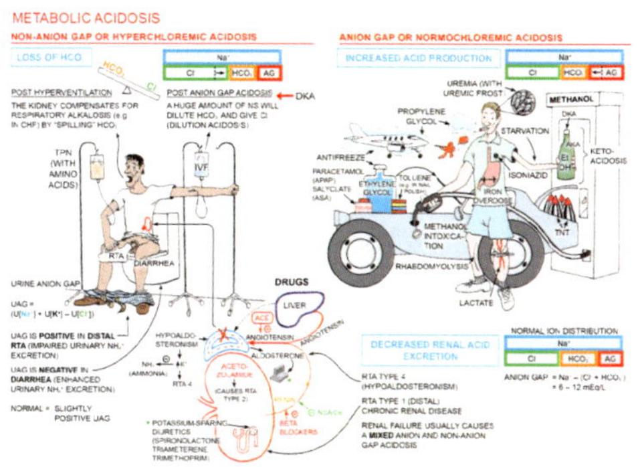
METABOLIC ACIDOSIS
NON-ANION GAP OR HYPERCHLOREMIC ACIDOSIS
LOSS OF HCO_3^-
Na⁺
Cl⁻
HCO_3^-
AG
POST HYPERVENTILATION
THE KIDNEY COMPENSATES FOR RESPIRATORY ALKALOSIS (e.g. IN CHF) BY "SPILLING" HCO_3^-
POST ANION GAP ACIDOSIS
DKA
A HUGE AMOUNT OF NS WILL DILUTE HCO_3^- AND GIVE Cl⁻ (DILUTION ACIDOSIS)
TPN (WITH AMINO ACIDS)
IVF
RTA
DIARRHEA
URINE ANION GAP
UAG = (U[Na⁺] + U[K⁺] − U[Cl⁻])
UAG IS POSITIVE IN DISTAL RTA (IMPAIRED URINARY NH_4^+ EXCRETION)
UAG IS NEGATIVE IN DIARRHEA (ENHANCED URINARY NH_4^+ EXCRETION)
NORMAL = SLIGHTLY POSITIVE UAG
DRUGS
LIVER
ACE
ANGIOTENSIN
HYPOALDOSTERONISM
ALDOSTERONE
NH_3 (AMMONIA)
RTA 4
ACETAZOLAMIDE (CAUSES RTA TYPE 2)
NSAIDs
BETA BLOCKERS
POTASSIUM-SPARING DIURETICS (SPIRONOLACTONE TRIAMETERENE TRIMETHOPRIM)
ANION GAP OR NORMOCHLOREMIC ACIDOSIS
INCREASED ACID PRODUCTION
UREMIA (WITH UREMIC FROST)
METHANOL
PROPYLENE GLYCOL
STARVATION
DKA
AKA
KETO-ACIDOSIS
ANTIFREEZE
PARACETAMOL (APAP)
SALYCLATE (ASA)
ETHYLENE GLYCOL
TOLUENE (e.g. IN NAIL POLISH)
ISONIAZID
IRON OVERDOSE
METHANOL INTOXICATION
TNT
RHABDOMYOLYSIS
LACTATE
NORMAL ION DISTRIBUTION
DECREASED RENAL ACID EXCRETION
ANION GAP = Na⁺ − (Cl⁻ + HCO_3^-) = 6 − 12 mEq/L
RTA TYPE 4 (HYPOALDOSTERONISM)
RTA TYPE 1 (DISTAL)
CHRONIC RENAL DISEASE
RENAL FAILURE USUALLY CAUSES A MIXED ANION AND NON-ANION GAP ACIDOSIS

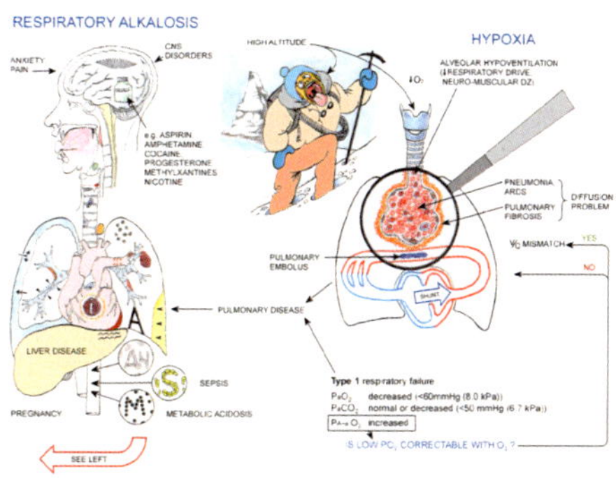
RESPIRATORY ALKALOSIS
ANXIETY PAIN
CNS DISORDERS
e.g. ASPIRIN AMPHETAMINE COCAINE PROGESTERONE METHYLXANTINES NICOTINE
LIVER DISEASE
SEPSIS
PREGNANCY
METABOLIC ACIDOSIS
SEE LEFT
PULMONARY DISEASE
HIGH ALTITUDE
HYPOXIA
↓O₂
ALVEOLAR HYPOVENTILATION (↓RESPIRATORY DRIVE NEURO-MUSCULAR DZ)
PNEUMONIA ARDS
PULMONARY FIBROSIS
DIFFUSION PROBLEM
V/Q MISMATCH
YES
NO
PULMONARY EMBOLUS
SHUNT
Type 1 respiratory failure
P_aO_2 decreased (<60mmHg (8.0 kPa))
P_aCO_2 normal or decreased (<50 mmHg (6.7 kPa))
$P_{A-a}O_2$ increased
IS LOW PO_2 CORRECTABLE WITH O_2 ?

"Simplicity is the ultimate sophistication."

Leonardo da Vinci

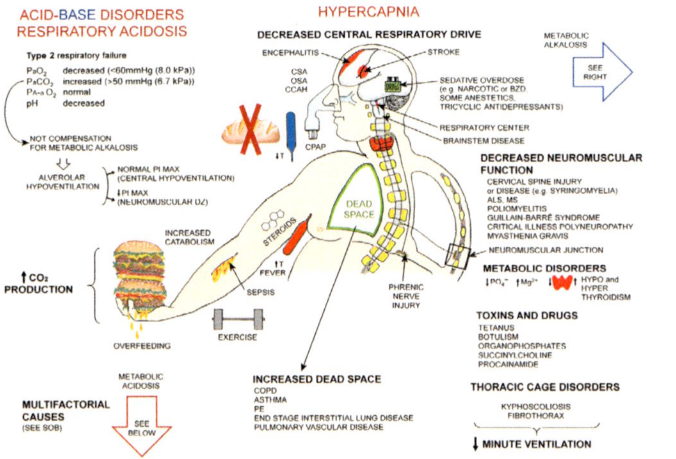
ACID-BASE DISORDERS
RESPIRATORY ACIDOSIS
Type 2 respiratory failure
PaO2 decreased (<60mmHg (8.0 kPa))
PaCO2 increased (>50 mmHg (6.7 kPa))
PA-a O2 normal
pH decreased
NOT COMPENSATION FOR METABOLIC ALKALOSIS
ALVEOLAR HYPOVENTILATION
NORMAL PI MAX (CENTRAL HYPOVENTILATION)
↓PI MAX (NEUROMUSCULAR DZ)
↑CO2 PRODUCTION
INCREASED CATABOLISM
OVERFEEDING
EXERCISE
SEPSIS
↑T FEVER
STEROIDS
↓T
CPAP
HYPERCAPNIA
DECREASED CENTRAL RESPIRATORY DRIVE
ENCEPHALITIS
STROKE
CSA
OSA
CCAH
SEDATIVE OVERDOSE (e.g. NARCOTIC or BZD SOME ANESTETICS, TRICYCLIC ANTIDEPRESSANTS)
RESPIRATORY CENTER
BRAINSTEM DISEASE
DEAD SPACE
PHRENIC NERVE INJURY
METABOLIC ALKALOSIS
SEE RIGHT
DECREASED NEUROMUSCULAR FUNCTION
CERVICAL SPINE INJURY or DISEASE (e.g. SYRINGOMYELIA)
ALS, MS
POLIOMYELITIS
GUILLAIN-BARRÉ SYNDROME
CRITICAL ILLNESS POLYNEUROPATHY
MYASTHENIA GRAVIS
NEUROMUSCULAR JUNCTION
METABOLIC DISORDERS
↓PO4 ↑Mg
HYPO and HYPER THYROIDISM
TOXINS AND DRUGS
TETANUS
BOTULISM
ORGANOPHOSPHATES
SUCCINYLCHOLINE
PROCAINAMIDE
THORACIC CAGE DISORDERS
KYPHOSCOLIOSIS
FIBROTHORAX
↓ MINUTE VENTILATION
METABOLIC ACIDOSIS
SEE BELOW
MULTIFACTORIAL CAUSES
(SEE SOB)
INCREASED DEAD SPACE
COPD
ASTHMA
PE
END STAGE INTERSTITIAL LUNG DISEASE
PULMONARY VASCULAR DISEASE

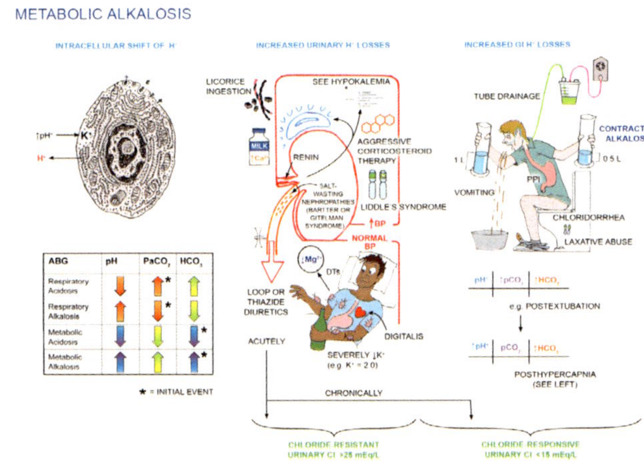
METABOLIC ALKALOSIS
INTRACELLULAR SHIFT OF H+
↑pH
K+
H+
ABG | pH | PaCO2 | HCO3
Respiratory Acidosis
Respiratory Alkalosis
Metabolic Acidosis
Metabolic Alkalosis
* = INITIAL EVENT
INCREASED URINARY H+ LOSSES
LICORICE INGESTION
MILK
SEE HYPOKALEMIA
RENIN
AGGRESSIVE CORTICOSTEROID THERAPY
SALT-WASTING NEPHROPATHIES (BARTTER OR GITELMAN SYNDROME)
LIDDLE'S SYNDROME
↑BP
NORMAL BP
Mg
DTs
LOOP OR THIAZIDE DIURETICS
DIGITALIS
SEVERELY ↓K+ (e.g. K+ = 2.0)
ACUTELY
CHRONICALLY
CHLORIDE RESISTANT URINARY Cl >25 mEq/L
INCREASED GI H+ LOSSES
TUBE DRAINAGE
CONTRACTION ALKALOSIS
1 L
0.5 L
VOMITING
PPI
CHLORIDORRHEA
LAXATIVE ABUSE
pH ↑pCO2 ↑HCO3
e.g. POSTEXTUBATION
↑pH pCO2 ↑HCO3
POSTHYPERCAPNIA (SEE LEFT)
CHLORIDE RESPONSIVE URINARY Cl <15 mEq/L

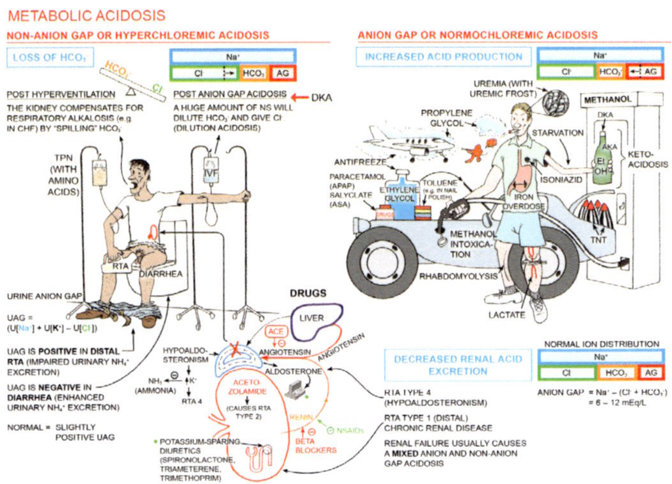
METABOLIC ACIDOSIS
NON-ANION GAP OR HYPERCHLOREMIC ACIDOSIS
LOSS OF HCO3
Na+
Cl
HCO3
AG
POST HYPERVENTILATION
THE KIDNEY COMPENSATES FOR RESPIRATORY ALKALOSIS (e.g. IN CHF) BY "SPILLING" HCO3
POST ANION GAP ACIDOSIS
DKA
A HUGE AMOUNT OF NS WILL DILUTE HCO3 AND GIVE Cl (DILUTION ACIDOSIS)
TPN (WITH AMINO ACIDS)
IVF
RTA
DIARRHEA
URINE ANION GAP
UAG = (U[Na+] + U[K+] – U[Cl])
UAG IS POSITIVE IN DISTAL RTA (IMPAIRED URINARY NH4+ EXCRETION)
UAG IS NEGATIVE IN DIARRHEA (ENHANCED URINARY NH4+ EXCRETION)
NORMAL = SLIGHTLY POSITIVE UAG
HYPOALDOSTERONISM
NH3 (AMMONIA)
K+
RTA 4
DRUGS
LIVER
ACE
ANGIOTENSIN
ANGIOTENSIN
ALDOSTERONE
ACETOZOLAMIDE (CAUSES RTA TYPE 2)
RENIN
NSAIDs
BETA BLOCKERS
POTASSIUM-SPARING DIURETICS (SPIRONOLACTONE, TRIAMETERENE, TRIMETHOPRIM)
ANION GAP OR NORMOCHLOREMIC ACIDOSIS
INCREASED ACID PRODUCTION
UREMIA (WITH UREMIC FROST)
PROPYLENE GLYCOL
STARVATION
METHANOL
DKA
AKA
EtOH
KETO-ACIDOSIS
ANTIFREEZE
PARACETAMOL (APAP)
SALYCLATE (ASA)
ETHYLENE GLYCOL
TOLUENE (e.g. IN NAIL POLISH)
ISONIAZID
IRON OVERDOSE
METHANOL INTOXICATION
TNT
RHABDOMYOLYSIS
LACTATE
DECREASED RENAL ACID EXCRETION
RTA TYPE 4 (HYPOALDOSTERONISM)
RTA TYPE 1 (DISTAL)
CHRONIC RENAL DISEASE
RENAL FAILURE USUALLY CAUSES A MIXED ANION AND NON-ANION GAP ACIDOSIS
NORMAL ION DISTRIBUTION
ANION GAP = Na+ – (Cl + HCO3) = 6 – 12 mEq/L

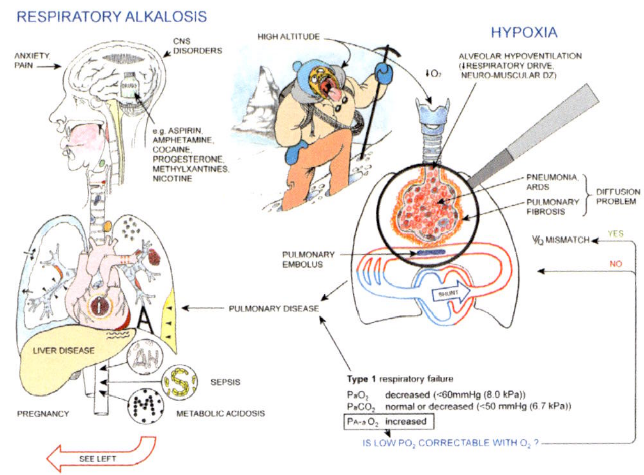
RESPIRATORY ALKALOSIS
ANXIETY PAIN
CNS DISORDERS
e.g. ASPIRIN, AMPHETAMINE, COCAINE, PROGESTERONE, METHYLXANTINES, NICOTINE
LIVER DISEASE
PREGNANCY
SEPSIS
METABOLIC ACIDOSIS
SEE LEFT
PULMONARY DISEASE
HYPOXIA
HIGH ALTITUDE
↓O2
ALVEOLAR HYPOVENTILATION (↓RESPIRATORY DRIVE, NEURO-MUSCULAR DZ)
PNEUMONIA, ARDS
PULMONARY FIBROSIS
DIFFUSION PROBLEM
V/Q MISMATCH
YES
NO
PULMONARY EMBOLUS
SHUNT
Type 1 respiratory failure
PaO2 decreased (<60mmHg (8.0 kPa))
PaCO2 normal or decreased (<50 mmHg (6.7 kPa))
PA-a O2 increased
IS LOW PO2 CORRECTABLE WITH O2 ?

RESPIRATORY ACIDOSIS

There are two underlying mechanisms of respiratory failure:

1. **Failure to oxygenate.** The patient's Partial pressure of oxygen (PaO_2) is less than 60 mmHg on room air.
2. **Failure to ventilate.** The patient's PaO_2 is greater than 50 mmHg.

There are two broad categories of respiratory failure, which reflect different underlying pathophysiological processes:

- Type 1 respiratory failure involves **hypoxemia** (PaO_2 <8 kPa / 60mmHg) with **normocapnia** (Partial pressure of carbon dioxide ($PaCO_2$) <6.0 kPa / 45mmHg)
- Type 2 respiratory failure involves **hypoxemia** (PaO_2 <8 kPa / 60mmHg) with **hypercapnia** ($PaCO_2$ >6.0 kPa / 45mmHg)

The causes of the respiratory failure could be remembered in a clockwise direction of the picture: on the top are central nervous system **(CNS) disorders**, on the right side **neuromuscular muscular disorders, chest wall disorders, and upper and lower airway obstructions**, on the bottom **disorders increasing dead space,** and on the left side are **conditions leading to excess carbon dioxide production.**

Phosphate, a high-energy substrate, is crucial for nerve function and muscle contraction.

Magnesium plays an essential role in nerve excitability. With magnesium levels exceeding 6.5 mEq/L, respiratory failure may be observed.

Both **hypothyroidism** and **hyperthyroidism** cause respiratory muscle weakness and decrease pulmonary function. Hypothyroidism reduces respiratory drive and can cause obstructive sleep apnea or pleural effusion, while hyperthyroidism increases respiratory drive and can cause dyspnea on exertion.

Hypothermia (shown as a thermometer) and **starvation** (shown as a crossed-out bread) can decrease central respiratory drive.

A continuous positive airway pressure (CPAP) mask symbolizes ventilatory support for obstructive sleep apnea (OSA), central sleep apnea (CSA) and congenital central alveolar hypoventilation (CCAH).

Increased carbon dioxide production can happen during fever, thyrotoxicosis, increased catabolism (sepsis, steroids), overfeeding, including total parenteral nutrition (TPN), exercise and metabolic acidosis.

Multifactorial causes can include: severe laryngeal or tracheal disorders (stenosis/tumors/angioedema/tracheomalacia), vocal cord paralysis, epiglottitis, foreign body aspiration, retropharyngeal disorders and obstructive goiter.[18]

---

18 Abbreviations: COPD: chronic obstructive pulmonary disease; PE: pulmonary embolism; PO4-: phosphorus; Mg2+: magnesium

ACID-BASE DISORDERS
RESPIRATORY ACIDOSIS

Type 2 respiratory failure

P_aO_2	decreased (<60mmHg (8.0 kPa))
P_aCO_2	increased (>50 mmHg (6.7 kPa))
$P_{A-a}\,O_2$	normal
pH	decreased

→ NOT COMPENSATION FOR METABOLIC ALKALOSIS

⇩

ALVEROLAR HYPOVENTILATION
- NORMAL PI MAX (CENTRAL HYPOVENTILATION)
- ↓PI MAX (NEUROMUSCULAR DZ)

HYPERCAPNIA

DECREASED CENTRAL RESPIRATORY DRIVE

METABOLIC ALKALOSIS ⇨ SEE RIGHT

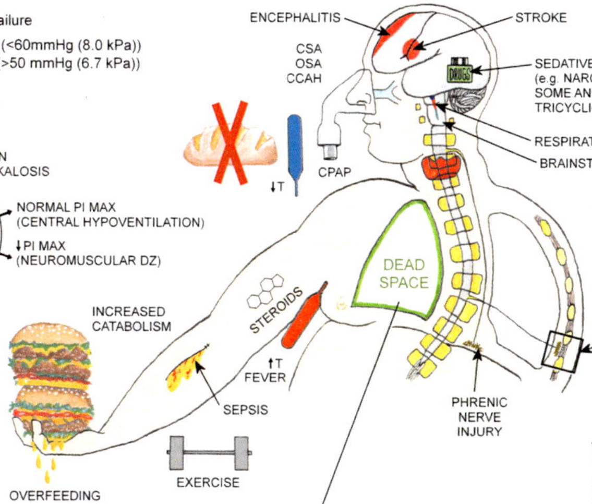

↑ CO_2 PRODUCTION

DECREASED NEUROMUSCULAR FUNCTION
- CERVICAL SPINE INJURY or DISEASE (e.g. SYRINGOMYELIA)
- ALS, MS
- POLIOMYELITIS
- GUILLAIN-BARRÉ SYNDROME
- CRITICAL ILLNESS POLYNEUROPATHY
- MYASTHENIA GRAVIS

METABOLIC DISORDERS

↓PO_4^- ↑Mg^{2+} ↓↑ HYPO and HYPER THYROIDISM

TOXINS AND DRUGS
- TETANUS
- BOTULISM
- ORGANOPHOSPHATES
- SUCCINYLCHOLINE
- PROCAINAMIDE

THORACIC CAGE DISORDERS
- KYPHOSCOLIOSIS
- FIBROTHORAX

↓ MINUTE VENTILATION

INCREASED DEAD SPACE
- COPD
- ASTHMA
- PE
- END STAGE INTERSTITIAL LUNG DISEASE
- PULMONARY VASCULAR DISEASE

MULTIFACTORIAL CAUSES
(SEE SOB)

METABOLIC ACIDOSIS ⇩ SEE BELOW

“Vision without action is a daydream.
Action without vision is a nightmare.”

Japanese proverb

ACID-BASE DISORDERS
RESPIRATORY ACIDOSIS

Type 2 respiratory failure

P_aO_2	decreased (<60mmHg (8.0 kPa))
P_aCO_2	increased (>50 mmHg (6.7 kPa))
$P_{A\text{-}a}O_2$	normal
pH	decreased

NOT COMPENSATION FOR METABOLIC ALKALOSIS

ALVEROLAR HYPOVENTILATION
- NORMAL PI MAX (CENTRAL HYPOVENTILATION)
- ↓PI MAX (NEUROMUSCULAR DZ)

HYPERCAPNIA

DECREASED CENTRAL RESPIRATORY DRIVE

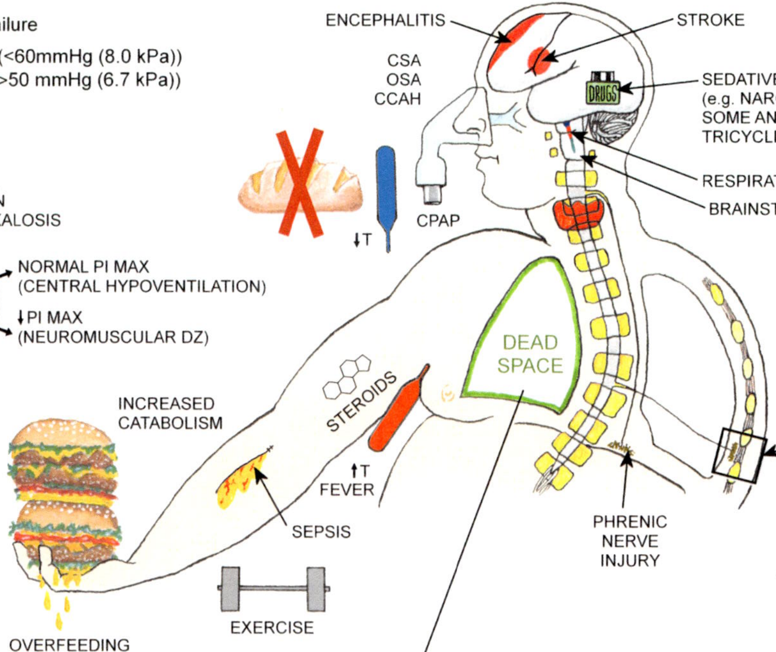

METABOLIC ALKALOSIS

SEE RIGHT

↑ CO_2 PRODUCTION

DECREASED NEUROMUSCULAR FUNCTION

CERVICAL SPINE INJURY or DISEASE (e.g. SYRINGOMYELIA)
ALS, MS
POLIOMYELITIS
GUILLAIN-BARRÉ SYNDROME
CRITICAL ILLNESS POLYNEUROPATHY
MYASTHENIA GRAVIS

METABOLIC DISORDERS

↓PO_4^- ↑Mg^{2+} ↓↑ HYPO and HYPER THYROIDISM

TOXINS AND DRUGS

TETANUS
BOTULISM
ORGANOPHOSPHATES
SUCCINYLCHOLINE
PROCAINAMIDE

THORACIC CAGE DISORDERS

KYPHOSCOLIOSIS
FIBROTHORAX

↓ MINUTE VENTILATION

INCREASED DEAD SPACE

COPD
ASTHMA
PE
END STAGE INTERSTITIAL LUNG DISEASE
PULMONARY VASCULAR DISEASE

MULTIFACTORIAL CAUSES
(SEE SOB)

METABOLIC ACIDOSIS

SEE BELOW

METABOLIC ACIDOSIS

Metabolic acidosis is a pathologic process due to reduced bicarbonate (HCO_3) concentration and/or increases in the hydrogen ion concentration in the body. The causes of metabolic acidosis are loss of bicarbonate, increased acid generation or diminished renal acid excretion.

Non-anion gap or hyperchloremic acidosis is caused by reduction in serum HCO_3^- which is matched by an equivalent increase in the serum chloride, resulting in hyperchloremia in the absence of an increase in the serum *anion gap*.

The primary pH buffer system in the human body is the HCO_3^-/CO_2 chemical equilibrium system: $H^+ + HCO_3^- \leftrightarrow H_2CO_3 \leftrightarrow CO_2 + H_2O$.

Therefore, **hyperventilation** (e.g., during congestive heart failure [CHF] pulmonary edema) will decrease carbon dioxide [CO_2] and will shift equilibrium toward the left, causing increases in bicarbonate [HCO_3^-], making blood more alkalotic. To maintain the acid-base balance the kidney will remove an extra HCO_3^-. When breathing normalizes, there still will be loss of HCO_3^- since it will take some time for the kidney to normalize the HCO_3^- level.

Post anion gap acidosis may happen in the treatment and recovery phases of diabetic keto acidosis (DKA).

Total parenteral nutrition (**TPN**) can cause metabolic acidosis due to the metabolism of cationic amino acids and amino acids containing sulfuric acid, thiamine deficiency and hypophosphatemia.

Healthy subjects typically have a **urine anion gap** of 0 to < 10 mEq/L. A urine anion gap (UAG) of more than 20 mEq/L is seen in metabolic acidosis when the kidneys are unable to excrete ammonia (such as renal tubular acidosis [RTA]). Urine anion gap is used to diagnose **metabolic acidosis** of a normal anion gap variety. However, pitfalls exist when using urine anion gap in the setting of **toluene** sniffing ("glue sniffing").

Hyperkalemia decreases proximal tubule ammonia generation and collecting duct ammonia transport, leading to impaired ammonia excretion and therefore metabolic acidosis.

Anion gap or normochloremic acidosis occurs when the body produces too much acid, or when the kidneys are not removing it enough. Uremic **frost** urea deposits can be found on the skin of those affected by chronic renal failure. **Ketoacidosis** includes acidosis due to starvation, alcohol, and diabetes mellitus. The hepatic generation of ketone bodies is the normal physiologic response to **fasting (starvation)**. **Ethanol** is rapidly oxidized, mainly in the liver, first to acetaldehyde and then to acetic acid. When there is not enough glucose due to a reduced insulin level, the body starts the catabolism of fatty acids for energy leading to ketones production. (The bottle cap represents a cube of sugar as a symbol of **DKA**).

Methanol was known as wood alcohol because it was once produced by the distillation of wood. Fuel producers blend methanol with gasoline. Methanol is occasionally used to fuel internal combustion engines. The patient's tourniquet in his leg is a symbol for ischemia with subsequent anaerobic condition and production of **lactic acid**, while a tag for exercising in his stomach is a symbol for **iron**.

Rhabdomyolysis (shown as a crushed muscle by a tire) is due to the release of protons and anions directly from the muscle. **Toluene** (like in the nail polish or in Trinitrotoluene [TNT]) industrial plant occupational exposure can also cause an acidosis and the anion gap may be **elevated or normal.** The acidosis caused by these toxins may sometimes present as a normal anion-gap hyperchloremic acidosis. **Antifreeze** from ethylene glycol has an arrow toward the windshield wiper. **Propylene glycol** is antifreeze for airplanes and is used in **e-cigarettes.**

METABOLIC ACIDOSIS

NON-ANION GAP OR HYPERCHLOREMIC ACIDOSIS

LOSS OF HCO_3^-

Na^+		
Cl^- →	HCO_3^-	AG

HCO_3^- / Cl^-

POST HYPERVENTILATION

THE KIDNEY COMPENSATES FOR RESPIRATORY ALKALOSIS (e.g. IN CHF) BY "SPILLING" HCO_3

POST ANION GAP ACIDOSIS ← DKA

A HUGE AMOUNT OF NS WILL DILUTE HCO_3^- AND GIVE Cl^-. (DILUTION ACIDOSIS)

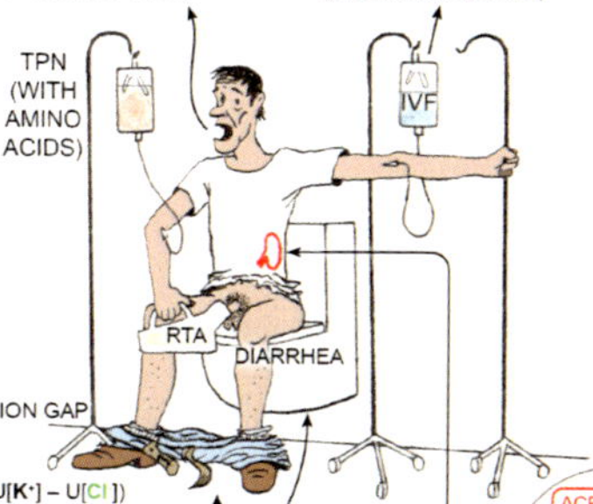

URINE ANION GAP

UAG = $(U[Na^+] + U[K^+] - U[Cl^-])$

UAG IS **POSITIVE** IN **DISTAL RTA** (IMPAIRED URINARY NH_4^+ EXCRETION)

UAG IS **NEGATIVE** IN **DIARRHEA** (ENHANCED URINARY NH_4^+ EXCRETION)

NORMAL = SLIGHTLY POSITIVE UAG

DRUGS

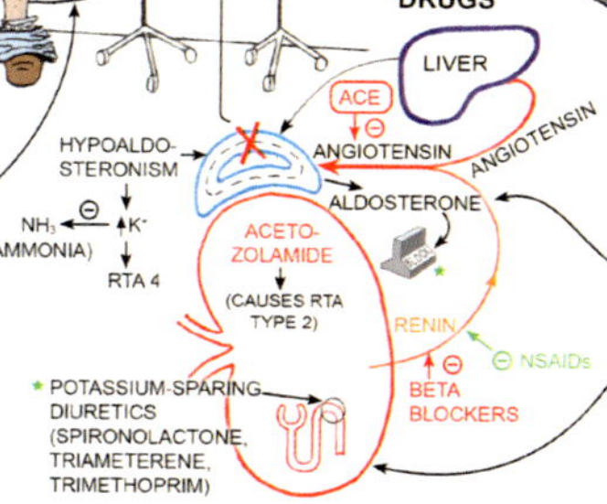

ANION GAP OR NORMOCHLOREMIC ACIDOSIS

INCREASED ACID PRODUCTION

Na^+		
Cl^-	HCO_3^-	← AG

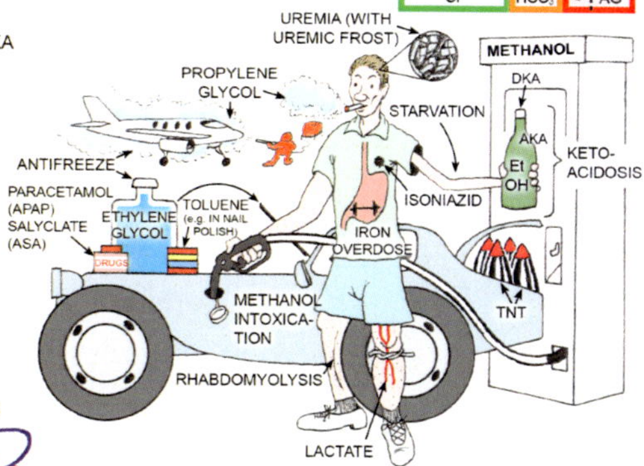

DECREASED RENAL ACID EXCRETION

RTA TYPE 4 (HYPOALDOSTERONISM)

RTA TYPE 1 (DISTAL)

CHRONIC RENAL DISEASE

RENAL FAILURE USUALLY CAUSES A **MIXED** ANION AND NON-ANION GAP ACIDOSIS

NORMAL ION DISTRIBUTION

Na^+		
Cl^-	HCO_3^-	AG

ANION GAP $= Na^+ - (Cl^- + HCO_3^-)$
$= 6 - 12$ mEq/L

"Illustrations are a visual language that can transcend barriers of culture and language."

Shaun Tan

METABOLIC ACIDOSIS

NON-ANION GAP OR HYPERCHLOREMIC ACIDOSIS

ANION GAP OR NORMOCHLOREMIC ACIDOSIS

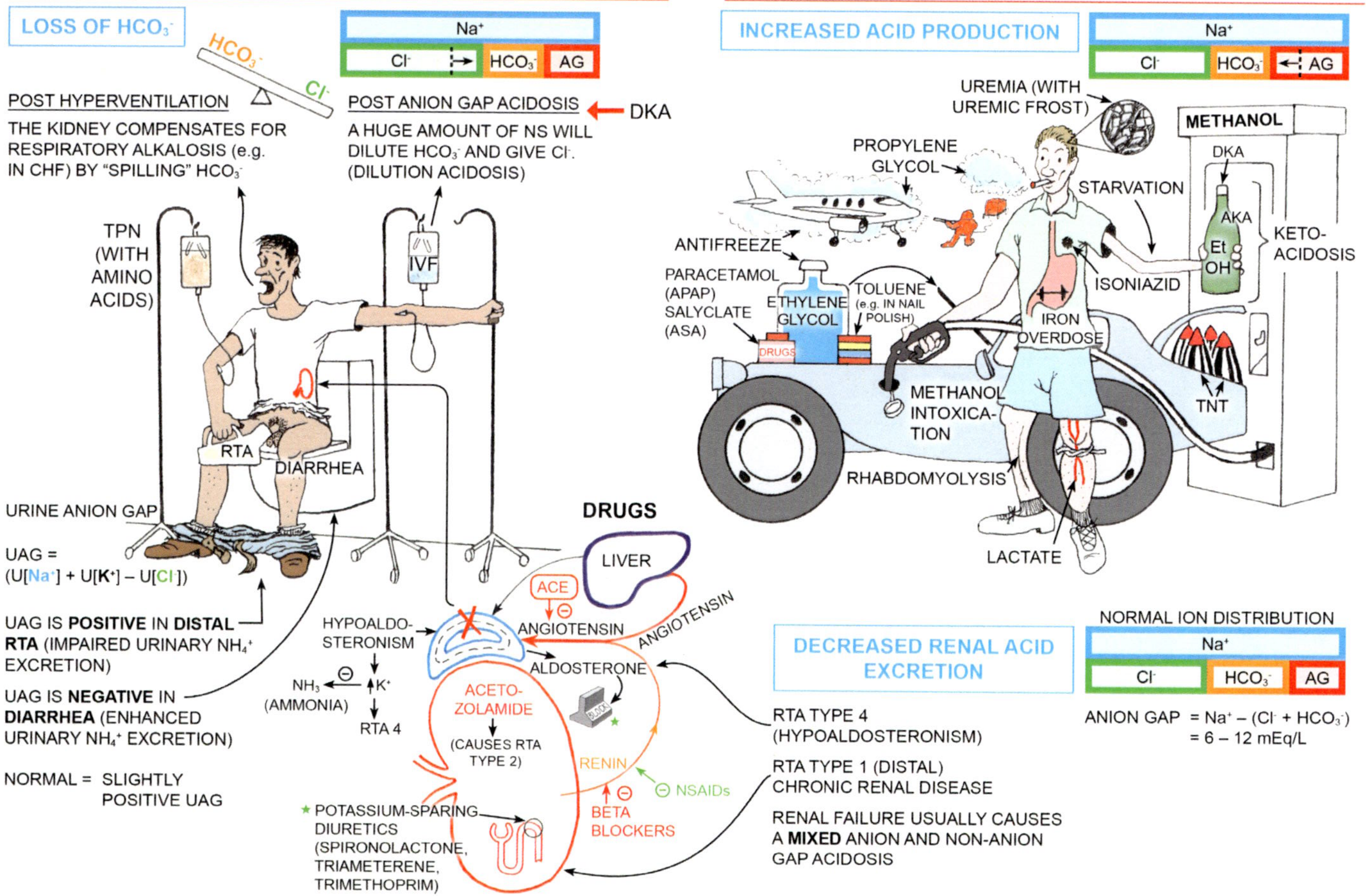

METABOLIC ALKALOSIS

Metabolic alkalosis, a disorder that elevates the serum bicarbonate, can result from several mechanisms: intracellular shift of hydrogen ions, excessive renal hydrogen ion loss, gastrointestinal loss of hydrogen ions, administration and retention of bicarbonate ions, or volume contraction around a constant amount of extracellular bicarbonate (**contraction alkalosis**).

Hypokalemia occurs frequently in patients with metabolic alkalosis. Potassium depletion causes potassium to move from cells into the extracellular fluid, and this transcellular potassium flux causes extracellular hydrogen ions to move into cells to maintain electroneutrality. As a consequence, plasma bicarbonate concentration increases and lowers the intracellular pH. Since this occurs also in renal tubular cells, the ensuing intracellular acidosis promotes hydrogen secretion into the lumen, which results in the addition of bicarbonate to the blood.

Hypokalemia also increases renal ammonia genesis and ammonium excretion, which can both generate and help to maintain metabolic alkalosis.

Milk-alkali syndrome (MAS), also known as **calcium-alkali syndrome**, is a condition characterized by elevated blood calcium levels, metabolic alkalosis, and acute kidney injury. (It is the **third most common cause of hypercalcemia**.) MAS occurs due to the excessive intake of **calcium** and **absorbable alkali**. Sources of calcium and alkali include dietary supplements taken for the prevention of osteoporosis or hyperparathyroidism, as well as antacids used for peptic ulcer disease. (If left untreated, milk-alkali syndrome may lead to kidney failure or even death.)

Consumption of excessive **licorice** (an herb with a sweet and distinctive flavor, which has many health benefits and risks) can lead to pseudo hyperaldosteronism with subsequent hypokalemia and metabolic alkalosis, and in some cases milk-alkali syndrome.

Potassium depletion with subsequent alkalosis occurs with **mineralocorticoid excess**. Inappropriate **hypersecretion of mineralocorticoids** is generally accompanied by hypertension and hypokalemia. By contrast, patients with secondary hyperaldosteronism due to reduced effective arterial blood volume (as in hypovolemia, heart failure, or cirrhosis) usually do not develop metabolic alkalosis or hypokalemia. However, administration of **loop or thiazide diuretics** (which elevate renin, angiotensin II, and aldosterone levels) to patients with secondary hyperaldosteronism markedly increases aldosterone levels and generates marked metabolic alkalosis and hypokalemia. (The picture shows the patient with alcoholic cirrhosis and delirium tremens with tactile hallucinations in the form of bugs crawling on him.)

Hypomagnesemia, frequently found in alcoholics, makes it difficult to successfully treat hypokalemia, and may contribute to alkalosis. Abbreviation DTs is for delirium tremens.

Post hypercapnic alkalosis — Chronic respiratory acidosis increases renal hydrogen excretion and bicarbonate reabsorption. If a chronically elevated PCO2 is rapidly lowered, usually by mechanical ventilation, the plasma bicarbonate concentration may remain elevated for a period of time, especially if the patient has a low effective arterial blood volume, has a reduced glomerular filtration rate, and/or is chloride deficient.

Chloride-resistant metabolic alkalosis cannot be corrected by the administration of a chloride-containing solution (e.g., normal saline). It is associated with inappropriate renal excretion of sodium chloride.

METABOLIC ALKALOSIS

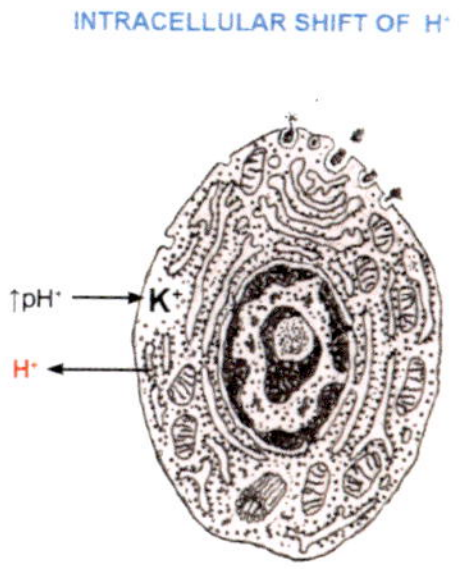

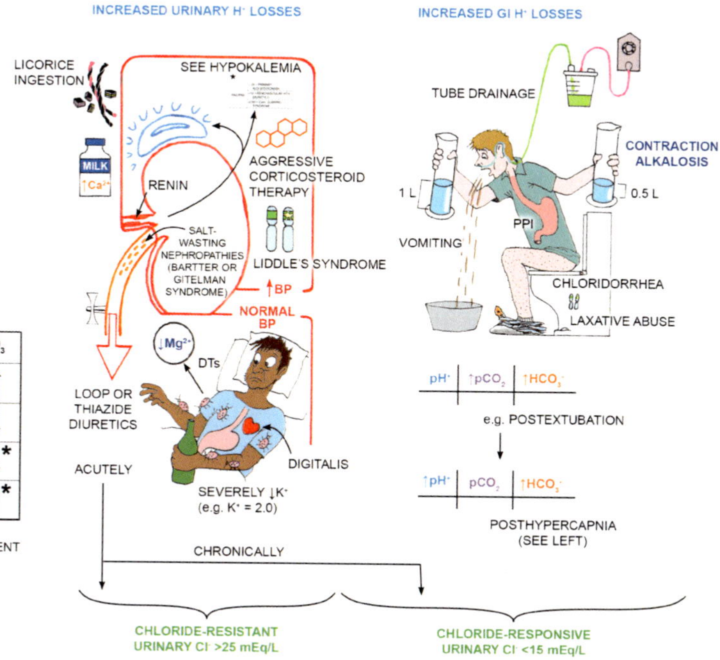

ABG	pH	$PaCO_2$	HCO_3
Respiratory Acidosis	↓	↑ *	↑
Respiratory Alkalosis	↑	↓ *	↓
Metabolic Acidosis	↓	↓	↓ *
Metabolic Alkalosis	↑	↑	↑ *

* = INITIAL EVENT

"Visual education is the most powerful tool for learning."

John Henrik Clarke

METABOLIC ALKALOSIS

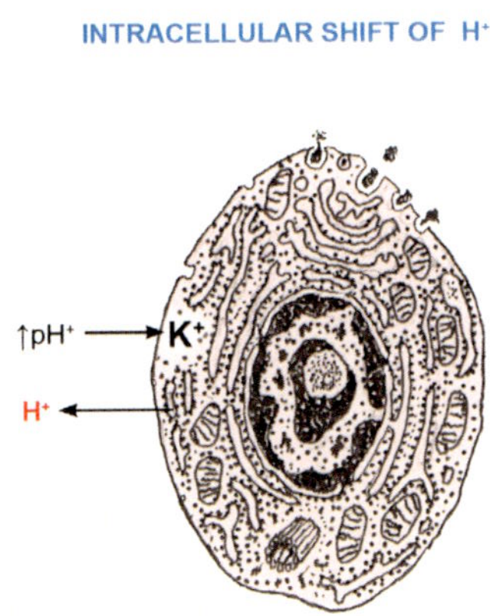

ABG	pH	$PaCO_2$	HCO_3
Respiratory Acidosis	↓	↑*	↑
Respiratory Alkalosis	↑	↓*	↓
Metabolic Acidosis	↓	↓	↓*
Metabolic Alkalosis	↑	↑	↑*

* = INITIAL EVENT

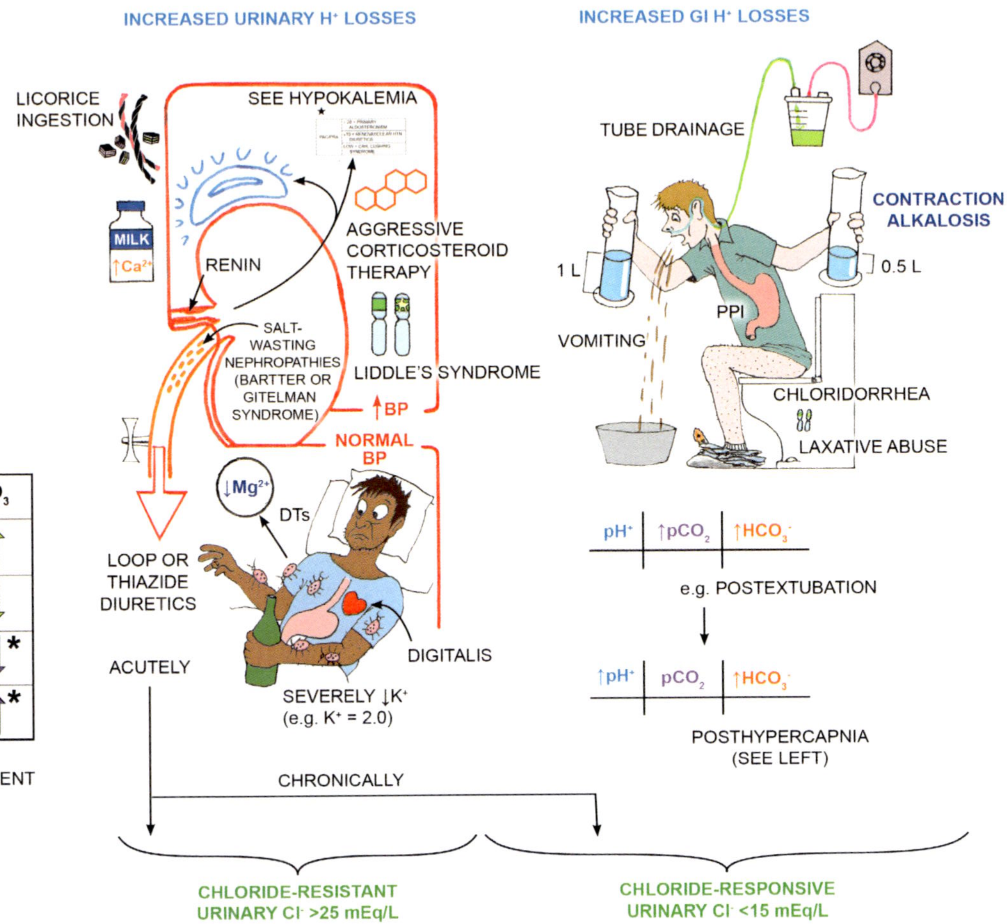

RESPIRATORY ALKALOSIS

In order to confirm the presence of hypoxemia, arterial blood is needed. A **normal** oxygen tension PaO_2 is **80-100 mmHg**. To determine the normal PA for a particular patient: subtract 1 mmHg for every decade of age; subtract 3 mmHg for every 1,000 feet altitude.

Some common causes of respiratory alkalosis include anxiety, hyperventilation, fever, pneumonia or high altitudes.

Ventilation-perfusion (V/Q) mismatch accounts for more than **95% of cases of hypoxemia**. V/Q mismatch examples are CHF, ARDS, pneumonia, atelectasis, and tumor field alveoli.

A clinical clue to the presence of **diffusion defect** is that often the patient will become much more hypoxemic with ambulation.

A **shunt** doesn't correct with 100% supplemental oxygen, unlike V/Q mismatch and diffusion defect.[19]

19 Abbreviations: PaO2: Partial pressure of oxygen; PaCO2: Partial pressure of carbon dioxide; A-a O2; the Alveolar–arterial gradient (or A–a gradient), is a measure of the difference between the **alveolar concentration** (A) of oxygen and the **arterial** (a) concentration of oxygen. The A-a gradient can help narrow the differential diagnosis for hypoxemia. **A-a Gradient = PAO2 – PaO2**.

RESPIRATORY ALKALOSIS

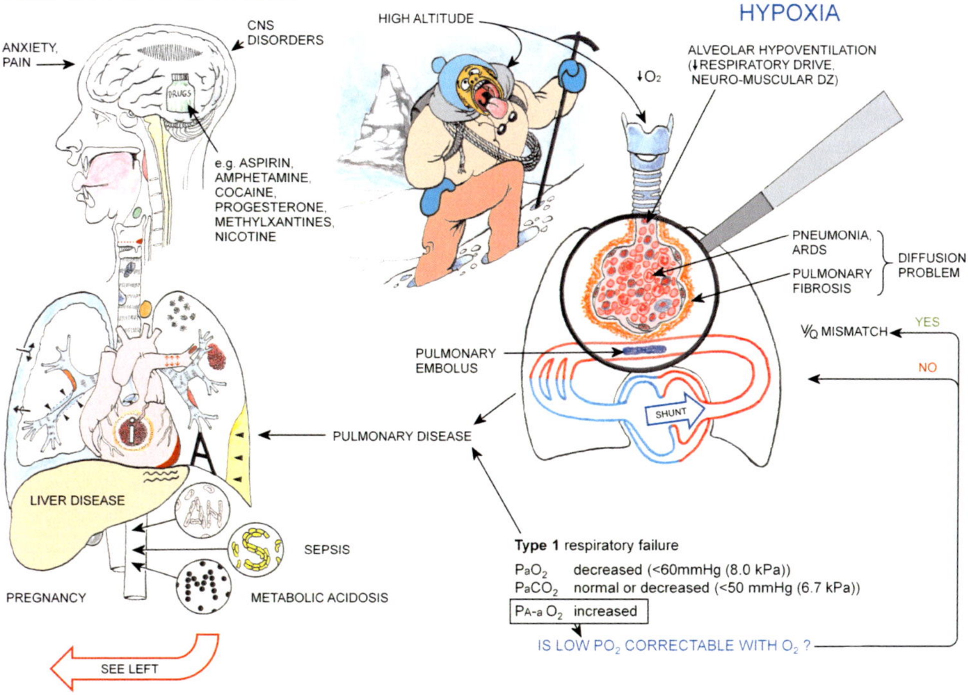

"Illustration is a visual approach to storytelling that can entice, excite, and entertain people of all ages."

Rebecca Green

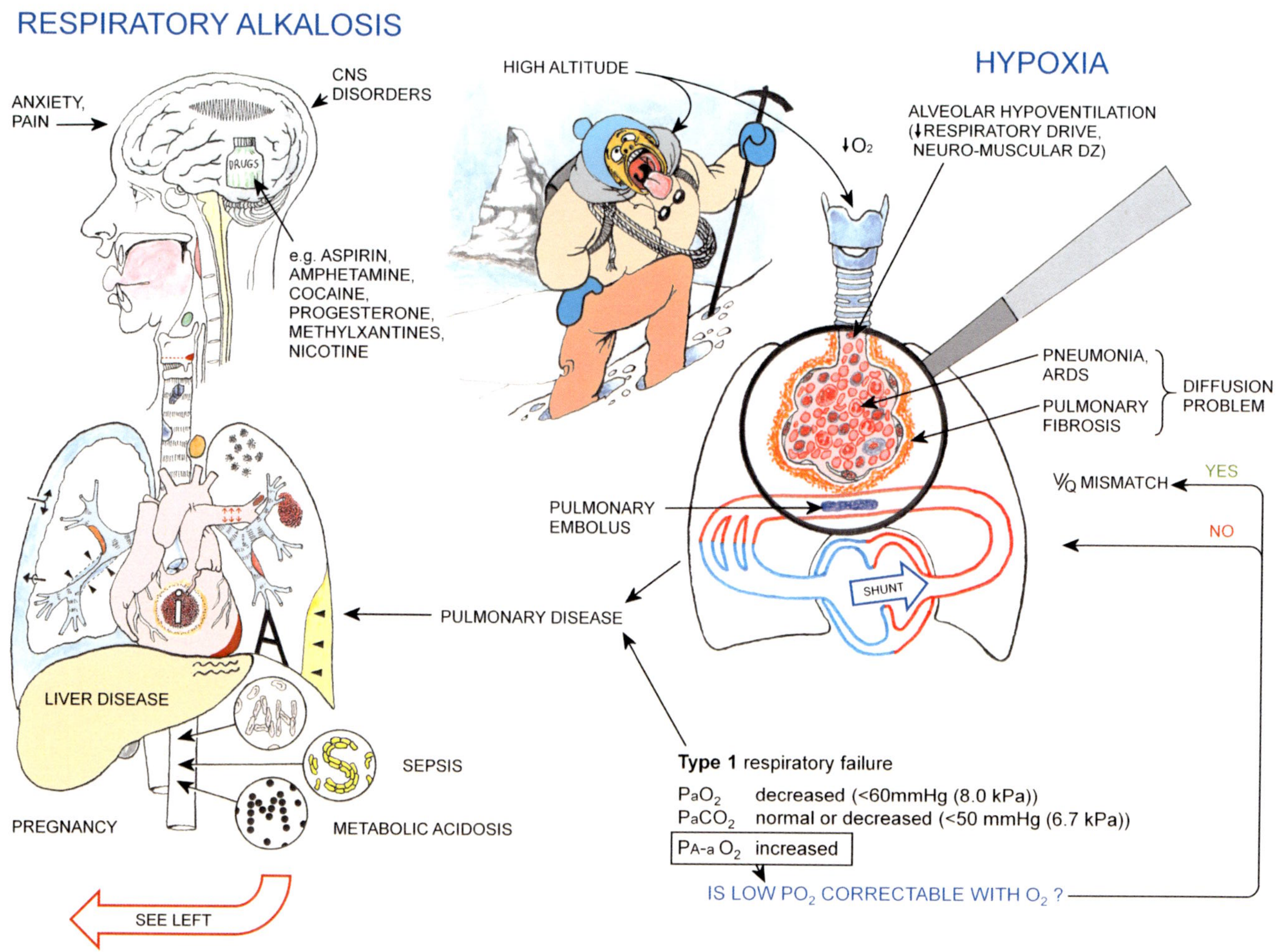
RESPIRATORY ALKALOSIS
ANXIETY, PAIN
CNS DISORDERS
DRUGS
e.g. ASPIRIN, AMPHETAMINE, COCAINE, PROGESTERONE, METHYLXANTINES, NICOTINE
HIGH ALTITUDE
HYPOXIA
↓O2
ALVEOLAR HYPOVENTILATION (↓RESPIRATORY DRIVE, NEURO-MUSCULAR DZ)
PNEUMONIA, ARDS
PULMONARY FIBROSIS
DIFFUSION PROBLEM
V/Q MISMATCH
YES
NO
PULMONARY EMBOLUS
SHUNT
PULMONARY DISEASE
LIVER DISEASE
SEPSIS
PREGNANCY
METABOLIC ACIDOSIS
Type 1 respiratory failure
PaO2 decreased (<60mmHg (8.0 kPa))
PaCO2 normal or decreased (<50 mmHg (6.7 kPa))
PA-a O2 increased
IS LOW PO2 CORRECTABLE WITH O2 ?
SEE LEFT

EXPECTED COMPENSATION FOR ACID-BASE DISTURBANCE

Metabolic Acidosis:	**1** $\downarrow HCO_3 \rightarrow$ **1** $\downarrow PCO_2$
Metabolic Alkalosis:	**10** $\uparrow HCO_3 \rightarrow$ **7** $\uparrow PCO_2$
Acute Respiratory Acidosis:	**10** $\uparrow PCO_2 \rightarrow$ **1** $\uparrow HCO_3$
Chronic Respiratory Acidosis:	**10** $\uparrow PCO_2 \rightarrow$ **4** $\uparrow HCO_3$
Acute Respiratory Alkalosis:	**10** $\downarrow PCO_2 \rightarrow$ **2** $\downarrow HCO_3$
Chronic Respiratory Alkalosis:	**10** $\downarrow PCO_2 \rightarrow$ **5** $\downarrow HCO_3$

Compensation in the context of acid-base disturbances refers to the body's attempt to restore the balance of pH by adjusting either the respiratory or renal systems.

Metabolic Acidosis occurs when the serum bicarbonate (HCO3) level falls below 24 mEq/L. The respiratory system compensates by **hyperventilation**, which leads to a decrease in arterial carbon dioxide (pCO2).

Metabolic Alkalosis occurs when the serum bicarbonate level exceeds 28 mEq/L. The respiratory system compensates by **hypoventilation**, leading to an increase in pCO2.

Respiratory Acidosis occurs when the arterial pCO2 exceeds 40 mm Hg (hypercapnia). The kidneys compensate by **retaining bicarbonate** (HCO3).

Respiratory Alkalosis occurs when the arterial pCO2 falls below 38 mm Hg (hypocapnia). The kidneys compensate by **excreting bicarbonate** (HCO3).

The numbers above represent the expected increase or decrease in certain units with respect to acid-base change.

An easy way to see whether acid-base changes are **respiratory** or **metabolic** is to look at the **directions of the changes of pH and** PCO_2. In respiratory disorders they are going in **opposite** directions while in metabolic ones they are in the **same** one. (See the table on the left in the picture of metabolic alkalosis.)

RESPIRATORY ACIDOSIS	METABOLIC ALKALOSIS
1	
4	10 for 7

METABOLIC ACIDOSIS	RESPIRATORY ALKALOSIS
1 for 1	2
	5

CLINICAL VIGNETTES – 1

73 yo admitted to the ER from extended care facility. He is confused and has a history of congestive heart failure (CHF) that has been treated with Thiazides and Digoxin for the last several years. He had cerebrovascular accident (CVA) two months ago, which has impaired his swallowing ability. He has a gastrostomy tube in place, and there is a moderate amount of thin, nonpurulent draining around the tube, with excoriation of the skin at the tube site. He was admitted for increased confusion and lethargy over the last two days. He has dry skin and mucous membranes, and his tongue is furrowed.

The patient appears to be hypovolemic, based on his appearance and vital signs, including orthostatic drop in blood pressure (BP). His metabolic alkalosis is severe due to hypovolemic effect of thiazide diuretics and GI loss of H^+. (The patient has a moderate amount of drainage around the GI tube. If the drainage contains gastric secretion, the loss of HCl can cause or contribute to metabolic alkalosis. The skin is excoriated around the tube system and this might be the result of contact with acidic fluid.)

---

24 yo anorexic patient with induced vomiting and subsequent asthma attack.

In the acid-base table in the picture of metabolic alkalosis, the first line shows respiratory acidosis which goes with ↓pH and ↑ Partial pressure of carbon dioxide ($PaCO_2$) and ↑bicarbonate (HCO_3^-). (Primary derangement is increased in $PaCO_2$ followed by compensatory increase in HCO_3.) In this case, however, there is ↓pH with ↑$PaCO_2$ and ↓HCO_3, indicating respiratory acidosis and metabolic acidosis.

Normal albumin levels in children or adults varies from 3.5 g/dl to 5.4g/dl.

AG metabolic acidosis is coming from starvation, while metabolic alkalosis from vomiting (loss of H^+ from the gastric content). An asthma attack is causing respiratory acidosis.

---

62 yo woman with severe kyphosis on diuretic for her legs' edema due to obesity.

Kyphosis (a restrictive lung disease) and obesity (causing obesity-hypoventilation syndrome [OHS]) are causing hypercarbia. Obesity is causing legs edema due to compression of the lymph nodes in the groin area, compromising the lymphatic system. Diuretic is causing alkalosis due to contraction of the extracellular fluid space caused by urinary losses of a relatively HCO_3-free fluid.

There is a sleep medicine pearl that calculated HCO3 > 27 mmol/L in obese people has 86% sensitivity and 90% specificity for diagnosis of OHS.

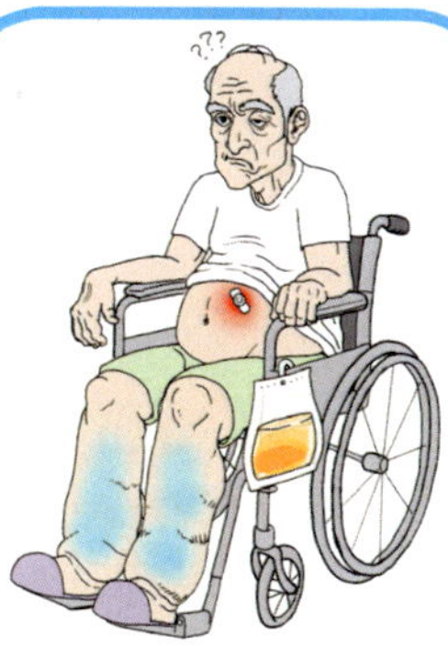

73 yo with CHF and CVA, two months ago admitted to the ER from an extended care facility for increased confusion and lethargy over the last two days.

pH	7.48
$PaCO_2$	47 mmHg
PaO_2	82 mmHg
HCO_3^-	34 mEq/L

BP	100/70 mmHg (supine) 70/50 mmHg (sitting)
HR	110 bpm and irregular
RR	12 bpm and shallow
T	36.5°C (97.8°F)

Acidemia or alkalemia? Alkalemia

Primary derangement? Metabolic alkalosis since pH and HCO_3^- are elevated

Compensation?
Expect ≈ 10 for 7 → pCO_2 increases by 7 for each increase in HCO_3^- by 10. $PaCO_2$ is appropriately increased.

Diagnosis: Metabolic alkalosis

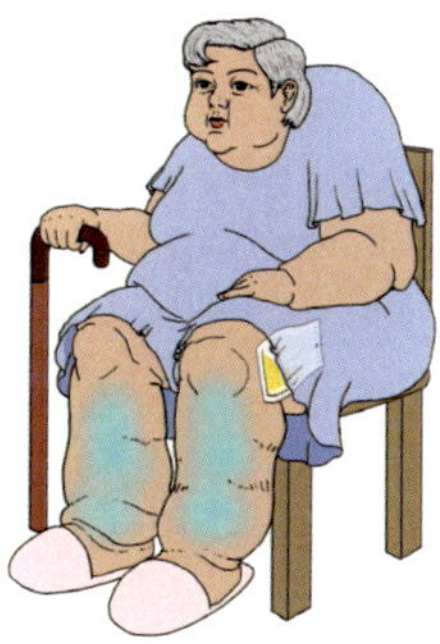

62 yo woman with severe kyphosis, on diuretic for her legs' edema due to obesity.

pH	7.43
$PaCO_2$	53 mmHg
HCO_3^-	33 mEq/L

Acidemia or alkalemia?
Normal pH but elevated pCO_2 and HCO_3^- indicate an acid base disturbance.

Primary derangement?
Normal pH suggests mixed disorder.

Compensation?
For chronic respiratory acidosis (due to patient's kyphosis), expect ≈ 10 for 4 → increases in HCO_3^- by 4 for each increase in pCO_2 by 10. HCO_3^- is inappropriately increased.

Diagnosis: Respiratory acidosis with metabolic alkalosis

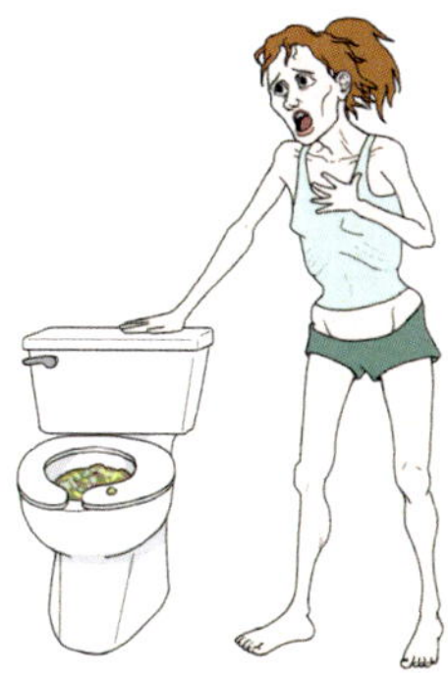

24 yo anorexic patient with induced vomiting and subsequent asthma attack.

pH	7.30	**Na^+**	141 mEq/L
$PaCO_2$	48 mmHg	**Cl^-**	108 mEq/L
HCO_3^-	21 mEq/L	**Albumin**	2 g/dL

141	108	BUN	Glucose
K^+	21	Cr	

Acidemia or alkalemia? Acidemia

Primary derangement? Respiratory acidosis and metabolic acidosis since $PaCO_2$ is high and HCO_3^- is low.

Is anion gap present?
Anion gap (AG) = $Na^+ - [Cl^- + HCO_3^-]$
Normal AG = **12**
141 – [108 + 21] = 12

AG is largely the result of negatively charged proteins.
Hypoalbuminemia reduced the expected normal values for the AG.
Adjustment for low albumin: AG decreases by 2.5 mEq/L for every 1 g/dL decrease in albumin. (Normal albumin is approximately 4 g/dL).
Expect an AG of **12** – (2 x 2.5) = 7
Observed AG of 12 is therefore increased.

Is there additional NG acidosis or metabolic alkalosis?
Change (Δ) AG = (AG – normal AG) = **12** – 7 = 5
Normal HCO_3^- = **24**
Change (Δ) HCO_3^- = **24** – HCO_3^- = **24** – 21 = 3

$$\frac{\Delta AG}{\Delta HCO_3^-} = \frac{5}{3}$$

If < 1 ← $\frac{\Delta AG}{\Delta HCO_3^-}$ → If > 1

Hidden Non-ANION GAP ACIDOSIS | **Hidden METABOLIC ALKALOSIS**

Diagnosis: AG Metabolic acidosis, metabolic alkalosis, and respiratory acidosis

“Visual education is more than a tool for communication, it’s the key to unlocking the full potential of knowledge.”

Daniel Tammet

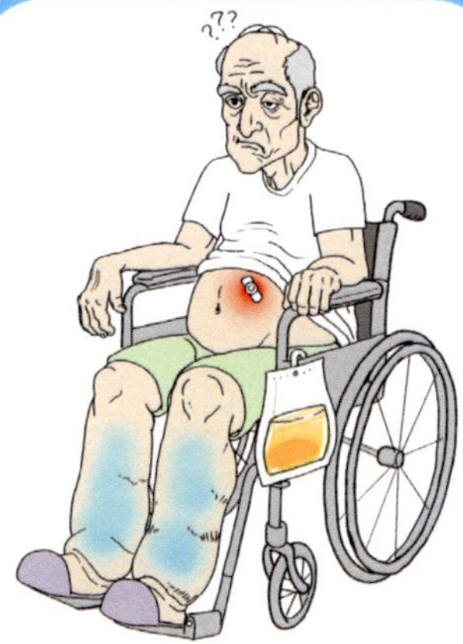

73 yo with CHF and CVA, two months ago admitted to the ER from an extended care facility for increased confusion and lethargy over the last two days.

pH 7.48
$PaCO_2$ 47 mmHg
PaO_2 82 mmHg
HCO_3^- 34 mEq/L

BP 100/70 mmHg (supine)
70/50 mmHg (sitting)
HR 110 bpm and irregular
RR 12 bpm and shallow
T 36.5°C (97.8°F)

Acidemia or alkalemia? Alkalemia

Primary derangement? Metabolic alkalosis since pH and HCO_3^- are elevated

Compensation?
Expect ≈ 10 for 7 → pCO_2 increases by 7 for each increase in HCO_3^- by 10. $PaCO_2$ is appropriately increased.

Diagnosis: Metabolic alkalosis

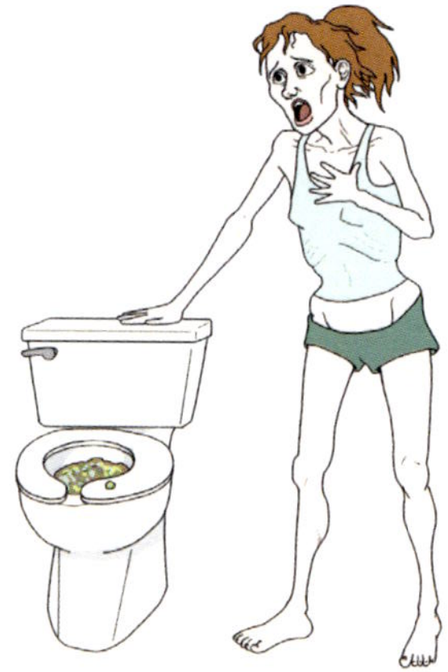

24 yo anorexic patient with induced vomiting and subsequent asthma attack.

pH 7.30
$PaCO_2$ 48 mmHg
HCO_3^- 21 mEq/L

Na^+ 141 mEq/L
Cl^- 108 mEq/L
Albumin 2 g/dL

141	108	BUN	Glucose
K^+	21	Cr	

Acidemia or alkalemia? Acidemia

Primary derangement? Respiratory acidosis and metabolic acidosis since $PaCO_2$ is high and HCO_3^- is low.

Is anion gap present?
Anion gap (AG) = Na^+ – [Cl^- + HCO_3^-]
Normal AG = 12
141 – [108 + 21] = 12

AG is largely the result of negatively charged proteins.
Hypoalbuminemia reduced the expected normal values for the AG.
Adjustment for low albumin: AG decreases by 2.5 mEq/L for every 1 g/dL decrease in albumin. (Normal albumin is approximately 4 g/dL).
Expect an AG of 12 – (2 x 2.5) = 7
Observed AG of 12 is therefore increased.

Is there additional NG acidosis or metabolic alkalosis?
Change (Δ) AG = (AG – normal AG) = 12 – 7 = 5
Normal HCO_3^- = 24
Change (Δ) HCO_3^- = 24 – HCO_3^- = 24 – 21 = 3

$\frac{\Delta AG}{\Delta HCO_3^-}$ = 5 / = 3

If < 1 ← $\frac{\Delta AG}{\Delta HCO_3^-}$ → If > 1

Hidden Non-ANION GAP ACIDOSIS | Hidden METABOLIC ALKALOSIS

Diagnosis: AG Metabolic acidosis, metabolic alkalosis, and respiratory acidosis

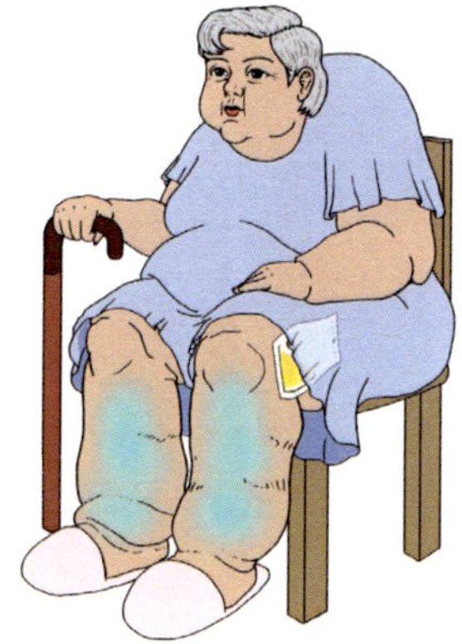

62 yo woman with severe kyphosis, on diuretic for her legs' edema due to obesity.

pH 7.43
$PaCO_2$ 53 mmHg
HCO_3^- 33 mEq/L

Acidemia or alkalemia?
Normal pH but elevated pCO_2 and HCO_3^- indicate an acid base disturbance.

Primary derangement?
Normal pH suggests mixed disorder.

Compensation?
For chronic respiratory acidosis (due to patient's kyphosis), expect ≈ 10 for 4 → increases in HCO_3^- by 4 for each increase in pCO_2 by 10. HCO_3^- is inappropriately increased.

Diagnosis: Respiratory acidosis with metabolic alkalosis

CLINICAL VIGNETTES – 2

18 yo man found at home by his parents. The patient was arousable but very lethargic with deep respirations. An almost empty bottle of Aspirin was found near him. His parents stated that he has been upset after breaking up with his girlfriend.

Respiratory alkalosis is caused by the direct effect salicylates have on the respiratory center. The stimulation of the respiratory center results in hyperventilation and hypocapnia. Low bicarbonate ($HCO3^-$) cannot be ascribed to renal compensation for a respiratory alkalosis since the patient's history clearly indicates that this was an acute disturbance. In addition, maximal renal compensation takes days to occur and does not cause $HCO3^-$–to fall below 15 or 18 mEq/L. The metabolic acidosis results from the effect of salicylates on cellular functioning, which increases production of organic acids, and to a lesser extent, from the organic acid generated from the salicylates themselves.

---

56 yo woman with 20-year history of alcohol abuse admitted for her hematemesis. She has not had any alcohol for two weeks.

The first column represents the patient's labs on admission, while the second one the labs on the day after admission.

In the **first column** respiratory alkalosis is chronic because renal compensation has occurred. The serum HCO_3^- has decreased from a normal 24 mEq/L to 20 mEq/L to compensate for the decrease in CO_2 level. Liver disease causes stimulation of the respiratory center, generating chronic respiratory alkalosis. The respiratory center is stimulated by ammonia and other metabolic byproducts that accumulate in liver disease. Renal compensation takes several days to occur, therefore the respiratory alkalosis must be chronic.

The **second column** represents the day after admission when the patient experienced massive upper GI hemorrhage from esophageal varices. She was given 10 units of blood over an 8-hour period. Banked blood usually has a preservative containing citrate that helps prevent coagulation. After the blood is transfused, the citrate is metabolized by the body to HCO_3^- . The blood was transfused so rapidly that her kidneys were unable to excrete the alkali load as quickly as it was given, and a metabolic alkalosis developed. The PaO_2 decreased from 30 mmHg (its chronic steady state) to 28 mmHg due to an increase in alveolar ventilation because of anxiety.

---

57 yo female two days after hysterectomy developed sudden left chest pain due to pulmonary embolus

PaO_2 of 64 mmHg is not responsible for hyperventilation because PaO_2 must decrease to 50-60 mmHg before the chemoreceptors stimulate the respiratory center to increase respirations. The pulmonary receptors (sensitive to irritation, congestion and stretch) in the lung, thorax, and small airways may be stimulating the respiratory center due to presence of pulmonary emboli. The pain and anxiety may also contribute to her hyperventilation.

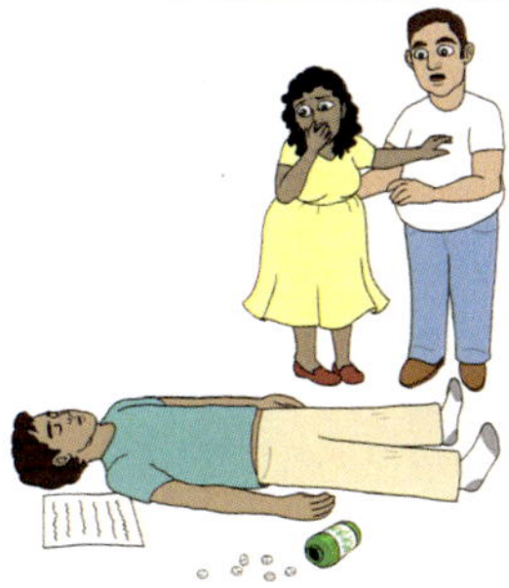

18 yo man found at home by his parents after overdosing on Aspirin.

pH	7.46
$PaCO_2$	14 mmHg
PaO_2	96 mmHg
HCO_3^-	10 mEq/L
Na^+	140 mEq/L
Cl^-	106 mEq/L
K^+	4.5 mEq/L
BP	110/60 mmHg
HR	84 bpm
RR	30 bpm deep and labored (Kussmaul respirations)

Acidemia or alkalemia? Alkalemia

Primary derangement? Respiratory alkalosis

Compensation? For acute respiratory alkalosis expect ≈ 10 for 2 → reduce in HCO_3^- by 2 for each reduction in pC02 by 10. HCO_3^- is inappropriately low.

Is an anion gap present?
Anion gap (AG) = $Na^+ - [Cl^- + HCO_3^-]$
Normal AG = 12   140 – [106 + 10] = 24

Diagnosis: Respiratory alkalosis with high AG metabolic acidosis

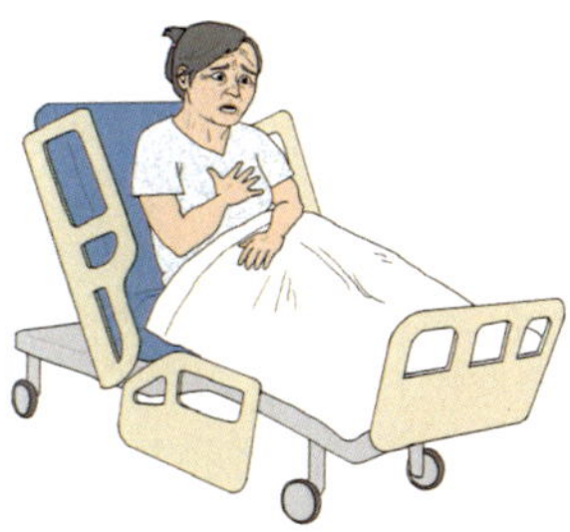

57 yo female two days after hysterectomy developed sudden left chest pain that increases with respiration. She feels breathless and is very anxious.

pH	7.49	**Na^+**	138 mEq/L	**BP**	140/86 mmHg
$PaCO_2$	29 mmHg	**Cl^-**	105 mEq/L	**HR**	124 bpm
PaO_2	64 mmHg	**K^+**	4.0 mEq/L	**RR**	28 bpm
HCO_3^-	22 mEq/L	**O_2**	87%	**T**	37°C

Acidemia or alkalemia? Alkalemia

Primary derangement? Acute respiratory alkalosis since pH is increased, while $PaCO_2$ and HCO_3^- are reduced.

Compensation? For acute respiratory alkalosis expect ≈ 10 for 2 → reduce in HCO_3^- by 2 for each reduction in pCO_2 by 10. HCO_3^- is appropriately reduced.

Is an anion gap present?
Anion gap (AG) = $Na^+ - [Cl^- + HCO_3^-]$
Normal AG = 12
138 – [105 + 22] = 11
AG is 11 which is within normal limits.
Therefore, no concurrent acid-base disturbance accompanies the acute respiratory alkalosis.

Diagnosis: Respiratory alkalosis

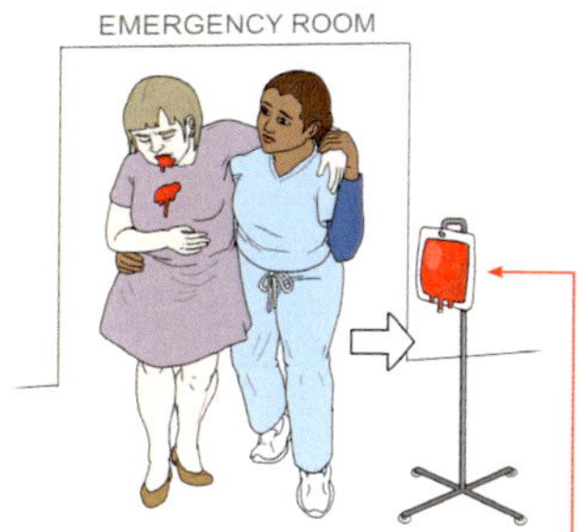

56 yo woman with 20-year history of alcohol abuse admitted for her hematemesis. She has not had any alcohol for two weeks.

Before transfusion:		**After transfusion:**	
pH	7.45	**pH**	7.59
$PaCO_2$	30 mmHg	**$PaCO_2$**	28 mmHg
PaO_2	93 mmHg	**PaO_2**	89 mmHg
HCO_3^-	20 mEq/L	**HCO_3^-**	26 mEq/L
Na+	138 mEq/L	**Na^+**	142 mEq/L
Cl^-	108 mEq/L	**Cl^-**	94 mEq/L

Acidemia or alkalemia? Alkalemia

Primary derangement? Metabolic alkalosis since pH and HCO_3^- are elevated.

Compensation? Expect ≈ 10 for 7 → pCO_2 increases by 7 for each increase in HCO_3^- by 10. $PaCO_2$ is lower than expected.

Diagnosis: Metabolic alkalosis and respiratory alkalosis

“The goal is to turn data into information,
and information into insight.”

Carly Fiorina

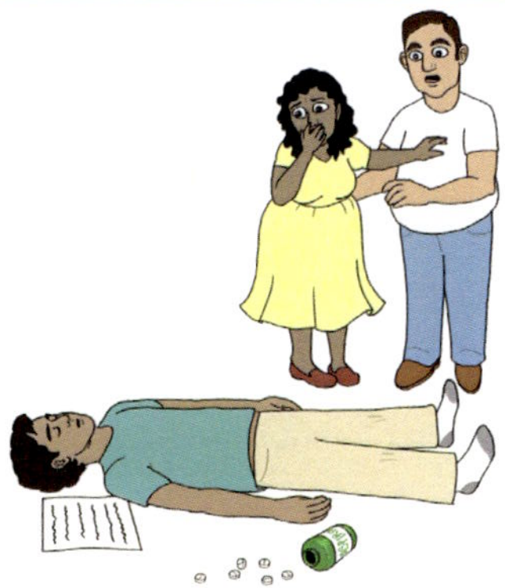

18 yo man found at home by his parents after overdosing on Aspirin.

pH	7.46
$PaCO_2$	14 mmHg
PaO_2	96 mmHg
HCO_3^-	10 mEq/L
Na^+	140 mEq/L
Cl^-	106 mEq/L
K^+	4.5 mEq/L
BP	110/60 mmHg
HR	84 bpm
RR	30 bpm deep and labored (Kussmaul respirations)

Acidemia or alkalemia? Alkalemia

Primary derangement? Respiratory alkalosis

Compensation? For acute respiratory alkalosis expect ≈ 10 for 2 → reduce in HCO_3^- by 2 for each reduction in pC02 by 10. HCO_3^- is inappropriately low.

Is an anion gap present?
Anion gap (AG) = $Na^+ - [Cl^- + HCO_3^-]$
Normal AG = **12** 140 – [106 + 10] = 24

Diagnosis: Respiratory alkalosis with high AG metabolic acidosis

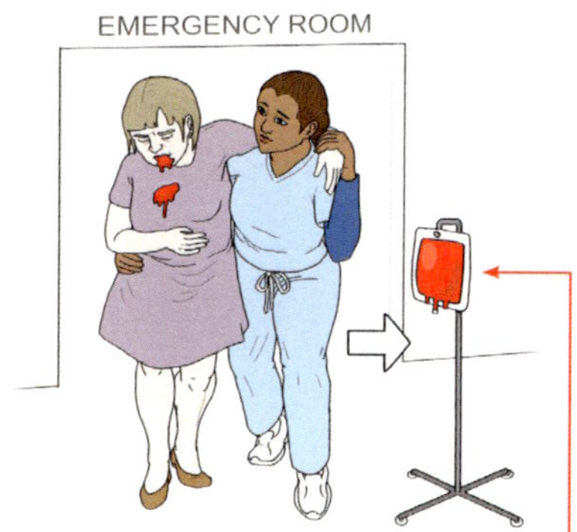

56 yo woman with 20-year history of alcohol abuse admitted for her hematemesis. She has not had any alcohol for two weeks.

Before transfusion:		**After transfusion:**	
pH	7.45	**pH**	7.59
$PaCO_2$	30 mmHg	**$PaCO_2$**	28 mmHg
PaO_2	93 mmHg	**PaO_2**	89 mmHg
HCO_3^-	20 mEq/L	**HCO_3^-**	26 mEq/L
Na+	138 mEq/L	**Na+**	142 mEq/L
Cl^-	108 mEq/L	**Cl^-**	94 mEq/L

Acidemia or alkalemia? Alkalemia

Primary derangement? Metabolic alkalosis since pH and HCO_3^- are elevated.

Compensation? Expect ≈ 10 for 7 → pCO_2 increases by 7 for each increase in HCO_3^- by 10. $PaCO_2$ is lower than expected.

Diagnosis: Metabolic alkalosis and respiratory alkalosis

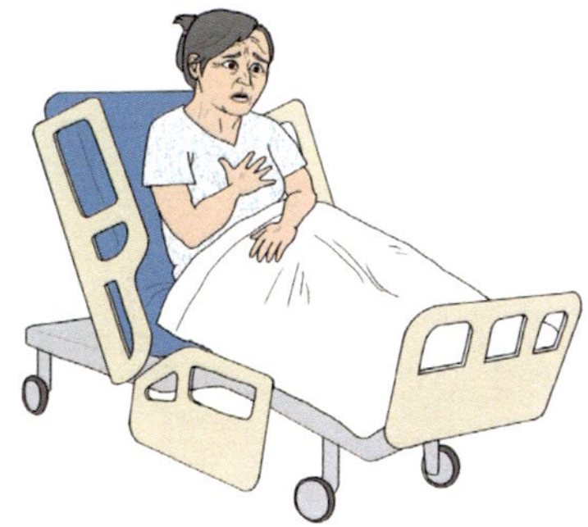

57 yo female two days after hysterectomy developed sudden left chest pain that increases with respiration. She feels breathless and is very anxious.

pH	7.49	**Na^+**	138 mEq/L	**BP**	140/86 mmHg
$PaCO_2$	29 mmHg	**Cl^-**	105 mEq/L	**HR**	124 bpm
PaO_2	64 mmHg	**K^+**	4.0 mEq/L	**RR**	28 bpm
HCO_3^-	22 mEq/L	**O_2**	87%	**T**	37°C

Acidemia or alkalemia? Alkalemia

Primary derangement? Acute respiratory alkalosis since pH is increased, while $PaCO_2$ and HCO_3^- are reduced.

Compensation? For acute respiratory alkalosis expect ≈ 10 for 2 → reduce in HCO_3^- by 2 for each reduction in pCO_2 by 10. HCO_3^- is appropriately reduced.

Is an anion gap present?
Anion gap (AG) = $Na^+ - [Cl^- + HCO_3^-]$
Normal AG = **12**
138 – [105 + 22] = 11
AG is 11 which is within normal limits.
Therefore, no concurrent acid-base disturbance accompanies the acute respiratory alkalosis.

Diagnosis: Respiratory alkalosis

CLINICAL VIGNETTES – 3

60 yo man was brought to the ER for progressively worsening dyspnea and 2+ legs edema. The ER physician auscultated crackles. The patient had MI two years ago. Tachycardia with PVCs caused pulmonary edema with hypoxia. When Partial pressure of oxygen (PaO_2) drops down to 50-60 mmHg, the respiratory center is stimulated, and hyperventilation occurs. Carbon dioxide (CO_2) is exchanged 20 times more readily than oxygen (O_2) so when CO_2 retention occurs, the PaO_2 on room air is usually markedly decreased. (If hypoxia not corrected, the further exhaustion of the respiratory drive would result in soon, in 1-2 days, CO_2 retention with $PaCO_2$ level of ≈ 50 mmHg or higher.)

A pH of 7.12 is life-threatening. Severe acidosis in this case is caused by combination of respiratory acidosis ($PaCO_2$ higher than expected) and metabolic acidosis (HCO_3^- 15 mEq/L). Hypoxia due to pulmonary edema results in anaerobic metabolism and the production of lactate, which can cause metabolic acidosis. A pH of 7.12 causes cardiac depression with decreased contractility and a tendency to develop ventricular dysrhythmias.

A 23 yo woman was brough to the ER by her roommate after found unresponsive with an empty bottle of secobarbital and a half empty bottle of wine near her. The patient's roommate said that she was depressed about her unemployment. Barbiturates lead to respiratory center depression, resulting in hypoventilation. The RR is 28 bpm, but the breaths are very shallow, leading to decreased minute volume and hypoventilation, which results in accumulation of CO_2.

The pH value is what is expected to be seen, since pH should decrease by 0.08 units for every 10 mmHg increase in $PaCO_2$. The $PaCO_2$ value is 25 mmHg greater than normal (40 mmHg). 25 x 0.08 = 0.20. 7.40-0.20 = 7.20.

Immediate tissue buffering (with no bicarbonate buffers) has occurred, which increased plasma HCO_3^- by 2-3 mEq/L. No renal compensation has occurred because not enough time has elapsed.

---

65 yo woman with advanced ovarian cancer. A tumor was surgically removed but evidence of microscopic disease remained. The patient received whole-abdomen irradiation. Two weeks after treatment she developed progressive diarrhea, refractory to outpatient medical management, necessitating hospital admission.

The stool contains a moderate amount of HCO_3^- which is lost with diarrhea. In addition, volume depletion due to diarrhea can cause hypoperfusion of tissue as the cardia output falls, with resultant generation of lactic acid, and thus metabolic acidosis.

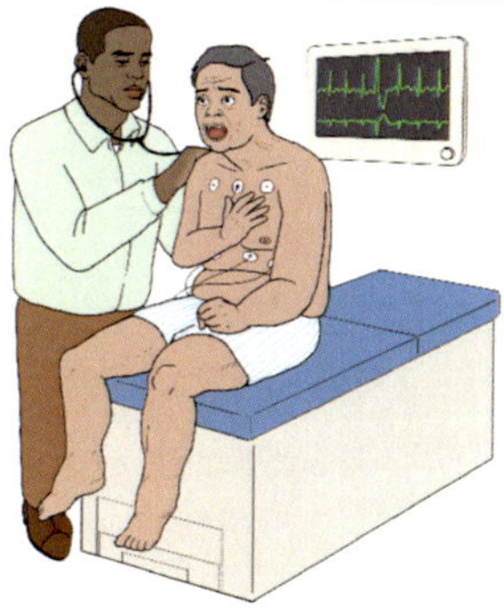

60 yo man with SOB and PVCs.

pH 7.12
$PaCO_2$ 35 mmHg
PaO_2 49 mmHg
HCO_3^- 15 mEq/L

BP 98/50 mmHg
HR 128 bpm
RR 28 bpm

Acidemia or alkalemia? Acidemia

Primary derangement? Metabolic acidosis since pH, $PaCO_2$ and HCO_3^- are low.

Compensation?
Expect ≈ 1 for 1; pCO_2 is higher than expected.

Diagnosis: Metabolic acidosis and respiratory acidosis

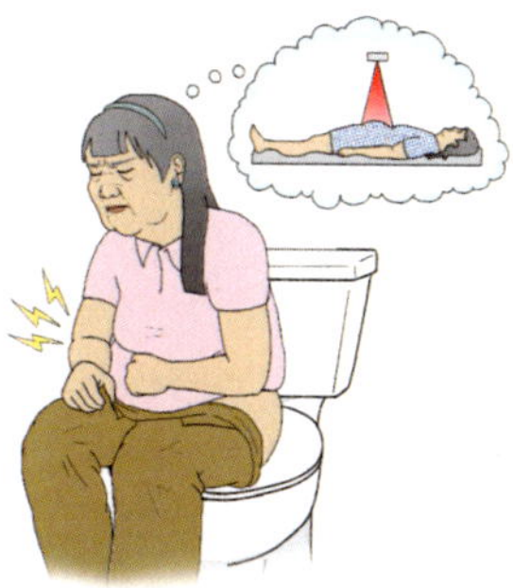

65 yo woman after whole-abdomen irradiation for advanced ovarian cancer.

pH 7.32
$PaCO_2$ 29 mmHg
PaO_2 90 mmHg
HCO_3^- 15 mEq/L

Acidemia or alkalemia? Acidemia

Primary derangement? Metabolic acidosis since pH, $PaCO_2$ and HCO_3^- are low.

Compensation?
Expect ≈ 1 for 1 → 1 pCO_2 decrease for each 1 decrease in HCO_3^-. $PaCO_2$ is appropriately decreased.

Diagnosis: Metabolic acidosis

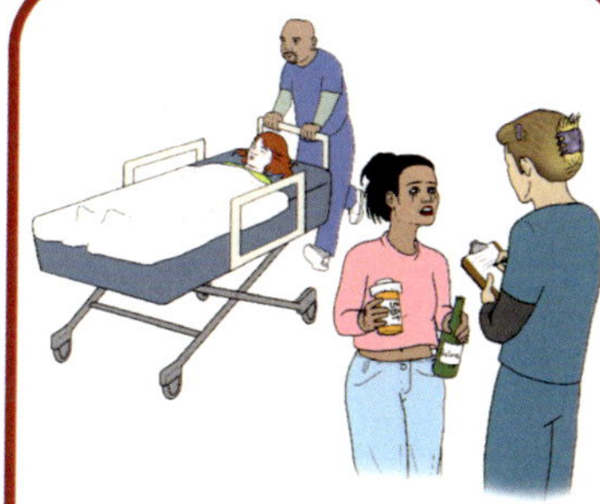

23 yo woman with decreased responsiveness.

pH 7.20
$PaCO_2$ 65 mmHg
PaO_2 45 mmHg
HCO_3^- 26 mEq/L

BP 70/40 mmHg
HR 120 bpm
RR 28 bpm

Acidemia or alkalemia? Acidemia

Primary derangement? Respiratory acidosis since pH is low, while $PaCO_2$ and HCO_3^- are high.

Compensation?
For acute respiratory acidosis, expect ≈ 1 HCO_3^- increase for every increase in pCO_2 by 10; HCO_3 is appropriately increased.

Diagnosis: Acute respiratory acidosis

"Data that is loved tends to survive."

Kurt Bollacker

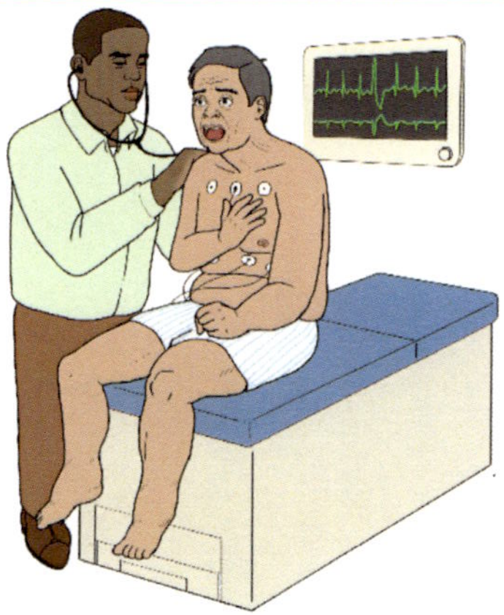

60 yo man with SOB and PVCs.

pH 7.12
$PaCO_2$ 35 mmHg
PaO_2 49 mmHg
HCO_3^- 15 mEq/L

BP 98/50 mmHg
HR 128 bpm
RR 28 bpm

Acidemia or alkalemia? Acidemia

Primary derangement? Metabolic acidosis since pH, $PaCO_2$ and HCO_3^- are low.

Compensation?
Expect ≈ 1 for 1; pCO_2 is higher than expected.

Diagnosis: Metabolic acidosis and respiratory acidosis

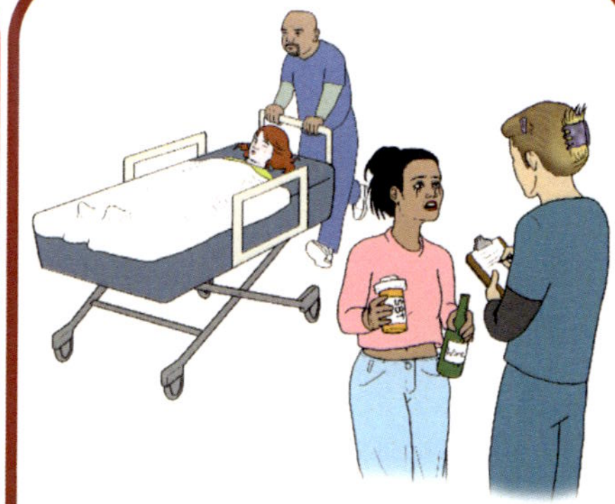

23 yo woman with decreased responsiveness.

pH 7.20
$PaCO_2$ 65 mmHg
PaO_2 45 mmHg
HCO_3^- 26 mEq/L

BP 70/40 mmHg
HR 120 bpm
RR 28 bpm

Acidemia or alkalemia? Acidemia

Primary derangement? Respiratory acidosis since pH is low, while $PaCO_2$ and HCO_3^- are high.

Compensation?
For acute respiratory acidosis, expect ≈ 1 HCO_3^- increase for every increase in pCO_2 by 10; HCO_3 is appropriately increased.

Diagnosis: Acute respiratory acidosis

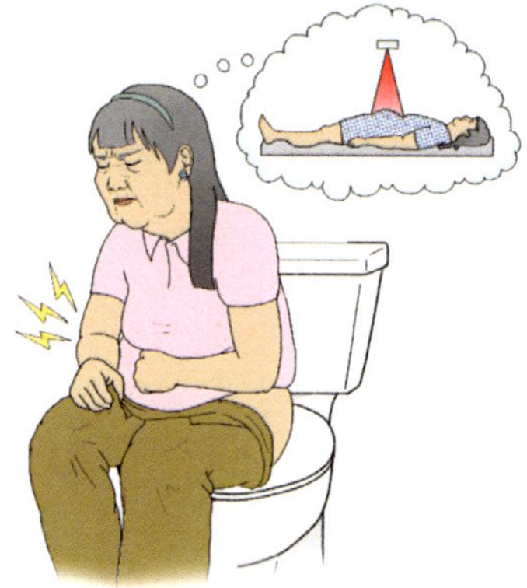

65 yo woman after whole-abdomen irradiation for advanced ovarian cancer.

pH 7.32
$PaCO_2$ 29 mmHg
PaO_2 90 mmHg
HCO_3^- 15 mEq/L

Acidemia or alkalemia? Acidemia

Primary derangement? Metabolic acidosis since pH, $PaCO_2$ and HCO_3^- are low.

Compensation?
Expect ≈ 1 for 1 → 1 pCO_2 decrease for each 1 decrease in HCO_3^-. $PaCO_2$ is appropriately decreased.

Diagnosis: Metabolic acidosis

CLINICAL VIGNETTES – 4

74 yo man, a heavy smoker, presented to his physician's office for his SOB that has become worse over the last several months. His cough is productive of thick, tenacious sputum and he states his feet swell occasionally, preventing him from getting his shoes on.

The pH of 7.39 reflects a mild acidosis, regardless of high $PaCO_2$ (62 mmHg). This is because of renal compensation (increased HCO_3^- of 34 mEq/L) for chronic respiratory acidosis.

The patient has predominant chronic bronchitis based on the history of severe dyspnea, copious, thick sputum production, and ABGs that reflect hypercapnia and hypoxemia. Smoking is common with both emphysema and chronic bronchitis, but patients with predominant emphysema usually are able to maintain their CO_2 at normal level and keep their PaO_2 in an acceptable range by increasing their minute volume via an increase in respiratory rate and respiratory effort until the end stage of their disease.

One week later, the patient is seen in the ER extremely confused SOB, and cyanotic. His sputum is thick and yellow, and his temperature is 38.5 C (101.4 F), his HR is 112 bpm and RR 20 bpm. CXR shows patchy infiltrates indicating pneumonia.

The pH of 7.39 was maintained when $PaCO_2$ was 62 mmHg. But, when $PaCO_2$ suddenly increased to 92 mmHg, the compensatory mechanism was inadequate to meet the increased demands for buffering and the ph decreased.

(The patient is in risk for oxygen-induced apnea since he has a long history of hypercapnia and his respiratory center has become insensitive to further increase in $PaCO_2$. The drive to breathe is now stimulated by hypoxemia, so if hypoxemia is suddenly corrected, the patient might stop breathing causing CO_2 narcosis. This patient requires oxygen because of dangerously low PaO_2, but it must be delivered cautiously (usually 1-2 l/min) with careful monitoring of patient's breathing effort, sensorium and ABGs. $PaCO_2$ should be also lowered slowly and only as far as the patient's baseline. If $PaCO_2$ suddenly normalized post *hypercapnic alkalosis* would occur because HCO_3^- would remain elevated until the kidneys could excrete the excess.

---

36 yo alcoholic man with vomiting.

HCO_3^- falls by 1 for every rise in the AG by 1.

If Δ/Δ is 1-2 (more precisely 1-1.6) -> pure AG metabolic acidosis

If Δ/Δ is < 1 -> AG metabolic acidosis is present with simultaneous non-anion gap metabolic acidosis.

If Δ/Δ is > 1 -> AG metabolic acidosis is present with simultaneous metabolic alkalosis.

Metabolic acidosis is coming from dehydration with subsequent lactic acidosis, while alkalosis is coming from vomiting (loss of H^+ from the gastric content).

---

40 yo dehydrated man from desert has diarrhea. His anion-gap acidosis is coming from his dehydration with subsequent increase in lactic acid and from his starvation, while his non-anion-gap acidosis is coming from his recent diarrhea (in the wilderness).

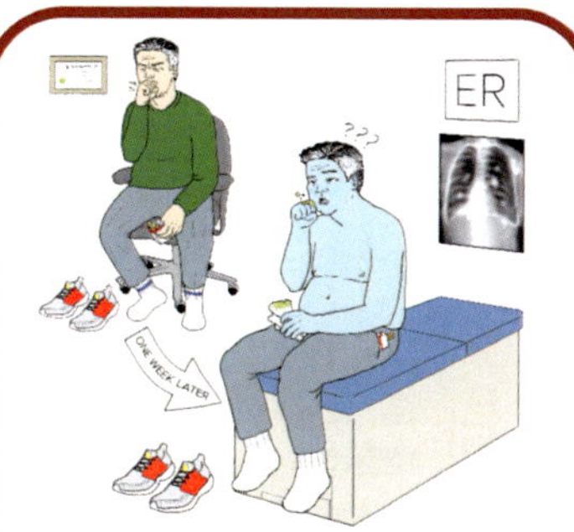

74 yo man, a heavy smoker, with worsening SOB and cough with productive sputum.

Doctor's visit:		**In the ER:**	
pH	7.39	**pH**	7.25
$PaCO_2$	62 mmHg	**$PaCO_2$**	92 mmHg
PaO_2	54 mmHg	**PaO_2**	33 mmHg
HCO_3^-	34 mEq/L	**HCO_3^-**	38 mEq/L

Acidemia or alkalemia? Acidemia

Primary derangement? Respiratory acidosis since pH is low, while $PaCO_2$ and HCO_3^- are high.

Compensation?
For <u>chronic</u> respiratory acidosis, expect ≈ 4 HCO_3^- increase for every increase in pCO_2 by 10; HCO_3^- is appropriately increased. Change in HCO_3^- is between expected change for acute and chronic respiratory acidosis.

Diagnosis: Acute on chronic respiratory acidosis

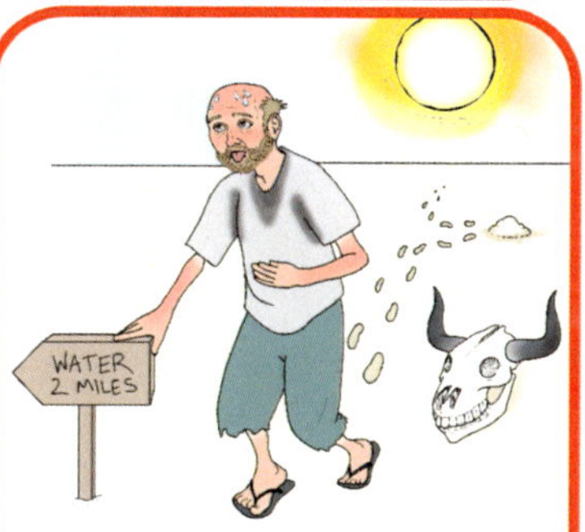

40 yo dehydrated man in desert after diarrhea.

pH	7.31	**Na^+**	151 mEq/L
$PaCO_2$	27 mmHg	**Cl^-**	121 mEq/L
HCO_3^-	11 mEq/L		

Acidemia or alkalemia? Acidemia

Primary derangement? Metabolic acidosis since pH, $PaCO_2$ and HCO_3^- are low.

Compensation?
Expect ≈ 1 for 1 pCO_2 decrease for each 1 decrease in HCO_3^-. $PaCO_2$ is appropriately decreased.

Is an anion gap present?
Anion gap (AG) = $Na^+ - [Cl^- + HCO_3^-]$
Normal AG = **12**
151 – [121 + 11] = 19

$$\frac{\Delta AG}{\Delta HCO_3^-} = \frac{7}{13}$$

Change (Δ) AG
= (AG – normal AG)
= 19 – **12** = 7

Normal HCO_3^- = **24**

Change (Δ) HCO_3^-
= **24** – HCO_3^-
= **24** – 11 = 13

$\frac{\Delta AG}{\Delta HCO_3^-}$: **If < 1** → **Hidden Non-ANION GAP ACIDOSIS**; **If > 1** → **Hidden METABOLIC ALKALOSIS**

Diagnosis: AG metabolic acidosis and non-AG metabolic acidosis

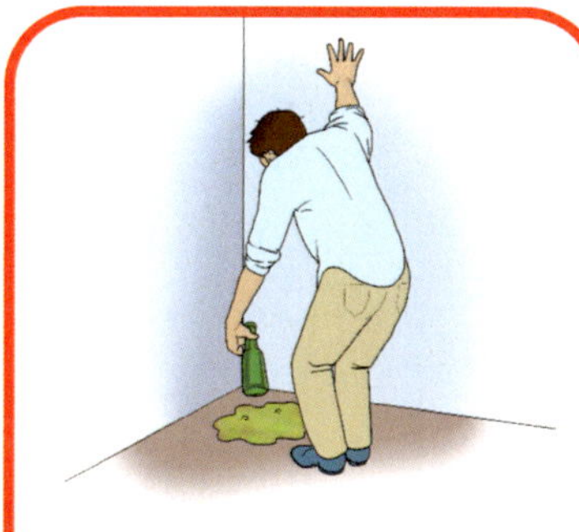

36 yo alcoholic man with vomiting.

pH	7.36	**Na+**	147 mEq/L
$PaCO_2$	30 mmHg	**Cl^-**	109 mEq/L
HCO_3^-	14 mEq/L	**Albumin**	4.5 mEq/L

Acidemia or alkalemia? Acidemia

Primary derangement? Metabolic acidosis since pH, $PaCO_2$ and HCO_3^- are low.

Compensation?
Expect ≈ 1 for 1 pCO_2 decrease for each 1 decrease in HCO_3^-. $PaCO_2$ is appropriately decreased.

Is an anion gap present?
Anion gap (AG) = $Na^+ - [Cl^- + HCO_3^-]$
Normal AG = **12**
147 – [109 + 14] = 24

$$\frac{\Delta AG}{\Delta HCO_3^-} = \frac{12}{10}$$

Change (Δ) AG
= (AG – normal AG)
= 24 – **12** = 12

Normal HCO_3^- = **24**

Change (Δ) HCO_3^-
= **24** – HCO_3^-
= **24** – 14 = 10

$\frac{\Delta AG}{\Delta HCO_3^-}$: **If < 1** → **Hidden Non-ANION GAP ACIDOSIS**; **If > 1** → **Hidden METABOLIC ALKALOSIS**

Diagnosis: AG metabolic acidosis and metabolic alkalosis

“Visual information is just as important
as verbal communication, if not more so.”

Robert Grant

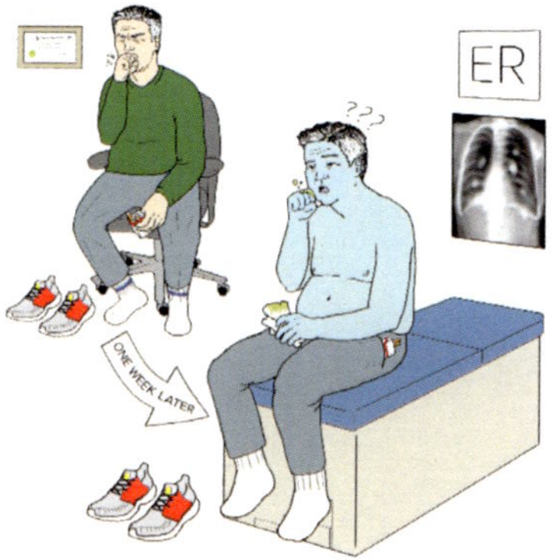

74 yo man, a heavy smoker, with worsening SOB and cough with productive sputum.

Doctor's visit:		In the ER:	
pH	7.39	**pH**	7.25
$PaCO_2$	62 mmHg	**$PaCO_2$**	92 mmHg
PaO_2	54 mmHg	**PaO_2**	33 mmHg
HCO_3^-	34 mEq/L	**HCO_3^-**	38 mEq/L

Acidemia or alkalemia? Acidemia

Primary derangement? Respiratory acidosis since pH is low, while $PaCO_2$ and HCO_3^- are high.

Compensation?
For chronic respiratory acidosis, expect ≈ 4 HCO_3^- increase for every increase in pCO_2 by 10; HCO_3^- is appropriately increased. Change in HCO_3^- is between expected change for acute and chronic respiratory acidosis.

Diagnosis: Acute on chronic respiratory acidosis

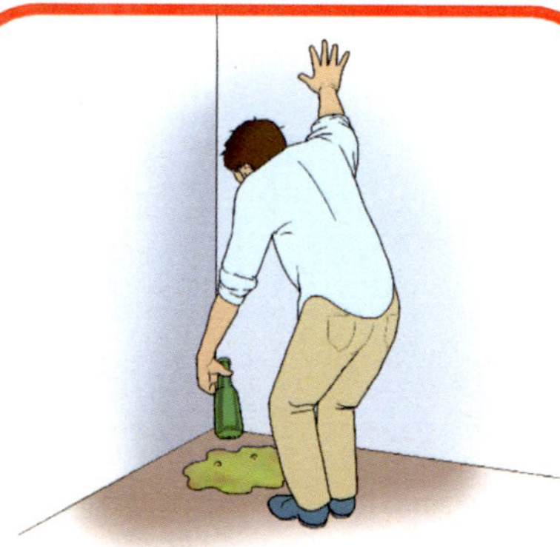

36 yo alcoholic man with vomiting.

pH	7.36	**Na+**	147 mEq/L
$PaCO_2$	30 mmHg	**Cl^-**	109 mEq/L
HCO_3^-	14 mEq/L	**Albumin**	4.5 mEq/L

Acidemia or alkalemia? Acidemia

Primary derangement? Metabolic acidosis since pH, $PaCO_2$ and HCO_3^- are low.

Compensation?
Expect ≈ 1 for 1 pCO_2 decrease for each 1 decrease in HCO_3^-. $PaCO_2$ is appropriately decreased.

Is an anion gap present?
Anion gap (AG) = $Na^+ - [Cl^- + HCO_3^-]$
Normal AG = **12**
147 – [109 + 14] = 24

$$\frac{\Delta AG}{\Delta HCO_3^-} \quad \begin{matrix} = 12 \\ = 10 \end{matrix}$$

Change (Δ) AG
= (AG – normal AG)
= 24 – **12** = 12

Normal HCO_3^- = **24**

Change (Δ) HCO_3^-
= **24** – HCO_3^-
= **24** – 14 = 10

If < 1 ← $\frac{\Delta AG}{\Delta HCO_3^-}$ → **If > 1**

Hidden Non-ANION GAP ACIDOSIS | **Hidden METABOLIC ALKALOSIS**

Diagnosis: AG metabolic acidosis and metabolic alkalosis

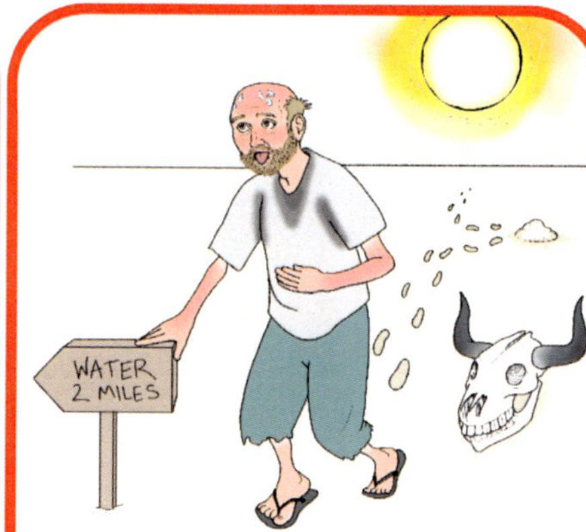

40 yo dehydrated man in desert after diarrhea.

pH	7.31	**Na^+**	151 mEq/L
$PaCO_2$	27 mmHg	**Cl^-**	121 mEq/L
HCO_3^-	11 mEq/L		

Acidemia or alkalemia? Acidemia

Primary derangement? Metabolic acidosis since pH, $PaCO_2$ and HCO_3^- are low.

Compensation?
Expect ≈ 1 for 1 pCO_2 decrease for each 1 decrease in HCO_3^-. $PaCO_2$ is appropriately decreased.

Is an anion gap present?
Anion gap (AG) = $Na^+ - [Cl^- + HCO_3^-]$
Normal AG = **12**
151 – [121 + 11] = 19

$$\frac{\Delta AG}{\Delta HCO_3^-} \quad \begin{matrix} = 7 \\ = 13 \end{matrix}$$

Change (Δ) AG
= (AG – normal AG)
= 19 – **12** = 7

Normal HCO_3^- = **24**

Change (Δ) HCO_3^-
= **24** – HCO_3^-
= **24** – 11 = 13

If < 1 ← $\frac{\Delta AG}{\Delta HCO_3^-}$ → **If > 1**

Hidden Non-ANION GAP ACIDOSIS | **Hidden METABOLIC ALKALOSIS**

Diagnosis: AG metabolic acidosis and non-AG metabolic acidosis

BLOOD UREA NITROGEN (BUN) AND CREATININE

BUN:Cr	Location	Mechanism
>20:1	Prerenal	BUN reabsorption is increased. BUN is disproportionately elevated relative to creatinine in serum. This may be indicative of **hypoperfusion of the kidneys** due to heart failure or dehydration, gastrointestinal hemorrhage or increased dietary protein.
12–20:1	Normal or Postrenal	Normal range. Can also be postrenal disease.
<12:1	Intrarenal	**Renal damage** causes reduced reabsorption of BUN, therefore lowering the BUN: creatinine (Cr) ratio. Decreased ratio indicates liver disease (due to decreased urea formation) or malnutrition.

During **pregnancy,** blood volume increases significantly. As a result, the concentration of various substances in the bloodstream decreases, including BUN and creatinine. Additionally, the increased blood flow to the kidneys during pregnancy helps to increase the glomerular filtration rate.

Malnutrition, often associated with a **low-protein diet** or **starvation**, can lead to decreased BUN levels. Additionally, impaired liver function due to liver disease may also result in lower BUN levels.

A variety of **drugs** (like cimetidine and trimethoprim) can affect the serum creatinine by competing with the secretion of creatinine at the level of the kidney tubule.

ACE inhibitor therapy should not be discontinued unless the serum creatinine level rises above 30% over baseline during the first 2 months after initiation of therapy or hyperkalemia (serum potassium level >or=5.6 mmol/L) develops.

BUN AND CREATININE

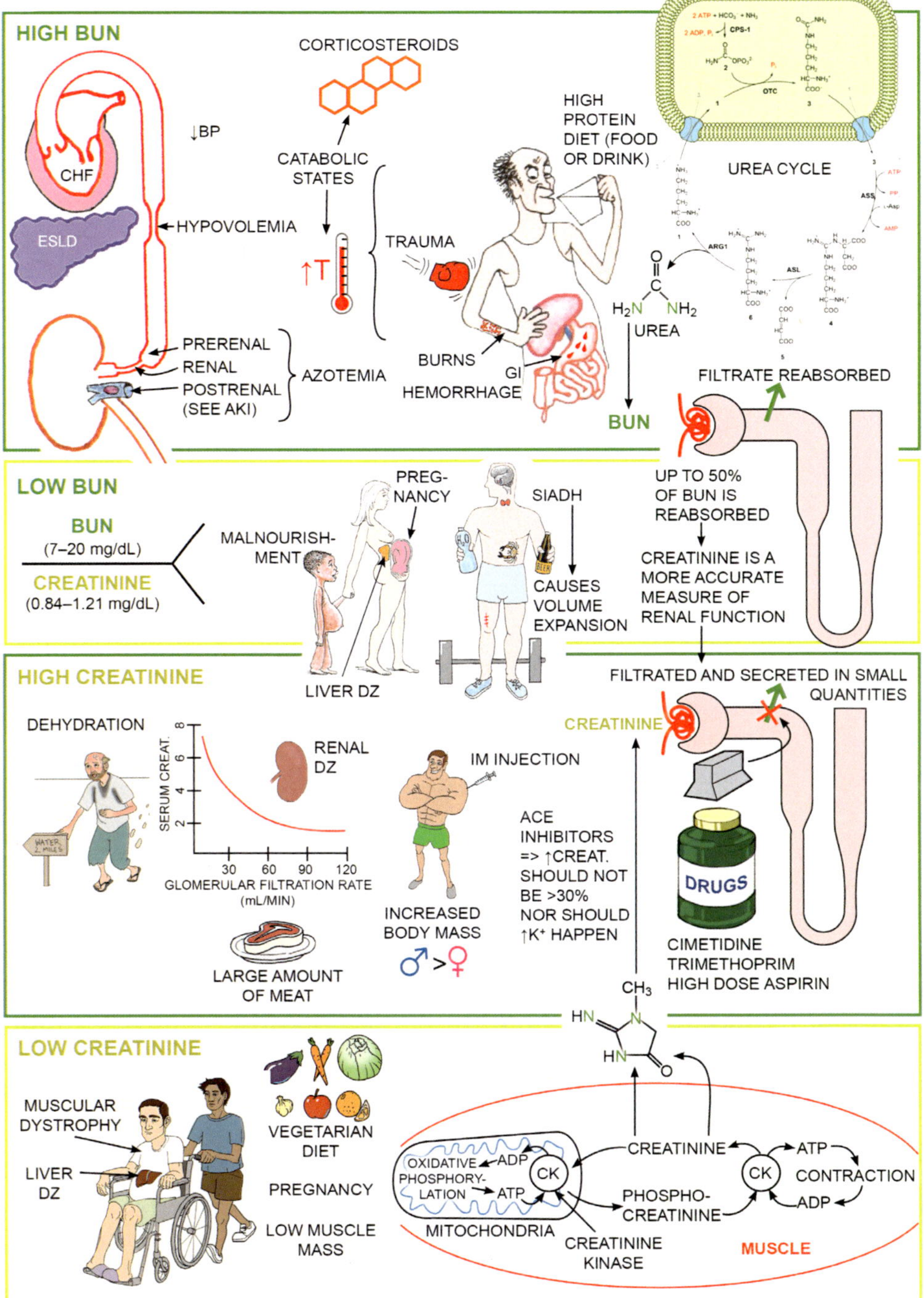

HYPER AND HYPOGLYCEMIA

Hyperglycemia may be caused by **diabetes** (illustrated by the patients who drink a lot of water due to polydipsia due to diabetes; diabetes mellitus [DM] which can lead to diabetic keto acidosis DKA, while DM II to hyperosmolar coma), **endocrine disorders** (**thyroid**, **adrena**l, **pancreatic**, and **pituitary** disorders), **hypoxia**, **hypotension/shock**, and **stressful conditions** like physical or psychological trauma, myocardial infarction, hypothermia. (In **hypothermia**, insulin secretion may be reduced, causing an increase in blood glucose levels. Additionally, hyperthermia can stimulate the body to release stress hormones).

With respect to endocrine disorders, **free T4** should be checked for possible **hyperthyroidism**, excessive **cortisol** and **ACTH** for possible **Cushing syndrome,** and **grow hormone (IGF-1)** for possible **acromegaly** (illustrated by the patient's large left hand). The **24-hour excessive catecholamine** level indicates **pheochromocytoma.** If all of the above endocrinological tests are normal, diabetes mellitus is usually the diagnosis, although some of the patients could have glucagonoma or pancreatic disease. Certain **drugs** can cause hyperglycemia.

Hypoglycemia could be caused by **drugs**, **critical illness** (hepatic, renal, or cardiac failure, sepsis, inanition), **hormone deficiency** (cortisol, glucagon, epinephrine), **nonislet cell tumor** and **endogenous hyperinsulinism. Ethanol** inhibits gluconeogenesis but not glycogenolysis. Thus, alcohol-induced hypoglycemia typically follows a several-day alcohol binge with hepatic glycogen depletion due to limited ingestion of food.

Glycogen storage disease (like **Pompe's disease)** is illustrated by the drawn DNA on the patient's leg.

Endogenous hyperinsulinism — Hyperinsulinemic hypoglycemia occurs when insulin secretion fails to fall appropriately in the setting of hypoglycemia. It is more likely in an **otherwise healthy individual** with no clinical clues suggesting other common causes of hypoglycemia. The diagnosis is often unrecognized for years. Hypoglycemia due to endogenous hyperinsulinism can be caused by:

- A **beta cell secretagogue**, such as a sulfonylurea (accidental, surreptitious, or malicious hypoglycemia).
- A beta cell tumor (**insulinoma**). (C-peptide level < 0.2 nmol/l [0.6 ng/ml] suggests hypoglycemia due to insulin administration).
- A functional beta cell disorder (nesidioblastosis) causes **noninsulinoma pancreatogenous hypoglycemia syndrome** (**NIPHS**). It is caused by **islet cell hypertrophy**, but not an islet cell tumor. In NIPHS, patients experience predominantly **postprandial hypoglycemia** (while in insulinoma symptoms typically occur during fasting).
- After **gastric bypass** or **Nissen fundoplication** when a mismatch occurs between postprandial glucose disappearance and the offset of insulin action. (**Functional hypoglycemia,** when blood glucose drops following a meal, in **younger women** doesn't need to be treated.)
- **Insulin autoimmune hypoglycemia** occurs in patients who have **antibodies** directed to endogenous **insulin** or to the **insulin receptor**. Insulin autoantibodies may be triggered by exposure to drugs or viruses, or they may manifest spontaneously. There are two types of autoimmune hypoglycemia. One is insulin autoimmune syndrome (IAS), which is characterized by hyperinsulinemic hypoglycemia, elevated insulin autoantibody (IAA) titers, no prior exposure to exogenous insulin, and no pathological abnormalities of the pancreatic islets. This condition is also known as "Hirata's disease". The other is type B insulin resistance syndrome (TBIRS), a rare autoimmune disorder resulting in a broad array of abnormalities in glucose homeostasis—from hypoglycemia to extremely insulin-resistant hyperglycemia—caused by the presence of insulin receptor autoantibodies (IRAbs).

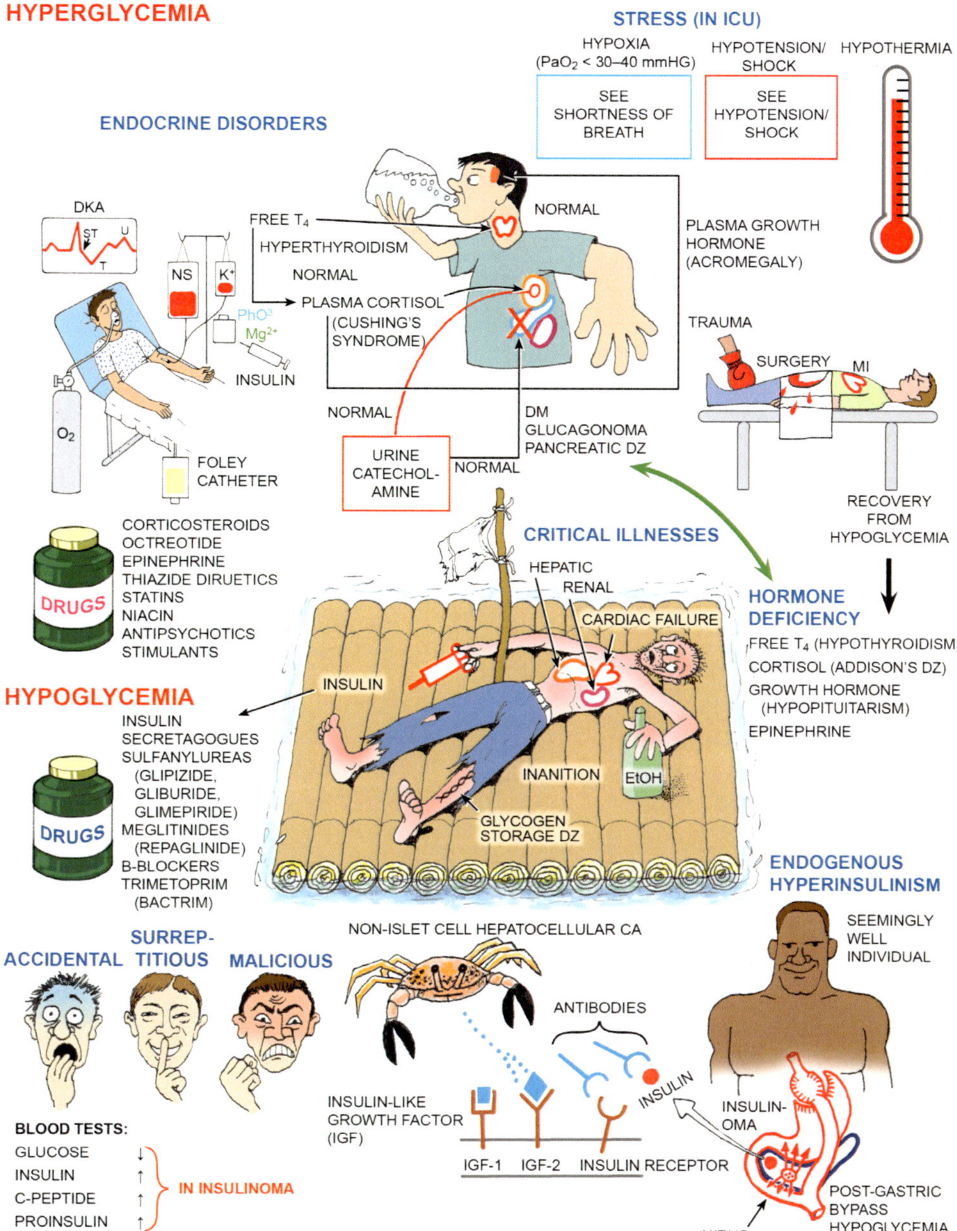

BLOOD TESTS:

GLUCOSE ↓
INSULIN ↑
C-PEPTIDE ↑
PROINSULIN ↑
} IN INSULINOMA

B-HYDROXYBUTIRATE (BHOB) ↓ IN INSULINOMA PATIENTS THAN IN NORMAL SUBJECTS

SULFONYLUREA AND MEGLITINIDE SCREEN → PRESENT IN THE PLASMA ONLY IN ORAL HYPOGLYCEMIA AGENT-INDUCED HYPOGLYCEMIA

COMPREHENSIVE METABOLIC PANEL (CMP)

1. LIVER FUNCTION TESTS (LFT) 1 and 2
2. HYPERCALCEMIA
3. HYPOCALCEMIA
4. HYPERMAGNESEMIA
5. HYPOMAGNESEMIA
6. HYPERPHOSPHATEMIA
7. HYPOPHOSPHATEMIA

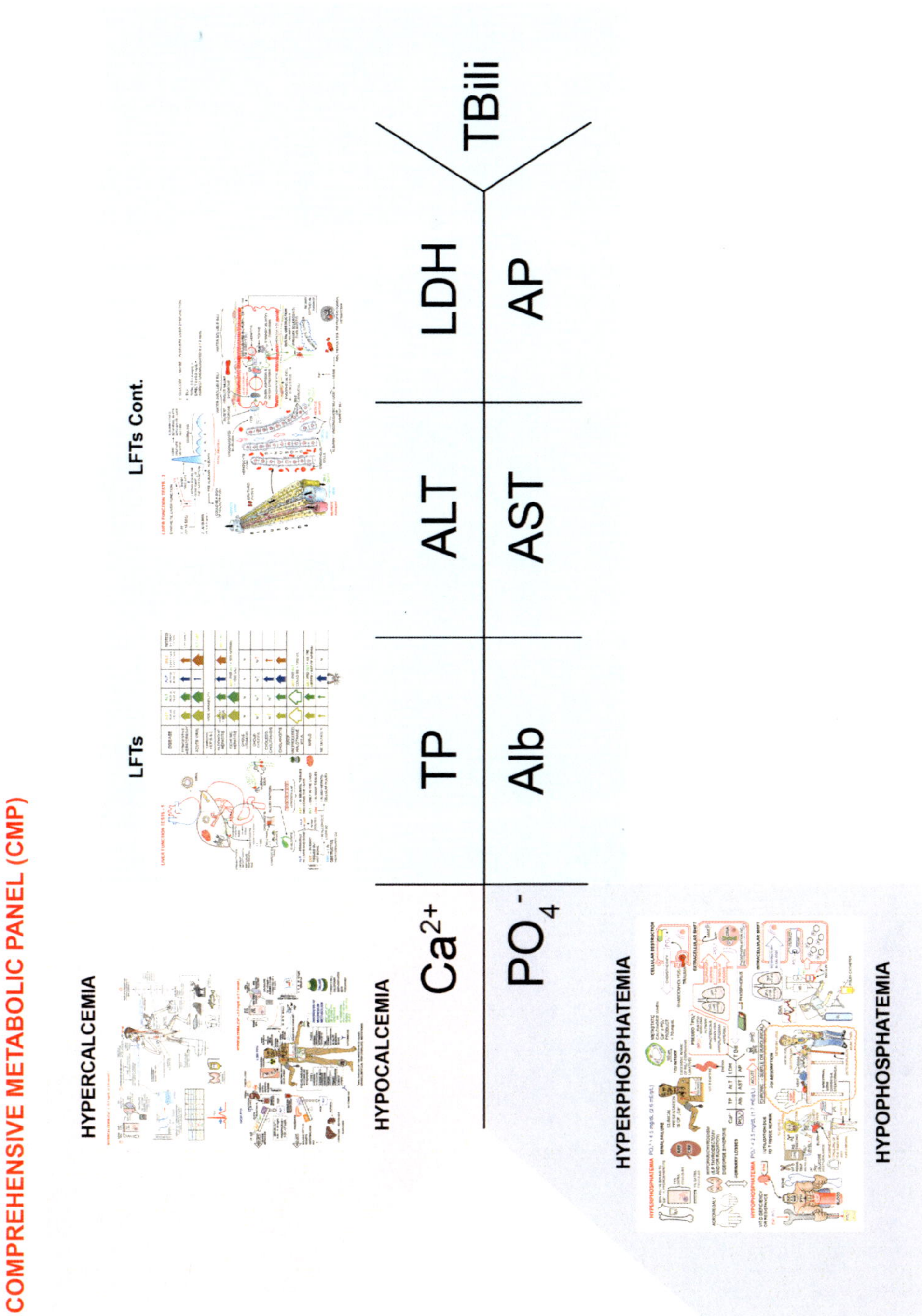

This picture is a compilation of the of pictures of hyper and hypocalcemia, hyper and hypophosphatemia and liver function tests (LFT) and LFT continuation. All of them exist as separate pictures on the separate pages. The purpose of this page was not to go into details of the picture (which are separately explained in detail on the bigger pages), but to show them all together on the comprehensive metabolic (CMP) panel grid.

LIVER FUNCTION TESTS (LFT) – 1

The two predominant patterns of liver injury are **cholestatic** and **hepatocellular.**

A cholestatic pattern is characterized by elevation of **alkaline phosphatase (ALP)** and **gamma glutamine transpeptidase (GGT).**

ALP is found primarily in liver and bone. It could also be found in the small intestine, kidney, placenta and leukocytes. In the liver, ALP is found primarily on the surface of the bile canalicular membrane. Disproportionate elevation of alkaline phosphatase occurs with any disease that obstructs bile flow (e.g., biliary stones, cholangitis, pathetic cancer) or diseases that infiltrated the liver causing microbe obstruction or damage (e.g., tuberculosis, sarcoidosis, metastatic cancer). Isolated ALP may suggest metastatic involvement of the liver.

GGT is an enzyme found in many tissues but notably not bone. Therefore, it is most useful for evaluating the course of an elevated alkaline phosphatase. If both enzymes are elevated, the liver is the likely source, whereas elevation of alkaline phosphatase within normal GGT suggests a bone source. GGT is also elevated in patients with alcoholic liver disease.

The hepatocellular pattern is associated with elevation in aspartate amino transferase (AST), alanine aminotransferase (ALT) and lactate dehydrogenase (LDH).

AST is an enzyme found in hepatocytes. It is also found in the cardiac muscle, renal, brain, pulmonary and pancreatic tissue, leukocytes and erythrocytes. AST is a sensitive indicator of hepatic injury but is not specific.

ALT is found only in the liver. ALT is a very specific indicator of hepatocellular injury.

LDH is found in many tissues. Its levels increase with any hepatocellular injury.

Increased **5'-Nucleotidase (5'-NT)** in the serum of patients with normal ALP identifies with high probability for the presence of liver disease, confirming that any increase in 5'-NT activity that is more than marginal is highly specific for **hepatobiliary disease**. The diagnostic value of 5'-NT has been shown to be superior to other liver enzymes, especially in liver metastasis. Raised levels of 5'-NT activities are found in 92% of patients with obstructive jaundice, 70% of patients with parenchymal liver disease and 81% of patients with hepatic metastasis.

Charcot's cholangitis triad is the combination of jaundice; fever, usually with rigors; and right upper quadrant abdominal pain. It occurs as a result of **ascending cholangitis.** When the presentation also includes low blood pressure and mental status changes, it is known as Reynolds' pentad.

Murphy's sign (also known as **Sweeney's sign**) is a maneuver during a physical examination as part of the abdominal examination. It is useful for differentiating pain in the right upper quadrant. Typically, it is **positive** in cholecystitis, but **negative** in choledocholithiasis, pyelonephritis, and ascending cholangitis.

Murphy's sign is elicited in patients with acute cholecystitis by asking the patient to take in and hold a deep breath while palpating the right subcostal area. If pain occurs on inspiration, when the inflamed gallbladder encounters the examiner's hand, **Murphy's sign** is positive.[20]

---

20 Abbreviations; N: normal; PT: prothrombin time

LIVER FUNCTION TESTS - 1

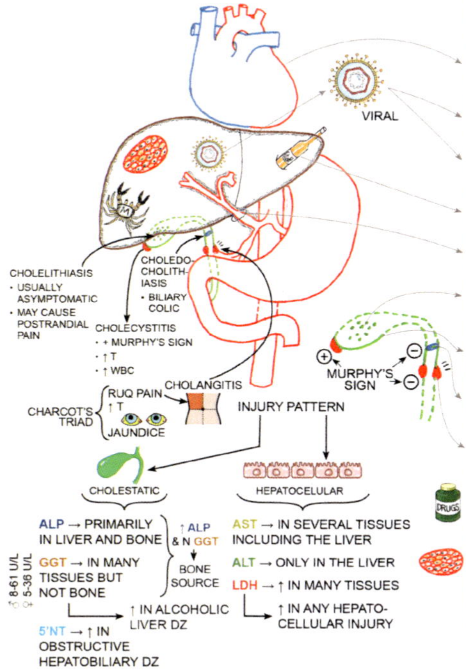

DISEASE	AST ♂ 10-40 U/L ♀ 9-32 U/L	ALT ♂ 29-33 U/L ♀ 19-25 U/L	ALP ♂ 45-115 U/L ♀ 30-100 U/L	BILI D: 0.0-0.3 mg/dL T: 0.0-1.4 mg/dL	NOTES D = DIRECT T = TOTAL
CONGESTIVE HEPATOPATHY	↑	↑	↑	↑	↑ PT EARLY
ACUTE VIRAL	↑	↑	↑	↑	ALT > AST
CHRONIC HEP B & C	WIDE VARIABILITY				
ALCOHOLIC HEPATITIS	USUALLY < 300 U/L	↑	↑	↑	AST > ALT
ISCHEMIC HEPATITIS	↑	↑	AST AND ALT > 50X NORMAL (> 1000 U/L)		
CHOLE-LITHIASIS	N	N	N	N	
CHOLE-CYSTITIS	N/↑	N/↑	N/↑	N/↑	
CHOLEDO-CHOLITHIASIS	N/↑	N/↑	↑	↑	
CHOLANGITIS	↑	↑	↑	↑	
APAP, VACPROCODED, HALOTHANE, VIT A	↑	↑	AST AND ALT COULD BE > 1000 U/L		
NAFLD	↑	↑	AST AND ALT < 4X THE UPPER LIMIT OF NORMAL		
METASTASES	↑	↑	↑	N	

Learning never exhausts the mind,"

Leonardo da Vinci.

LIVER FUNCTION TESTS - 1

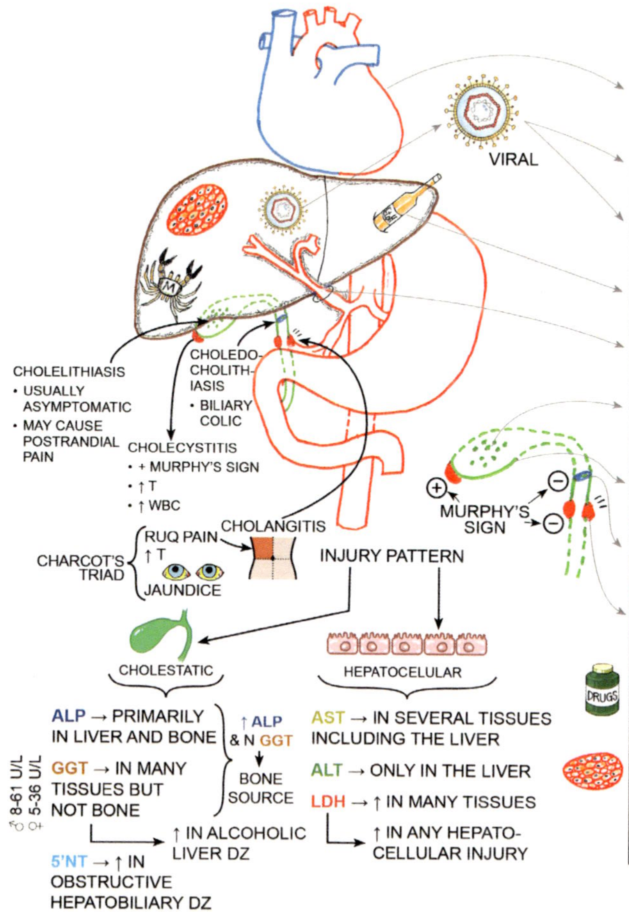

DISEASE	AST ♂ 10-40 U/L ♀ 9-32 U/L	ALT ♂ 29-33 U/L ♀ 19-25 U/L	ALP ♂ 45-115 U/L ♀ 30-100 U/L	BILI D: 0.0-0.3 mg/dL T: 0.0-1.4 mg/dL	NOTES D = DIRECT T = TOTAL
CONGESTIVE HEPATOPATHY	↑	↑	↑	↑	↑ PT EARLY
ACUTE VIRAL	↑	↑	↑	↑	ALT > AST
CHRONIC HEP B & C	WIDE VARIABILITY				
ALCOHOLIC HEPATITIS	USUALLY < 300 U/L	↑	↑	↑	AST > ALT
ISCHEMIC HEPATITIS	↑	↑	AST AND ALT > 50X NORMAL (> 1000 U/L)		
CHOLE-LITHIASIS	N	N	N	N	
CHOLE-CYSTITIS	N/↑	N/↑	N/↑	N/↑	
CHOLEDO-CHOLITHIASIS	N/↑	N/↑	↑	↑	
CHOLANGITIS	↑	↑	↑	↑	
APAP, VACPROCODED, HALOTHANE, VIT A	⇧	⇧	AST AND ALT COULD BE > 1000 U/L		
NAFLD	↑	↑	AST AND ALT < 4X THE UPPER LIMIT OF NORMAL		
METASTASES	↑	↑	↑	N	

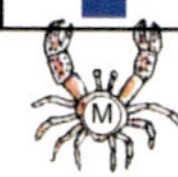

LIVER FUNCTION TESTS (LFT) – 2

Synthetic function of the liver could be assessed by levels of **albumin**, **prothrombin time** (**PT**), total **bilirubin** levels and **glucose** levels.

1) The liver is an important site of protein synthesis. Assessment of **albumin** levels can tell us how well delivery is making proteins in general. If dietary intake is constant and delivery fails, it can take several weeks for albumin levels to fall. Therefore, in a patient that is acutely with failure, the albumin level may be normal.
2) **PT** is a function of plasma levels and the activity of factors I, II, V, VII, and X. The half-lives of some of these proteins are much shorter than the half-life of albumin. Therefore, the PT increases within hours of a significant decrease in the synthetic function of the liver.
3) Clinical jaundice is usually apparent with **bilirubin** levels that exceed 3 mg/dl. Elevation of bilirubin could be predominantly **unconjugated** or **conjugated**. Most are a mix of both.

Total bilirubin = direct bilirubin + indirect bilirubin

Levels of **unconjugated bilirubin** increase if production increases (e.g., in hemolysis or hematoma) or hepatic uptake or conjugation decreases (as seen in Gilbert syndrome or Crigler-Najjar syndrome).

Levels of **conjugated bilirubin** increase with decreased secretion of bilirubin into bile canaliculi (as seen in Dubin-Johnson syndrome and Rotor's syndrome). Biliary epithelial damage (as a result of hepatitis, toxins or cirrhosis) or ductal obstruction (as a result of biliary stones, cholangitis, or pancreatic cancer) can also increase conjugated bilirubin levels.

4) **Glucose** levels may be decreased in patients with severe liver dysfunction. [21]

21 Abbreviations: ALP: alkaline phosphatase

LIVER FUNCTION TESTS - 2

SYNTHETIC LIVER FUNCTION

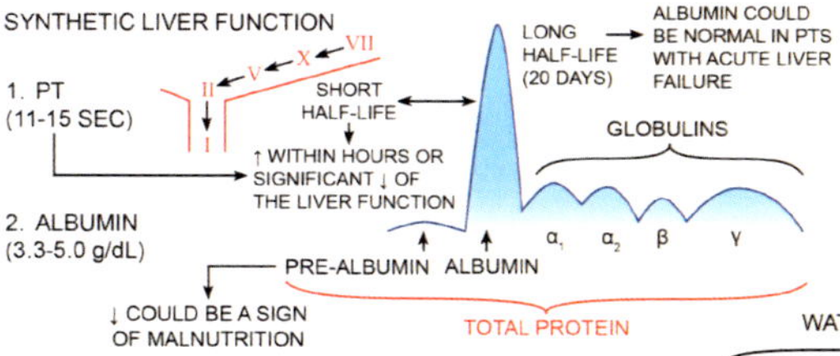

3. GLUCOSE → MAYBE ↓ IN SEVERE LIVER DYSFUNCTION

4. BILI

TOTAL 0.0-1.4 mg/dL =
DIRECT 0.0-0.3 mg/dL +
INDIRECT (UNCONJUGATED) 0.2-1.2 mg/dL

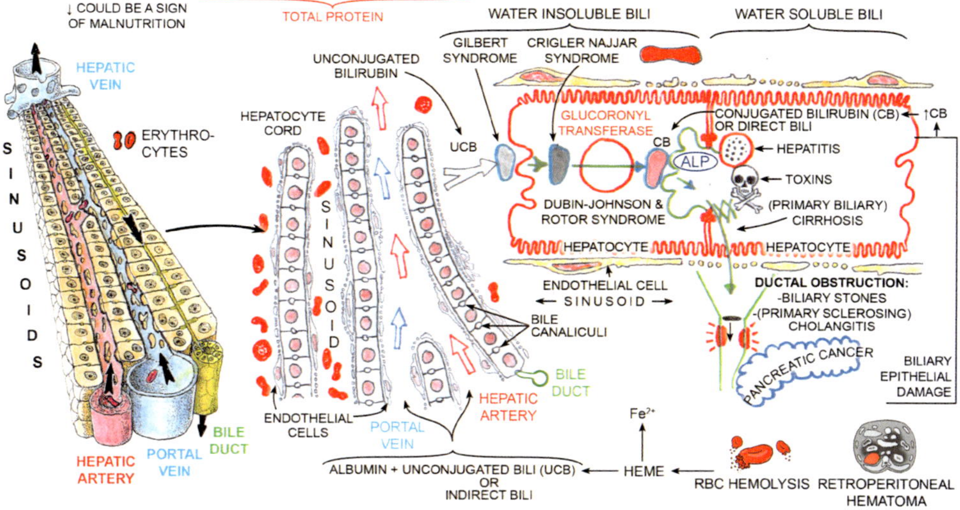

"Information is the oil of the 21st century,
and analytics is the combustion engine."

Peter Sondergaard

LIVER FUNCTION TESTS - 2

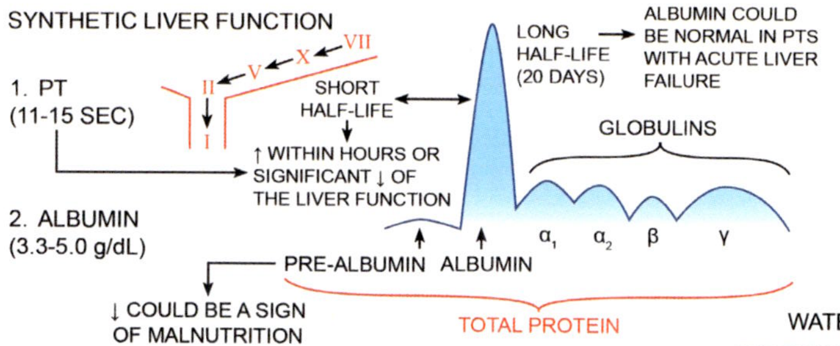

3. GLUCOSE → MAYBE ↓ IN SEVERE LIVER DYSFUNCTION

4. BILI

TOTAL 0.0-1.4 mg/dL =
DIRECT 0.0-0.3 mg/dL +
INDIRECT (UNCONJUGATED) 0.2-1.2 mg/dL

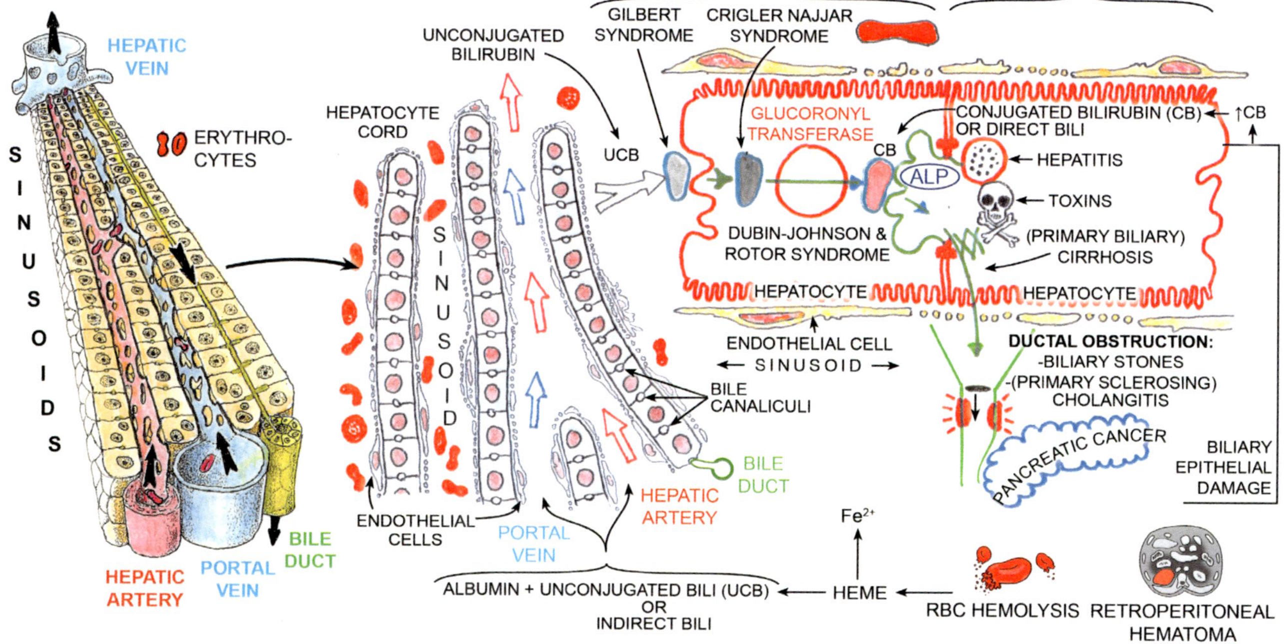

HYPERCALCEMIA

Among all causes of hypercalcemia, **primary hyperparathyroidism** and **malignancy** are the most common, accounting for greater than **90% of cases**. Therefore, the diagnostic approach to hypercalcemia typically involves distinguishing between the two. However, the first step in evaluation of hypercalcemia is to check albumin levels because hypercalcemia is due to ionized (or free) calcium concentration, while 40 to 45% of the calcium in serum is bound to protein, principally albumin.

For every 1 mg increase in albumin (the normal albumin level is 4 mg/dl), you must decrease the calcium level by 0.8 mg/dl. The converse is true for hypoalbuminemia. For example, if the serum calcium is 11 mg/dl and the albumin is 5 mg/dl, the corrected calcium is 10.2 mg/dl and the patient is not hypercalcemic.

A frankly elevated **parathyroid hormone (PTH)** concentration in the setting of hypercalcemia is highly likely to be the result of **primary hyperparathyroidism (PHPT)**. "Bones, stones, and psychic overtones" is a mnemonic used by medical students to remember the symptoms of hypercalcemia, which can be caused by PHPT. 10-20% of patients with PHPT have a serum PTH concentration in the **upper end of the normal range.** Such a "normal" level is also virtually diagnostic of PHPT since it is still inappropriately high considering the presence of hypercalcemia. However, in this circumstance, the diagnosis of **familial hypocalciuric hypercalcemia (FHH)** also should be considered, and urinary calcium excretion (24-hour urinary calcium or calcium-to-creatinine ratio) should be measured (since the patients with FHH have **abnormally high levels of calcium in the blood** [hypercalcemia] and **low to moderate levels of calcium in urine** [hypocalciuric]). It is shown in the picture as a crossed line from kidney to urethra. People with FHH usually do not exhibit any symptoms and are often diagnosed incidentally during routine blood tests. However, some individuals with FHH may experience weakness, fatigue, concentration issues, and polydipsia.

In **secondary hyperparathyroidism**, the parathyroid glands produce extra PTH due to a specific condition elsewhere in the body. Common causes are **vitamin D deficiency** and **renal failure**. **Tertiary hyperparathyroidism** occurs in patients who have undergone **kidney transplants**. After prolonged abnormal function during kidney failure and dialysis, the parathyroid glands may never return to normal. (The goal is to protect the transplanted kidney from any negative effects of excess PTH and the patients with tertiary hyperparathyroidism are usually referred for **parathyroid surgery**.)

A **low** or **low-normal serum intact PTH** level (below 20 pg/mL) is most consistent with non-PTH-mediated hypercalcemia. In such cases, vitamin D metabolites should be measured to assess for **vitamin D intoxication** and **PTH-related protein (PTHrP)** to assess for hypercalcemia of **malignancy**. The presence of **low serum levels of PTH, PTHrP, and low or normal vitamin D** metabolites suggests some other source for the hypercalcemia such as bone resorption (as with **multiple myeloma, thyrotoxicosis, immobilization, or vitamin A toxicity**) or **milk-alkali syndrome** (see Metabolic alkalosis).

Vitamin A is a fat soluble. Eskimo nutrition provides abundant sources of vitamin A and lays the probable basis in some individuals for **hypervitaminosis A** through ingestion of livers, kidneys, and fat of arctic fish and mammals, where the vitamin often is stored in poisonous quantities. (Excessive intake of Vitamin A can lead to increased bone resorption and elevated calcium level.)

HYPERCALCEMIA (Ca^{2+} > 10.5 mg/dL or 2.6 mmol/L)

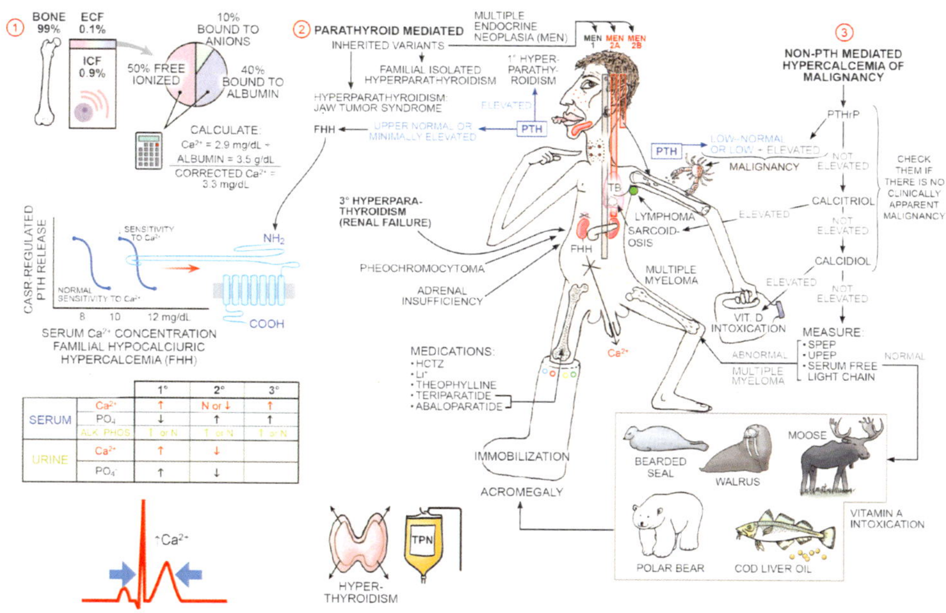

		1°	2°	3°
SERUM	Ca^{2+}	↑	N or ↓	↑
	PO_4	↓	↑	↑
	ALK. PHOS	↑ or N	↑ or N	↑ or N
URINE	Ca^{2+}	↑	↓	
	PO_4	↑	↓	

"The power of visualization is that it gives you answers to questions you didn't know you had."

Ben Fry

HYPERCALCEMIA (Ca^{2+} > 10.5 mg/dL or 2.6 mmol/L)

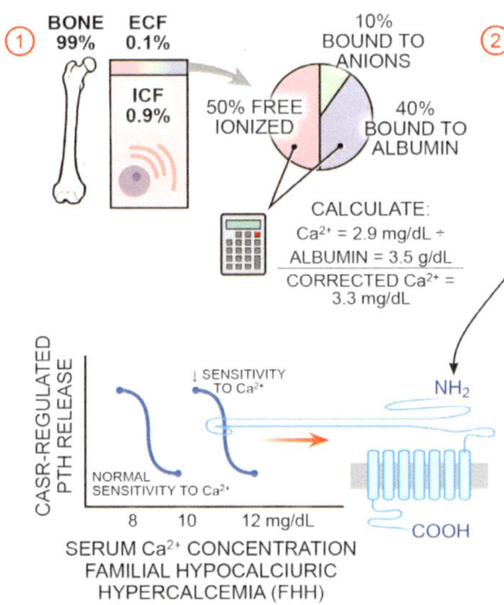

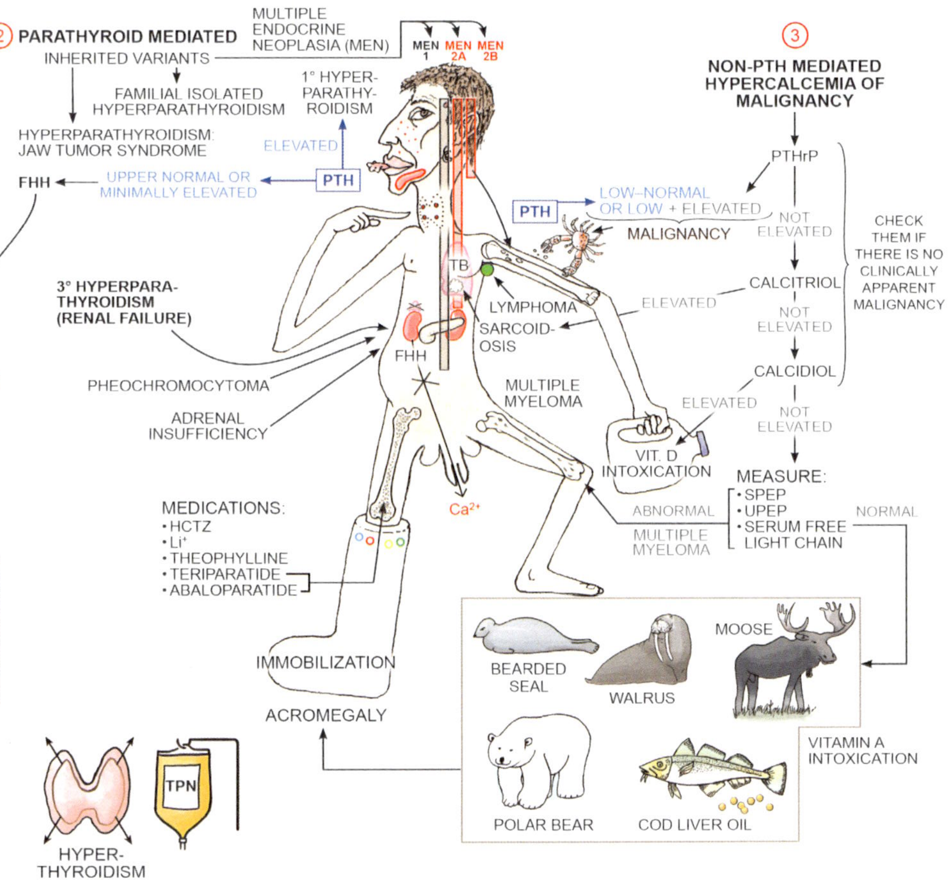

		1°	2°	3°
SERUM	Ca^{2+}	↑	N or ↓	↑
	PO_4^-	↓	↑	↑
	ALK. PHOS.	↑ or N	↑ or N	↑ or N
URINE	Ca^{2+}	↑	↓	
	PO_4^-	↑	↓	

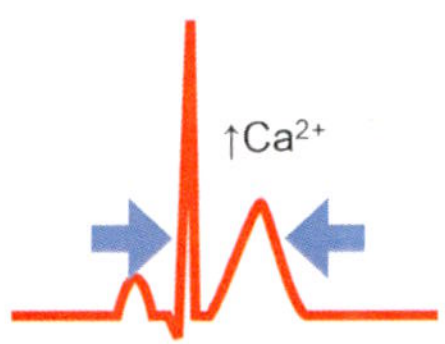

CALCIUM METABOLISM

Calcium and phosphorus have an inverse relationship: as blood calcium levels rise, phosphate levels drop, and vice versa. The parathyroid hormone (PTH) plays a critical role in maintaining this balance. If calcium levels are low, PTH prompts the kidneys to produce more active vitamin D, leading to increased calcium and phosphorus absorption from the intestines. Conversely, if calcium levels are high, PTH reduces phosphorus reabsorption in the kidneys.

The builder who is squeezing the nephron and the bone is a **PTH**.

PTH in kidneys decreases calcium excretion in urine and increases phosphorus excretion, in intestines enhances the production of active vitamin D, which aids in calcium absorption from the intestines, and in bones signals bones to release calcium and phosphorus into the bloodstream.

Problems with calcium, phosphorus, and PTH can occur in individuals with kidney failure. These issues typically start when kidney function drops to less than 40% of normal (or eGFR of 40 ml/min). Symptoms may or may not be present initially, but over time, irreversible damage to bones, the heart, or blood vessels can occur.

Rhabdomyolysis can lead to hypocalcemia. This occurs due to calcium loss from serum entering damaged muscle cells. Hyperphosphatemia is observed in rhabdomyolysis. Rhabdomyolysis can cause renal tubular obstruction when myoglobin precipitates in the glomerular filtrate, potentially leading to AKI. During the recovery phase, serum calcium levels may rebound to significantly elevated levels due to the release of calcium from injured muscle, mild secondary hyperparathyroidism, and an increase in calcitriol (1,25-dihydroxyvitamin D).

CALCIUM METABOLISM

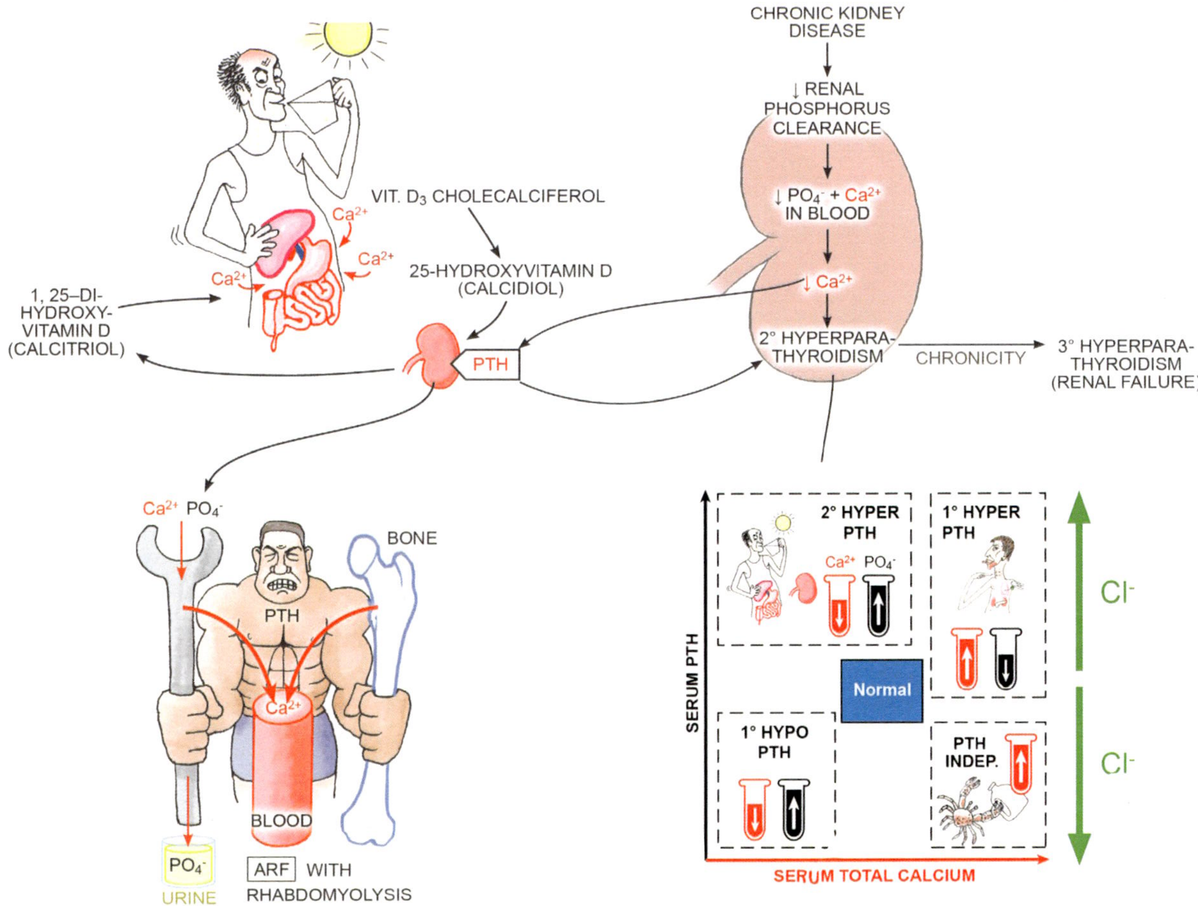

HYPOCALCEMIA

Hypocalcemia is most often caused by **vitamin D deficiency, hypoparathyroidism, chronic kidney disease, malnutrition alkalosis, and certain medications,** such as diuretics or antiepileptic drugs.

For every 1 mg <u>decrease</u> in albumin (the normal albumin level is 4 mg/dl), you must <u>increase</u> the calcium level by 0.8 mg/dl. The converse is true for hypoalbuminemia. For example, if the serum calcium is 7.5 mg/dl and the albumin is 2 mg/dl, the corrected calcium is 9.1 mg/dl and the patient is not hypocalcemic.

In hypocalcemia with high parathyroid hormone (**PTH**), the PTH is increased in response to low serum calcium concentrations. It is caused by **vitamin D deficiency or resistance**, **chronic kidney disease, and PTH resistance (pseudohypoparathyroidism).** PTH resistance represents unresponsiveness to PTH due to an alteration in the postreceptor PTH signaling pathway. It is characterized by <u>hypocalcemia</u>, <u>hyperphosphatemia</u> and, in contrast to hypoparathyroidism, <u>elevated</u> rather than reduced PTH concentrations.

In hyperparathyroidism PTH can stimulate bone turnover and lead to increased alkaline phosphatase levels (ALP). Therefore, a high PTH in combination with **elevated ALP** please suggests ARF, while elevated PTH and **normal ALP** suggests pseudohypoparathyroidism.

Tumor lysis syndrome can develop in some cancer patients and can lead to <u>hyperkalemia</u>, <u>hyperuricemia</u> and <u>hypocalcemia.</u> Occasional patients with widespread **osteoblastic metastases**, particularly those with breast or prostate cancer, have hypocalcemia.

Hypocalcemia is also a frequent finding in patients with **acute pancreatitis**, where it is associated with <u>precipitation of calcium soaps</u> in the abdominal cavity. Hypocalcemia is associated with **low phosphorus** levels when there is a **functional deficiency of vitamin D (malabsorption, rickets, osteomalacia).**

Hypocalcemia with low PTH occurs when there is decreased secretion of PTH due to <u>destruction</u> of the parathyroid glands (autoimmune, postsurgical, hemochromatosis, Wilson disease, granulomas, or metastatic cancer), <u>abnormal parathyroid gland development</u>, or altered regulation of <u>PTH production and secretion</u> (autosomal dominant or autosomal recessive hypoparathyroidism due to mutations in the signal peptide sequence of preproparathyroid hormone [preproPTH], which impair the normal processing of preproPTH to PTH and therefore lead to decreased PTH secretion and low circulating concentrations).

Polyglandular autoimmune syndromes are a group of rare conditions in which multiple autoimmune endocrine disorders occur simultaneously. <u>Acquired hypoparathyroidism not related to surgery is most often an autoimmune disease.</u> Permanent hypoparathyroidism can result from immune-mediated destruction of the parathyroid glands. Alternatively, hypoparathyroidism may result from activating antibodies to the calcium-sensing receptor (CASR) that decrease PTH secretion.

Hungry bone syndrome causes **persistent hypocalcemia**. It can also lead to **decreased phosphorus** levels and **low magnesium**. It most often happens after parathyroid or thyroid removal surgery but can happen in metastatic prostate cancer as well.

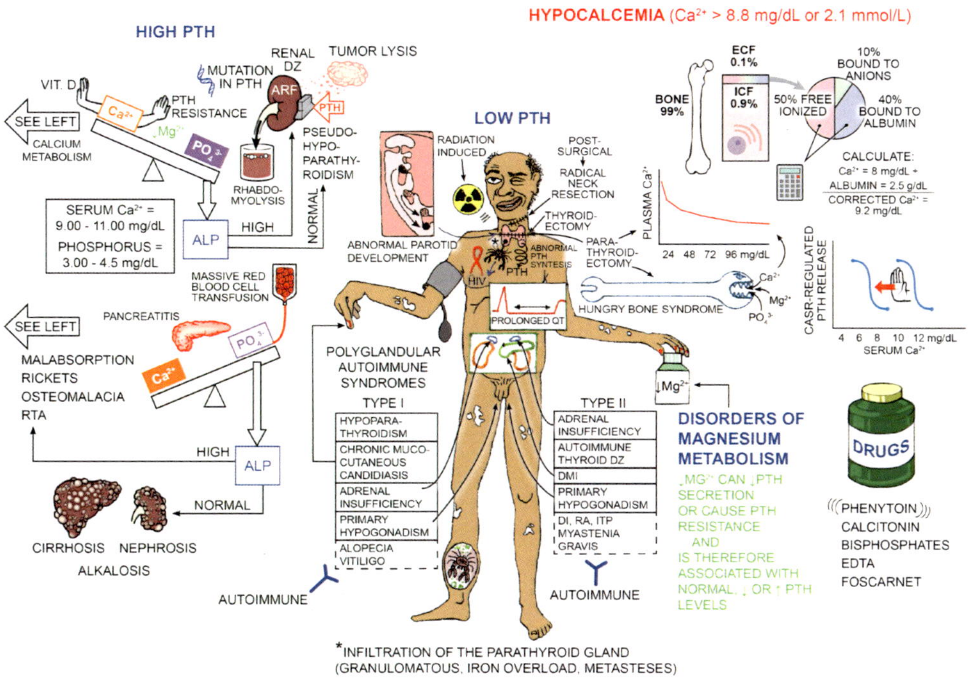
HYPOCALCEMIA (Ca^{2+} > 8.8 mg/dL or 2.1 mmol/L)
HIGH PTH
VIT. D
Ca^{2+}
PTH RESISTANCE
Mg^{2+}
PO_4^{3-}
SEE LEFT
CALCIUM METABOLISM
MUTATION IN PTH
RENAL DZ
ARF
TUMOR LYSIS
PTH
RHABDO-MYOLYSIS
PSEUDO-HYPO-PARATHY-ROIDISM
SERUM Ca^{2+} = 9.00 - 11.00 mg/dL
PHOSPHORUS = 3.00 - 4.5 mg/dL
ALP
HIGH
NORMAL
MASSIVE RED BLOOD CELL TRANSFUSION
PANCREATITIS
SEE LEFT
MALABSORPTION
RICKETS
OSTEOMALACIA
RTA
Ca^{2+}
PO_4^{3-}
HIGH
ALP
NORMAL
CIRRHOSIS
NEPHROSIS
ALKALOSIS
LOW PTH
RADIATION INDUCED
ABNORMAL PAROTID DEVELOPMENT
POST-SURGICAL
RADICAL NECK RESECTION
THYROID-ECTOMY
PARA-THYROID-ECTOMY
ABNORMAL PTH SYNTESIS
HIV
PTH
PROLONGED QT
HUNGRY BONE SYNDROME
Ca^{2+}
Mg^{2+}
PO_4^{3-}
PLASMA Ca^{2+}
24 48 72 96 mg/dL
POLYGLANDULAR AUTOIMMUNE SYNDROMES
TYPE I
HYPOPARA-THYROIDISM
CHRONIC MUCO-CUTANEOUS CANDIDIASIS
ADRENAL INSUFFICIENCY
PRIMARY HYPOGONADISM
ALOPECIA VITILIGO
AUTOIMMUNE
TYPE II
ADRENAL INSUFFICIENCY
AUTOIMMUNE THYROID DZ
DMI
PRIMARY HYPOGONADISM
DI, RA, ITP MYASTENIA GRAVIS
AUTOIMMUNE
↓Mg^{2+}
BONE 99%
ECF 0.1%
ICF 0.9%
10% BOUND TO ANIONS
50% FREE IONIZED
40% BOUND TO ALBUMIN
CALCULATE:
Ca^{2+} = 8 mg/dL +
ALBUMIN = 2.5 g/dL
CORRECTED Ca^{2+} = 9.2 mg/dL
CASR-REGULATED PTH RELEASE
4 6 8 10 12 mg/dL
SERUM Ca^{2+}
DISORDERS OF MAGNESIUM METABOLISM
↓Mg^{2+} CAN ↓PTH SECRETION OR CAUSE PTH RESISTANCE AND IS THEREFORE ASSOCIATED WITH NORMAL, ↓ OR ↑ PTH LEVELS
DRUGS
PHENYTOIN
CALCITONIN
BISPHOSPHATES
EDTA
FOSCARNET
*INFILTRATION OF THE PARATHYROID GLAND (GRANULOMATOUS, IRON OVERLOAD, METASTESES)

"Medicine is a science of uncertainty and an art of probability."

Dr. William Osler

HYPOCALCEMIA (Ca²⁺ > 8.8 mg/dL or 2.1 mmol/L)

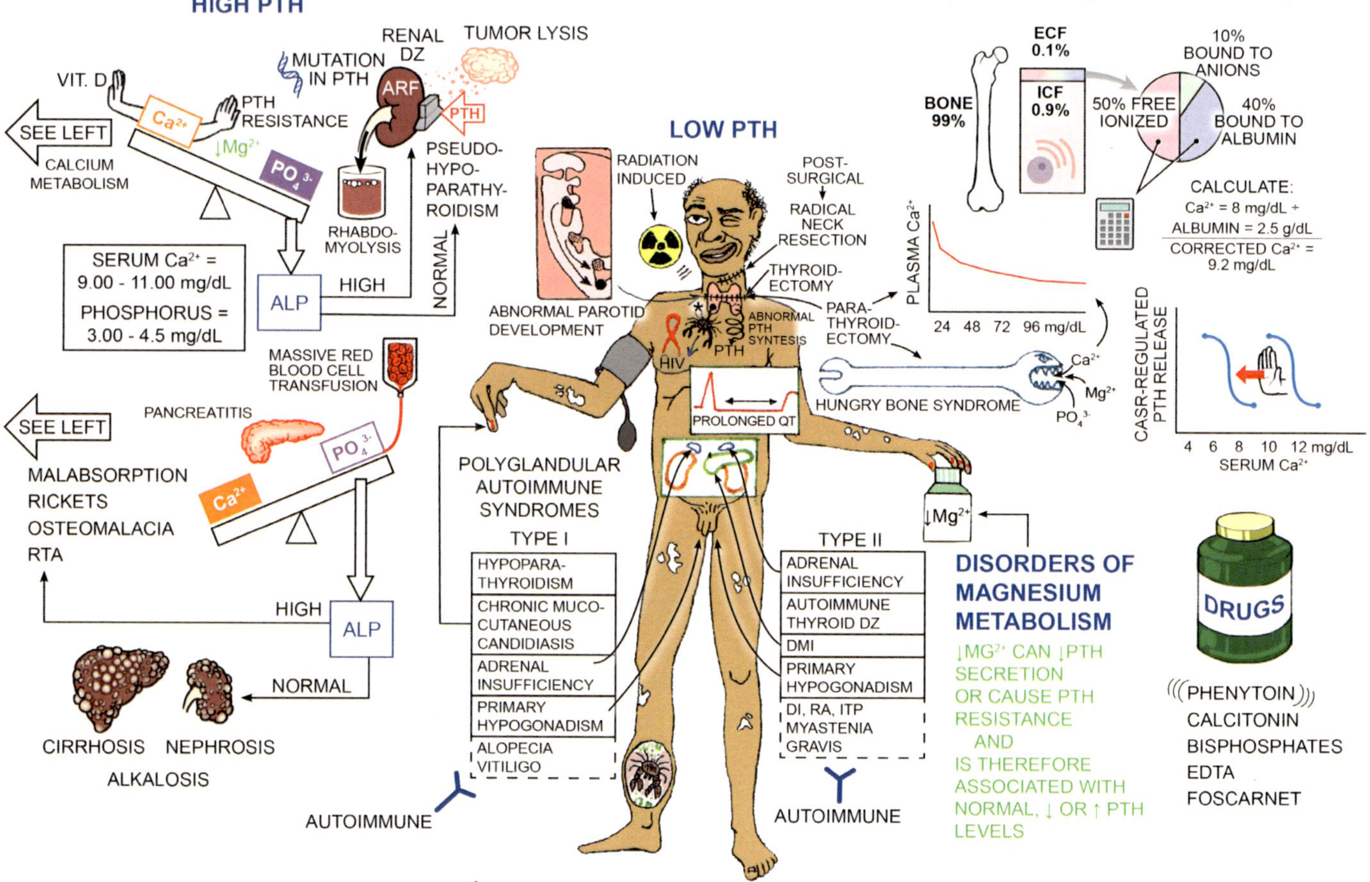

*INFILTRATION OF THE PARATHYROID GLAND (GRANULOMATOUS, IRON OVERLOAD, METASTESES)

"Learning never exhausts the mind."

Leonardo da Vinci

CALCIUM METABOLISM

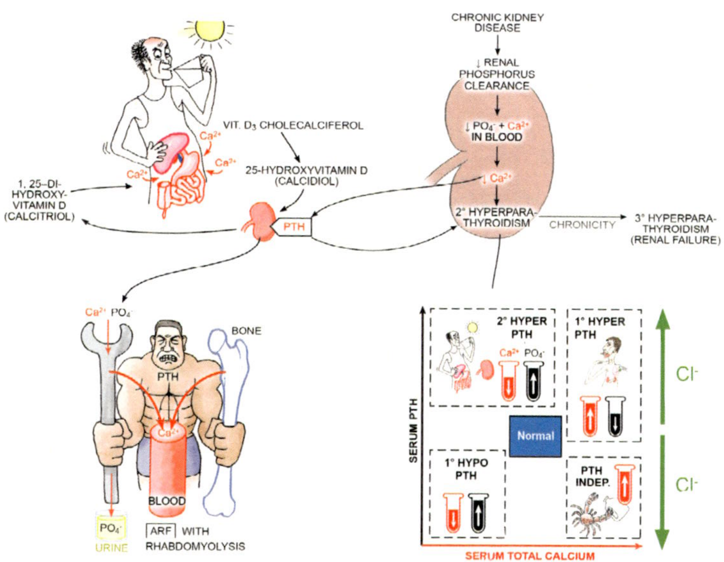

HYPOCALCEMIA (Ca^{2+} > 8.8 mg/dL or 2.1 mmol/L)

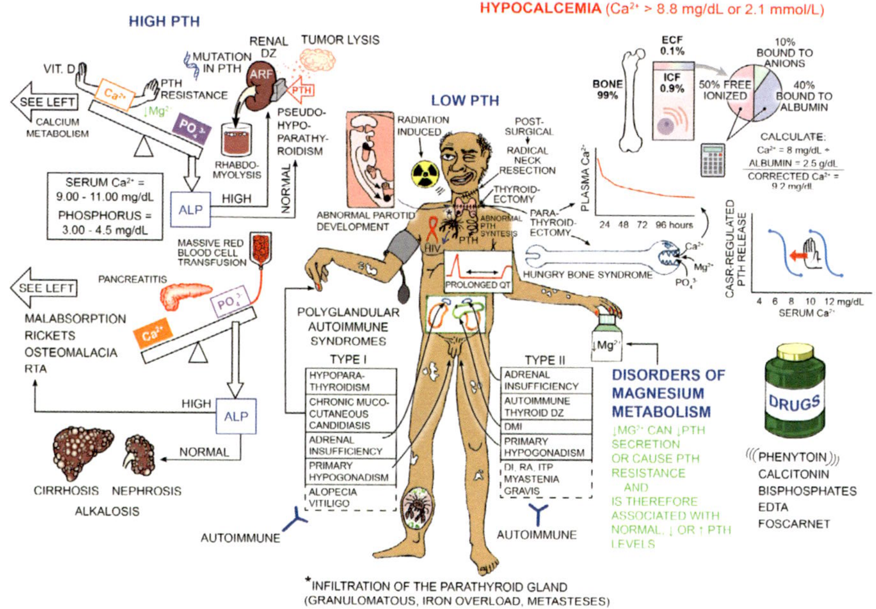

“Kindness in words creates confidence. Kindness in thinking creates profoundness. Kindness in giving creates love.”

Lao Tzu

HYPERCALCEMIA (Ca^{2+} > 10.5 mg/dL or 2.6 mmol/L)

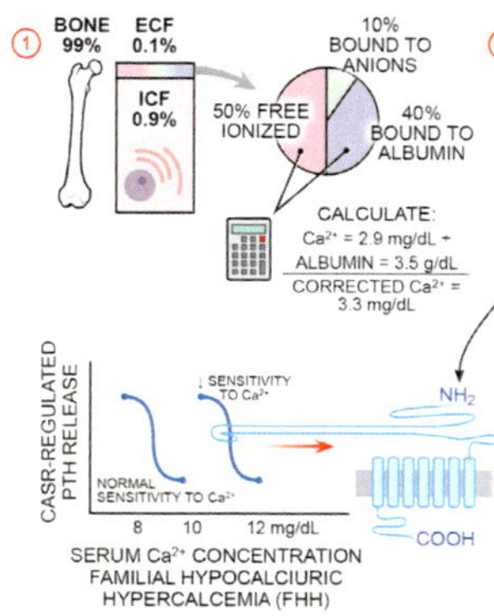

		1°	2°	3°
SERUM	Ca^{2+}	↑	N or ↓	↑
	PO_4^-	↓	↑	↑
	ALK. PHOS	↑ or N	↑ or N	↑ or N
URINE	Ca^{2+}	↑	↓	
	PO_4^-	↑	↓	

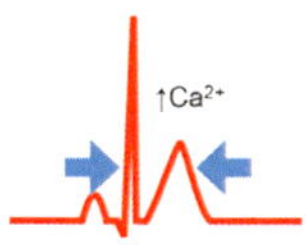

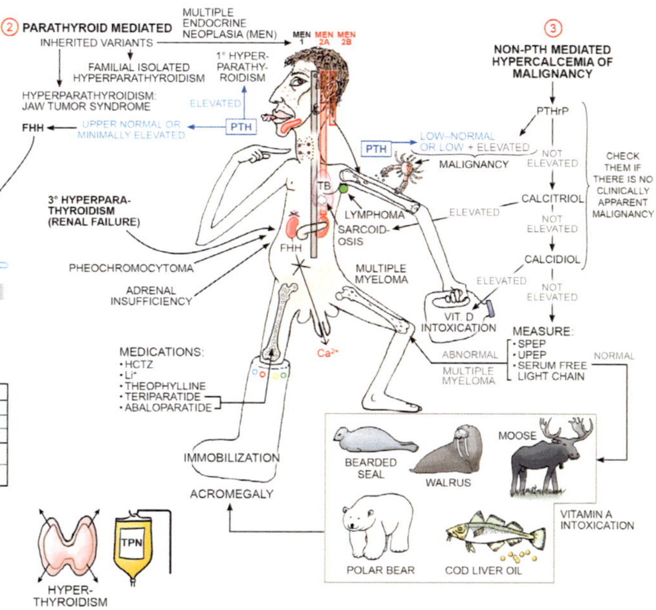

HYPOCALCEMIA (Ca^{2+} > 8.8 mg/dL or 2.1 mmol/L)

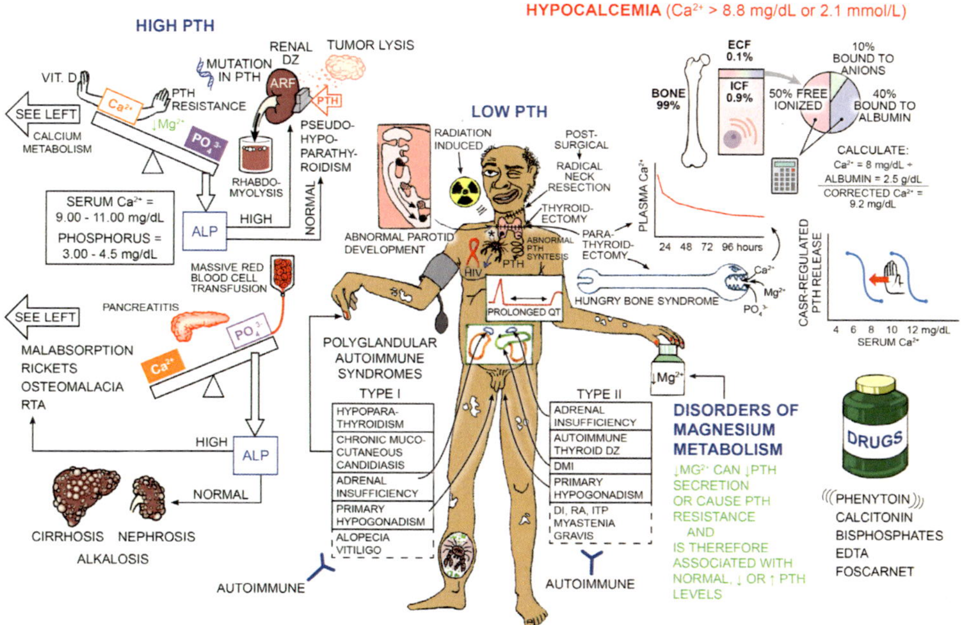

*INFILTRATION OF THE PARATHYROID GLAND (GRANULOMATOUS, IRON OVERLOAD, METASTESES)

HYPERMAGNESEMIA

The kidney is crucial in maintaining normal plasma magnesium concentration. Hypermagnesemia is an uncommon problem in the absence of **magnesium administration** or **kidney failure**. When it occurs, the elevation in the plasma magnesium concentration is usually mild (<3 mEq/L, 3.6 mg/dL, or 1.5 mmol/L) and the patient is asymptomatic. However, clinical symptoms may be seen when the plasma magnesium concentration exceeds 4 mEq/L (4.8 mg/dL or 2 mmol/L).

Hypermagnesemia can be seen in 10% to 15% of hospitalized patients, usually in the setting of **kidney failure** (illustrated in the picture as a hemodialysis machine).

Parenteral magnesium is commonly used to decrease neuromuscular excitability in pregnant women with severe preeclampsia or eclampsia. **Glutamate** is the most abundant **excitatory** neurotransmitter in the brain. One of the main neurological functions of magnesium is to **block** the calcium channel in the N-methyl-d-aspartate (NMDA) receptor. The NMDA receptor is part of a family of ionotropic **glutamate** receptors, alongside the α-amino-3-hydroxy-5-methyl-4-isoxazolepropionic acid receptor (AMPA) and kainate receptors.

Loss of deep tendon reflexes (DTR) is an early sign of hypermagnesemia and occurs at serum magnesium concentrations of 5 to 6 mEq/L. This loss of reflexes may be utilized in obstetrics to titrate magnesium sulfate infusions used in the treatment of preeclampsia.

Massive oral ingestion can occasionally exceed renal excretory capacity, particularly if there is underlying renal insufficiency. Such hypermagnesemia could happen with over-the-counter products, such as Epsom salts and laxatives, and during treatment of a variety of drug overdoses using magnesium as a cathartic.

Substantial quantities of magnesium can be absorbed from the large bowel following a **magnesium enema**. For Familial hypocalciuric hypercalcemia **(FHH)** see Hypercalcemia. For **Milk-Alkali syndrome** see Metabolic alkalosis.

Adrenal insufficiency leads to hypermagnesemia probably due to volume depletion and hemoconcentration. **Primary hyperparathyroidism** can cause increased calcium level in the blood, which can lead to increased excretion of magnesium in the urine, potentially leading to hypomagnesemia. Kidney impairment and elevated ketone levels (metabolic acidosis) in **DKA** can lead to hypermagnesemia. **Lithium therapy** causes hypermagnesemia by **decreasing urinary excretion**. (Sinusoidal line below lithium represents mood swing due to mania and depression.)

Tumor lysis syndrome is a hypercatabolic state, in which magnesium is released from the cells.

HELIX syndrome – Mild hypermagnesemia has been described as part of a familial syndrome associated with **hypohidrosis**, **electrolyte imbalance** (hypocalciuria and hypokalemic metabolic alkalosis), **lacrimal gland dysfunction** (crossed on the picture), and **xerostomia** (HELIX syndrome). It is caused by mutations in *CLDN10*, which encodes the tight junction protein, claudin-10, which likely functions as a paracellular sodium channel in the thick ascending limb of Henle.

HYPERMAGNESEMIA

KIDNEY IMPAIRMENT

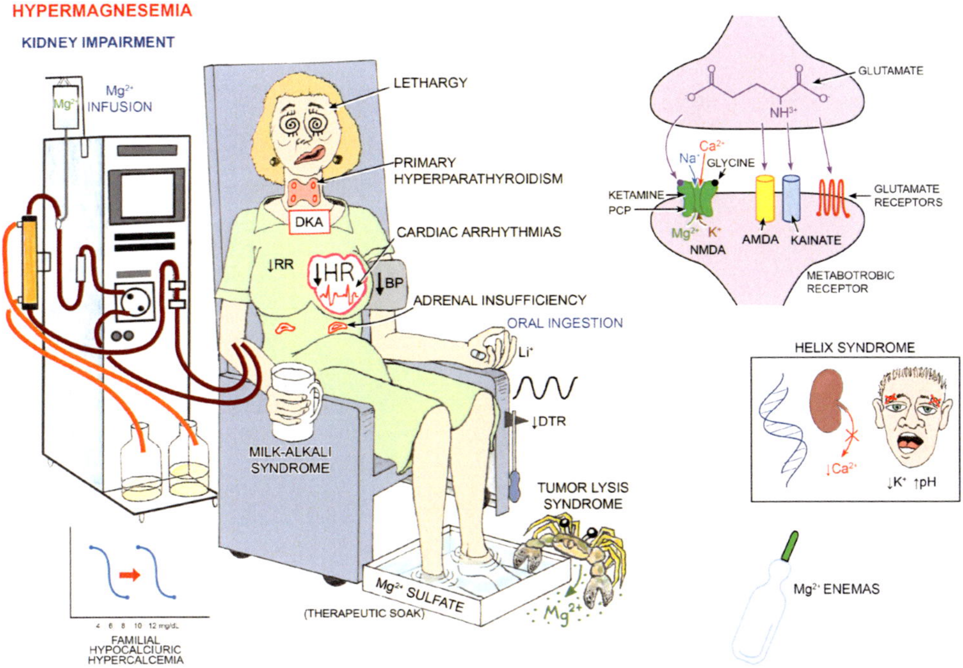

"Smooth seas do not make skillful sailors."

African proverb

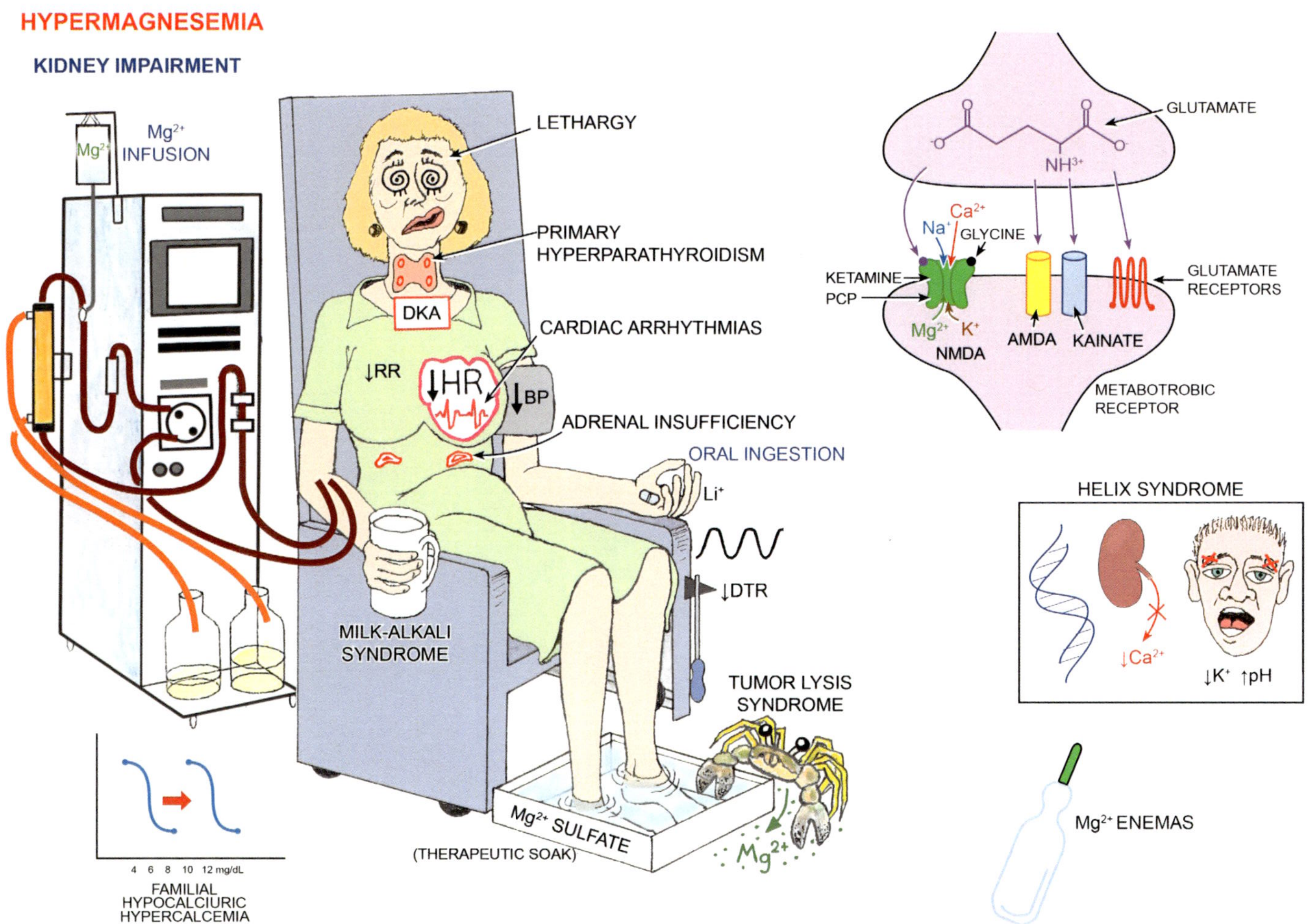

HYPERMAGNESEMIA
KIDNEY IMPAIRMENT
Mg2+ INFUSION
Mg2+
LETHARGY
PRIMARY HYPERPARATHYROIDISM
DKA
CARDIAC ARRHYTHMIAS
↓RR
↓HR
↓BP
ADRENAL INSUFFICIENCY
ORAL INGESTION
Li+
↓DTR
MILK-ALKALI SYNDROME
TUMOR LYSIS SYNDROME
Mg2+ SULFATE
(THERAPEUTIC SOAK)
Mg2+
4 6 8 10 12 mg/dL
FAMILIAL HYPOCALCIURIC HYPERCALCEMIA
GLUTAMATE
NH3+
Ca2+
Na+
GLYCINE
KETAMINE
PCP
Mg2+
K+
NMDA
AMDA
KAINATE
GLUTAMATE RECEPTORS
METABOTROBIC RECEPTOR
HELIX SYNDROME
↓Ca2+
↓K+ ↑pH
Mg2+ ENEMAS

HYPOMAGNESEMIA

Most of the body's magnesium stores are **intracellular**, principally within bone. In the extracellular fluid, magnesium can be ionized (free), bound to anions, or bound to protein.

The plasma magnesium concentration is not usually measured as part of routine blood tests. Thus, the identification of patients with hypomagnesemia often requires clinical suspicion in patients with risk factors for hypomagnesemia (e.g., **chronic diarrhea, proton pump inhibitor therapy, alcohol use disorder, diuretic use**) or with clinical manifestations of hypomagnesemia (e.g., **unexplained hypocalcemia, refractory hypokalemia, neuromuscular disturbances, ventricular arrhythmias**).

Magnesium deficiency may contribute to **sugar cravings**. This could be because magnesium plays a role in insulin secretion and glucose regulation in the body. **PPI** may interfere with magnesium absorption in the intestine, leading to hypomagnesemia.

When hypomagnesemia occurs, it is associated with **serious cardiac arrhythmias and aggravation of hypertension.** Magnesium influences blood vessel tone by relaxing smooth muscle cells in the arterial walls. When magnesium is deficient, blood vessels may constrict more easily, leading to increased blood pressure.

In acute pancreatitis, hypomagnesemia and hypocalcemia may occur alone or in combination, presumably due in part to **deposition of these cations in areas of fat necrosis.**

Hypomagnesemia with secondary hypocalcemia is a **genetic condition** due to the **TRPM6 gene** which is characterized by the body's inability to absorb and retain magnesium from the diet.

Restless leg syndrome (RLS) may be caused by a magnesium deficiency, and magnesium supplements can reduce RLS symptoms. Low levels of magnesium may cause **numbness and tingling**, especially in the legs and hands. Numbness may cause reduced sensation with propensity for injury. **Chronic diarrhea** (which can lead to magnesium loss) may contribute to both hypomagnesemia and steatorrhea.

Renal loss of magnesium can be caused by:

- Alcohol use disorder
- Uncontrolled diabetes
- Inherited kidney tubular disorders, such as Gitelman and Barter syndrome, East syndrome and Familial primary hypomagnesemia with hypercalciuria and nephrocalcinosis **(FHHNC)**
- Diuretic drugs (hydrochlorothiazide, chlorthalidone, furosemide, bumetanide)
- Antibiotics known to cause renal loss of magnesium including gentamicin, tobramycin, amikacin, plazomicin, streptomycin, neomycin, and paromomycin (**antibiotics** can also cause hypomagnesemia by causing antibiotic-related diarrhea)

Magnesium deficiency has been associated with a faster decline in the kidney function in people with CKD and those with diabetes.

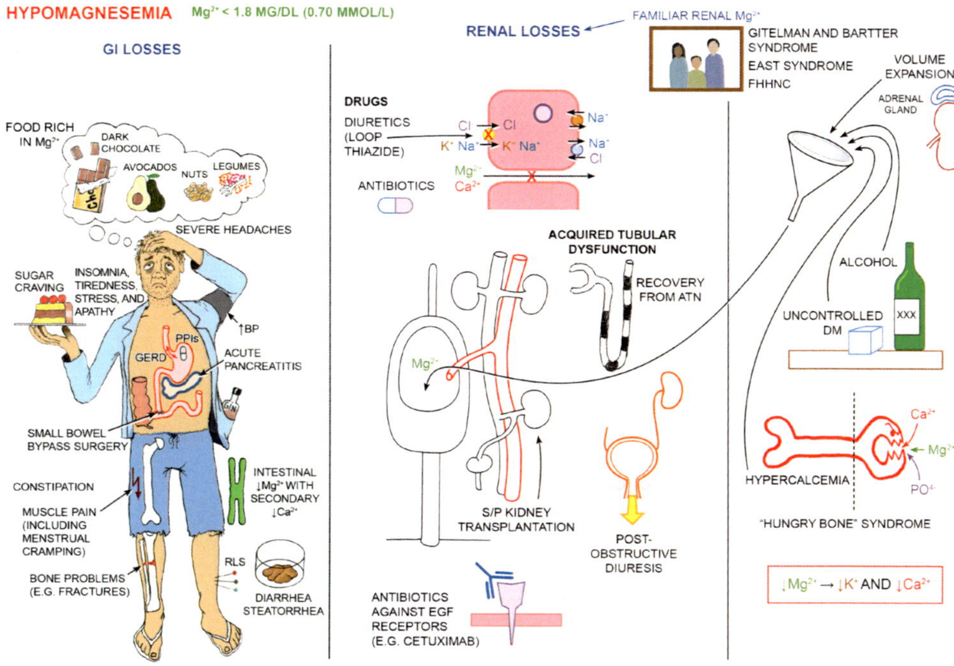

HYPOMAGNESEMIA
Mg2+ < 1.8 MG/DL (0.70 MMOL/L)
GI LOSSES
FOOD RICH IN Mg2+
DARK CHOCOLATE
AVOCADOS
NUTS
LEGUMES
SEVERE HEADACHES
SUGAR CRAVING
INSOMNIA, TIREDNESS, STRESS, AND APATHY
↑BP
PPIs
GERD
ACUTE PANCREATITIS
SMALL BOWEL BYPASS SURGERY
CONSTIPATION
MUSCLE PAIN (INCLUDING MENSTRUAL CRAMPING)
BONE PROBLEMS (E.G. FRACTURES)
INTESTINAL ↓Mg2+ WITH SECONDARY ↓Ca2+
RLS
DIARRHEA STEATORRHEA
RENAL LOSSES
FAMILIAR RENAL Mg2+
GITELMAN AND BARTTER SYNDROME
EAST SYNDROME
FHHNC
DRUGS
DIURETICS (LOOP THIAZIDE)
ANTIBIOTICS
Cl
K+ Na+
Na+
Mg2+
Ca2+
ACQUIRED TUBULAR DYSFUNCTION
RECOVERY FROM ATN
S/P KIDNEY TRANSPLANTATION
POST-OBSTRUCTIVE DIURESIS
ANTIBIOTICS AGAINST EGF RECEPTORS (E.G. CETUXIMAB)
VOLUME EXPANSION
ADRENAL GLAND
ALCOHOL
XXX
UNCONTROLLED DM
HYPERCALCEMIA
Ca2+
Mg2+
PO4-
"HUNGRY BONE" SYNDROME
↓Mg2+ → ↓K+ AND ↓Ca2+

"A small key opens the big doors."

Serbian proverb

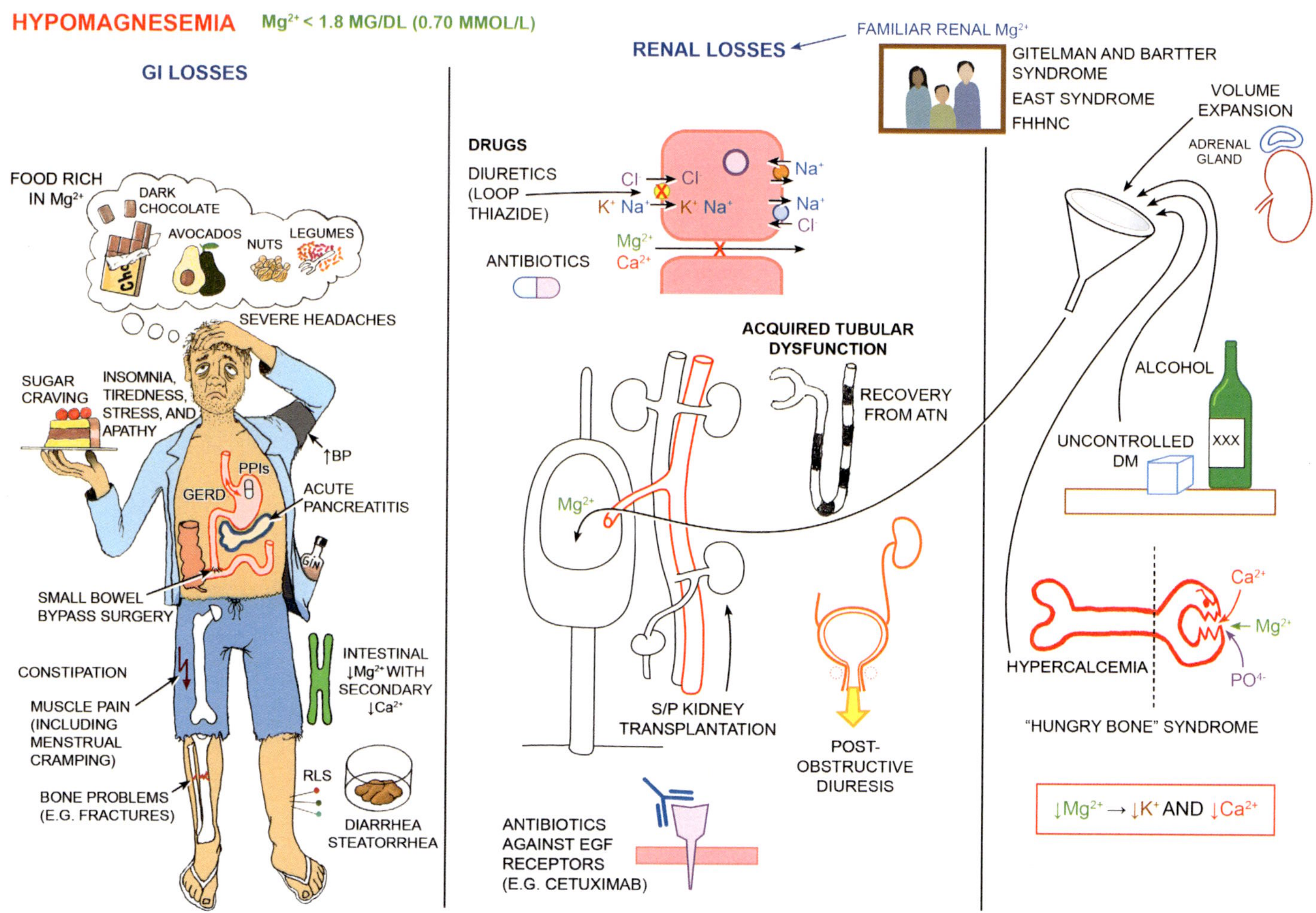

HYPOMAGNESEMIA
Mg2+ < 1.8 MG/DL (0.70 MMOL/L)
GI LOSSES
FOOD RICH IN Mg2+
DARK CHOCOLATE
AVOCADOS
NUTS
LEGUMES
SEVERE HEADACHES
SUGAR CRAVING
INSOMNIA, TIREDNESS, STRESS, AND APATHY
↑BP
PPIs
GERD
ACUTE PANCREATITIS
SMALL BOWEL BYPASS SURGERY
CONSTIPATION
MUSCLE PAIN (INCLUDING MENSTRUAL CRAMPING)
BONE PROBLEMS (E.G. FRACTURES)
INTESTINAL ↓Mg2+ WITH SECONDARY ↓Ca2+
RLS
DIARRHEA STEATORRHEA
RENAL LOSSES
FAMILIAR RENAL Mg2+
GITELMAN AND BARTTER SYNDROME
EAST SYNDROME
FHHNC
DRUGS
DIURETICS (LOOP THIAZIDE)
ANTIBIOTICS
Cl-
K+ Na+
Na+
Cl-
Mg2+
Ca2+
ACQUIRED TUBULAR DYSFUNCTION
RECOVERY FROM ATN
Mg2+
S/P KIDNEY TRANSPLANTATION
POST-OBSTRUCTIVE DIURESIS
ANTIBIOTICS AGAINST EGF RECEPTORS (E.G. CETUXIMAB)
VOLUME EXPANSION
ADRENAL GLAND
ALCOHOL
XXX
UNCONTROLLED DM
HYPERCALCEMIA
Ca2+
Mg2+
PO4-
"HUNGRY BONE" SYNDROME
↓Mg2+ → ↓K+ AND ↓Ca2+

HYPERPHOSPHATEMIA

The clinical presentation of hyperphosphatemia relates to hypocalcemia because phosphorus binds to calcium. The patient with hypocalcemia is shown with the **Chvostek** sign (abnormal twitching of muscles innervated by the facial nerve) and **Trousseau's** sign (a carpopedal spasm of the hand and wrist which occurs after an individual wears a blood pressure cuff inflated over their systolic blood pressure for 2 to 3 minutes).

Metastatic calcification is deposition of calcium salts in the presence of abnormal serum calcium and phosphorus levels. Calcium deposition occurs when the calcium phosphate product exceeds 70 mg/dL. These abnormal levels precipitate the calcium salts and resolve with correction of the calcium and phosphorus levels.

Pseudohyperphosphatemia is a laboratory artifact characterized by falsely elevated serum phosphate (mostly due to paraprotein interference on the conventional automated analyzer) in the absence of severely impaired renal function and clinical manifestation of hyperphosphatemia.

(Acute) phosphate nephropathy occurs after the ingestion of sodium-phosphate laxatives (solution or tablets) as bowel preparation for a colonoscopy. It causes acute renal failure and subsequent chronic renal failure.

In **respiratory acidosis** the increased H^+ ions can lead to **phosphate retention.**

In **metabolic acidosis**, the body produces excess non-carbonic acids (e.g., lactic acid, ketoacids) which can directly affect renal function, leading to **phosphate retention.**

Hypoparathyroidism, acromegaly, and **thyrotoxicosis** enhance **renal phosphate reabsorption** resulting in hyperphosphatemia.

Vitamin D increases intestinal phosphate and calcium absorption.

A **phosphate enema** may be used to relieve occasional constipation.

The 15th element in the periodic table, phosphorus, is one of the most important elements in the human body. It plays a crucial role in the biochemistry of all life. It's so reactive that it never exists in its free form. Adenosine triphosphate (ATP), a fundamental molecule in energy transfer, relies on phosphorus. It contains high-energy phosphoanhydride bonds.

A match head is made of phosphorus. [22]

---

22 Abbreviations: GI: gastrointestinal; PO4-: phosphorus; Ca2+: calcium; pO2: partial pressure of oxygen

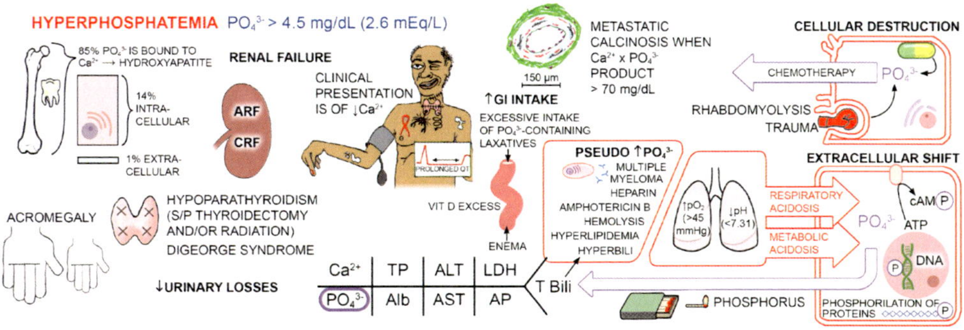

HYPERPHOSPHATEMIA PO_4^{3-} > 4.5 mg/dL (2.6 mEq/L)
85% PO_4^{3-} IS BOUND TO Ca^{2+} → HYDROXYAPATITE
14% INTRA-CELLULAR
1% EXTRA-CELLULAR
RENAL FAILURE
ARF
CRF
CLINICAL PRESENTATION IS OF ↓Ca^{2+}
PROLONGED QT
150 µm
METASTATIC CALCINOSIS WHEN Ca^{2+} x PO_4^{3-} PRODUCT > 70 mg/dL
↑GI INTAKE
EXCESSIVE INTAKE OF PO_4^{3-}-CONTAINING LAXATIVES
VIT D EXCESS
ENEMA
CELLULAR DESTRUCTION
CHEMOTHERAPY
PO_4^{3-}
RHABDOMYOLYSIS
TRAUMA
PSEUDO ↑PO_4^{3-}
MULTIPLE MYELOMA
HEPARIN
AMPHOTERICIN B
HEMOLYSIS
HYPERLIPIDEMIA
HYPERBILI
↑pO_2 (>45 mmHg)
↓pH (<7.31)
RESPIRATORY ACIDOSIS
METABOLIC ACIDOSIS
EXTRACELLULAR SHIFT
cAMP
ATP
PO_4^{3-}
DNA
PHOSPHORILATION OF PROTEINS
ACROMEGALY
HYPOPARATHYROIDISM (S/P THYROIDECTOMY AND/OR RADIATION)
DIGEORGE SYNDROME
↓URINARY LOSSES
Ca^{2+}
TP
ALT
LDH
PO_4^{3-}
Alb
AST
AP
T Bili
PHOSPHORUS

HYPOPHOSPHATEMIA

Inappropriately high phosphate excretion — Urinary 24-hour phosphate excretion **above** 100 mg/day or a fractional excretion of filtered phosphate (FEPO4) **above** 5% is indicative of **renal** phosphate wasting in patients with hypophosphatemia.

Phosphate excretion can be measured either from a 24-hour urine collection or by calculation of the fractional excretion of filtered phosphate (FEPO4) from a random urine specimen.

FEPO4 = [UPO4 x PCr x 100] ÷ [PPO4 x UCr]

where U and P refer to the urine and plasma concentrations of phosphate (PO4) and creatinine (Cr).

Inappropriately high phosphate excretion is usually due to **hyperparathyroidism**, increased activity of phosphatonins such as fibroblast **growth factor 23** (a hormone produced by osteoblasts/osteocytes in bone that acts on the kidney to regulate phosphate and vitamin D metabolism. A major consequence of persistently elevated serum FGF23 and the resulting phosphaturia is defective bone mineralization [osteomalacia], or **generalized proximal tubule dysfunction** [Fanconi syndrome]). All of these conditions reduce renal tubule phosphate absorption by diminishing the activity of the sodium-phosphate cotransporters. It could also be due to **vitamin D deficiency or resistance (**children with certain genetic mutations**), hereditary hypophosphatemic rickets, oncogenic osteomalacia, and acetazolamide, tenofovir, IV iron, chemotherapeutic agents. Hypomagnesemia** is often associated with **hypokalemia and hypocalcemia.** Hypocalcemia is a major stimulus for hypersecretion of PTH.

When insulin is secreted in response to **hypoglycemia**, it can cause the shift of phosphate from the extracellular fluid to the intracellular space, leading to a decrease in serum level phosphate.

A 24-hour urine phosphate excretion **less** than 100 mg or a FEPO4 **less** than 5% indicates appropriately low renal phosphate excretion, suggesting that the hypophosphatemia is caused by **internal redistribution** (e.g., **increased insulin secretion, particularly during refeeding syndrome** [when a malnourished person begins eating again]), **acute respiratory alkalosis,** (**hungry bone syndrome**) or **decreased intestinal absorption** (e.g., **inadequate intake,** shown as the anorexic women in the picture who stopped eating food rich in phosphorus), **chronic antacid therapy, steatorrhea and chronic diarrhea** (shown as a toilet behind the anorexic woman).

An **acute and severe deficiency of phosphate** in the blood can be **lethal** for several reasons, including respiratory failure, cardiac arrhythmias and heart failure, seizures, confusion and disorientation, and coma.

Hypophosphatemia from **respiratory alkalosis** can be attributed to an **intracellular shift of phosphate stores**. The hypophosphatemia rapidly improves without need for supplementation when hyperventilation resolves.

In diabetic keto acidosis (**DKA**)**,** net (urinary) loss of phosphate occurs because of a <u>transcellular shift</u>, <u>osmotic diuresis</u> and <u>reduced renal phosphate reabsorption</u> by the Na-Pi transporters in the renal proximal tubule (due to acidosis and hyperglycemia).

HYPOPHOSPHATEMIA $PO_4^{3-} < 2.5$ mg/dL (1.7 mEq/L)

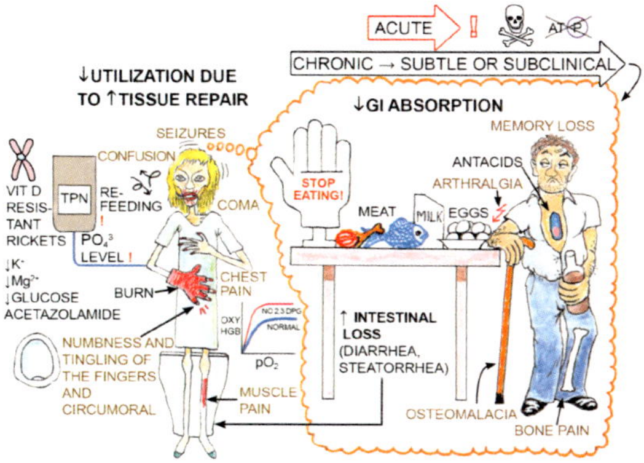

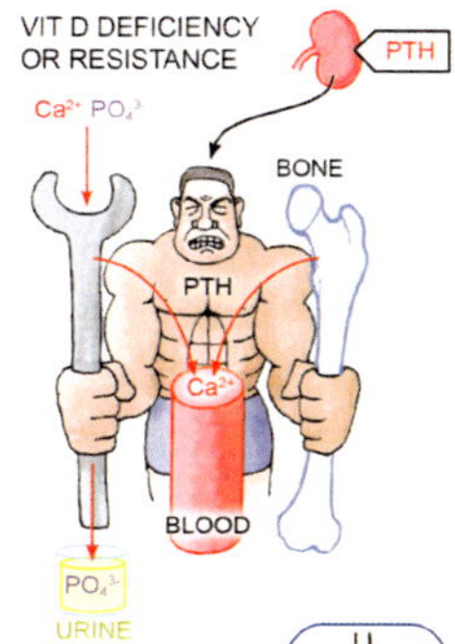

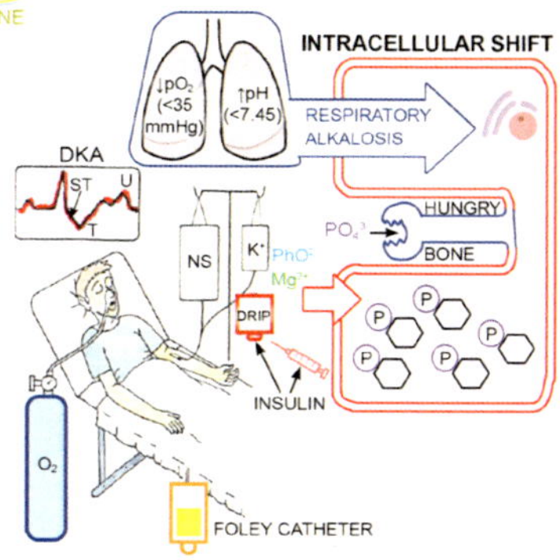

"A rising tide lifts all boats."

Folk saying

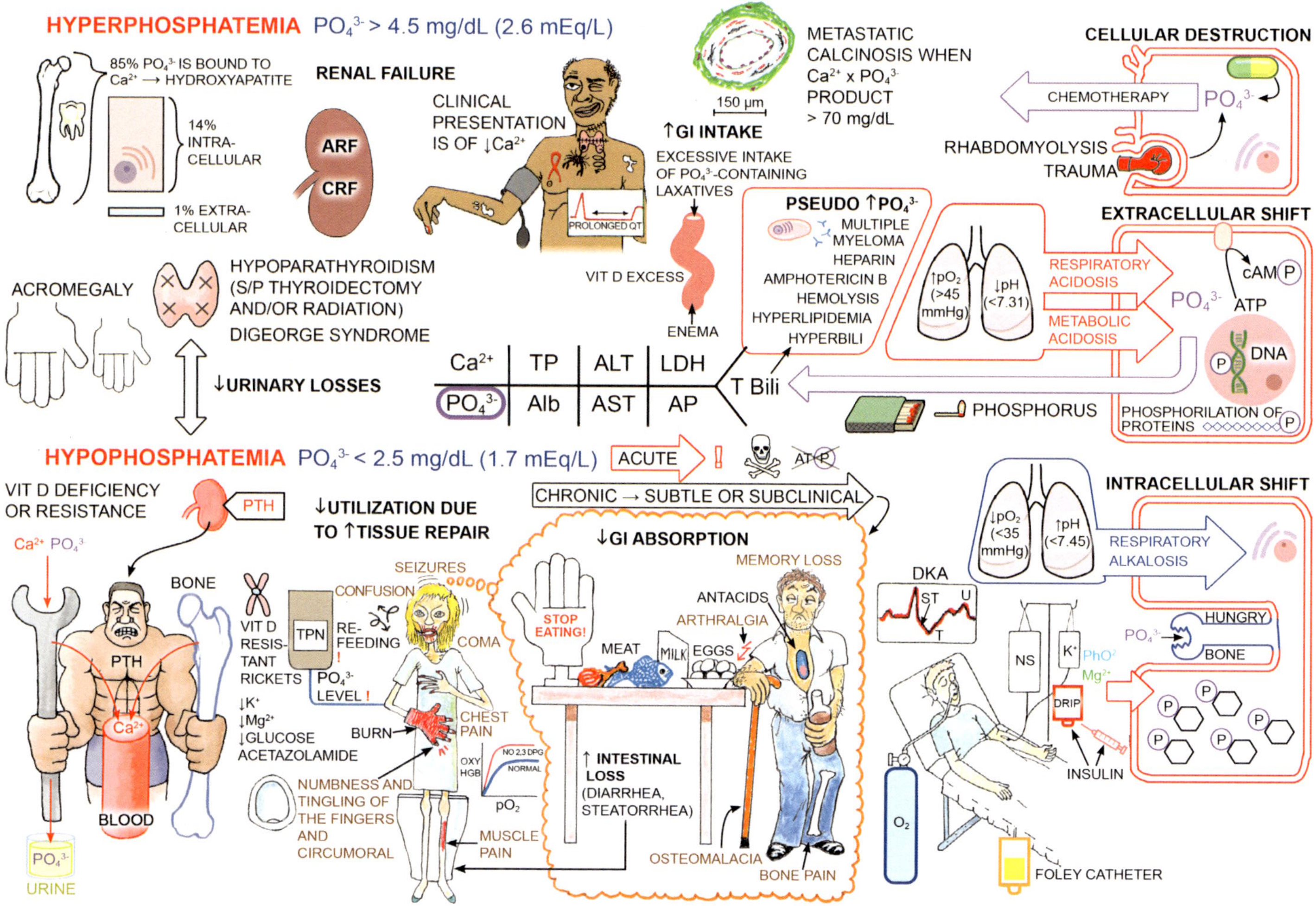

HYPERPHOSPHATEMIA PO4 3- > 4.5 mg/dL (2.6 mEq/L)
85% PO4 3- IS BOUND TO Ca2+ → HYDROXYAPATITE
14% INTRA-CELLULAR
1% EXTRA-CELLULAR
RENAL FAILURE
ARF
CRF
CLINICAL PRESENTATION IS OF ↓Ca2+
PROLONGED QT
↑GI INTAKE
EXCESSIVE INTAKE OF PO4 3- -CONTAINING LAXATIVES
VIT D EXCESS
ENEMA
150 μm
METASTATIC CALCINOSIS WHEN Ca2+ x PO4 3- PRODUCT > 70 mg/dL
CELLULAR DESTRUCTION
CHEMOTHERAPY
PO4 3-
RHABDOMYOLYSIS
TRAUMA
ACROMEGALY
HYPOPARATHYROIDISM (S/P THYROIDECTOMY AND/OR RADIATION)
DIGEORGE SYNDROME
↓URINARY LOSSES
PSEUDO ↑PO4 3-
MULTIPLE MYELOMA
HEPARIN
AMPHOTERICIN B
HEMOLYSIS
HYPERLIPIDEMIA
HYPERBILI
EXTRACELLULAR SHIFT
↑pO2 (>45 mmHg)
↓pH (<7.31)
RESPIRATORY ACIDOSIS
METABOLIC ACIDOSIS
PO4 3-
cAMP
ATP
DNA
PHOSPHORILATION OF PROTEINS
Ca2+ | TP | ALT | LDH
PO4 3- | Alb | AST | AP
T Bili
PHOSPHORUS
HYPOPHOSPHATEMIA PO4 3- < 2.5 mg/dL (1.7 mEq/L)
ACUTE
ATP
CHRONIC → SUBTLE OR SUBCLINICAL
VIT D DEFICIENCY OR RESISTANCE
PTH
Ca2+ PO4 3-
PTH
BONE
Ca2+
BLOOD
PO4 3-
URINE
↓UTILIZATION DUE TO ↑TISSUE REPAIR
VIT D RESISTANT RICKETS
↓K+
↓Mg2+
↓GLUCOSE
ACETAZOLAMIDE
TPN
RE-FEEDING !
PO4 3- LEVEL !
SEIZURES
CONFUSION
COMA
CHEST PAIN
BURN
NUMBNESS AND TINGLING OF THE FINGERS AND CIRCUMORAL
OXY HGB
NO 2,3 DPG
NORMAL
pO2
MUSCLE PAIN
↓GI ABSORPTION
STOP EATING!
MEAT
MILK
EGGS
ANTACIDS
ARTHRALGIA
MEMORY LOSS
↑ INTESTINAL LOSS (DIARRHEA, STEATORRHEA)
OSTEOMALACIA
BONE PAIN
INTRACELLULAR SHIFT
↓pO2 (<35 mmHg)
↑pH (<7.45)
RESPIRATORY ALKALOSIS
DKA
ST
U
T
NS
K+
PhO2
Mg2+
DRIP
INSULIN
O2
FOLEY CATHETER
HUNGRY
BONE
PO4 3-

"Drop by drop fills the pot."

Indian proverb

THYROID STIMULATING HORMONE (TSH)

1. HYPERTHYROIDISM
2. SUBCLINICAL HYPERTHYROIDISM
3. HYPOTHYROIDISM

HYPERTHYROIDISM

Serum TSH	Serum free T4	Serum T3	Assessment
Normal	Normal	Normal	Euthyroid
Normal hypothalamic-pituitary function			
Low	High (or normal)	High	Hyperthyroidism
	Normal	High	T3 toxicosis
	High	Normal	T4 toxicosis
Low	Normal	Normal	Subclinical hyperthyroidism
Abnormal hypothalamic-pituitary function			
Normal or high	High	High	TSH-mediated hyperthyroidism
Low	Normal	Low or normal	Euthyroid with nonthyroidal illness or hyperthyroidism in a critically ill patient. Consider hyperthyroidism in a critically ill patient when TSH is lower[#] and free T4 and T3 are higher than expected in nonthyroidal illness*.

Thyroid tests must be interpreted in conjunction with clinical presentation.

[#] In critically ill hyperthyroid patients, the TSH is typically very low (e.g., <0.01 mU/L). In contrast, detectable but subnormal TSH values (eg, 0.1 to 0.4 mU/L) are more consistent with nonthyroidal illness.

* Euthyroid patients with nonthyroidal illness may have low serum TSH and low-normal or low free thyroxine (T4); Triiodothyronine (T3) is usually low. Some patients with central hypothyroidism have low serum TSH and normal (but usually low-normal) or low free T4 and T3 concentrations.

For mnemonic purposes, the lobe on the left of the thyroid gland in the middle of the picture represents **hyperthyroidism with a normal or high radioiodine uptake**, while the right one **hyperthyroidism with a near absent radioiodine uptake** (subacute granulomatous [de Quervain's] thyroiditis, painless thyroiditis [silent thyroiditis], lymphocytic thyroiditis, postpartum thyroiditis, amiodarone induced hyperthyroidism, radiation thyroiditis, and palpation thyroiditis).

<u>Metastatic follicular thyroid cancer</u> is illustrated as a humerus because it can metastasize to be bone. **Amiodarone** has 37% iodine in itself and inhibits extrathyroidal conversion of T4 to T3 in all patients. **Intentional suppressive therapy** is a treatment approach for certain types of thyroid cancer, in which the patient is given a high dose of thyroid hormone replacement medication to suppress the production of TSH. This therapy is used to minimize the chances of the cancer returning after surgery. The goal is to keep the TSH levels low, which may help prevent the growth of any remaining cancer cells. In **factitious hyperthyroidism** (like in Munchausen syndrome) a person intentionally takes high doses of thyroid hormone medication to produce symptoms of hyperthyroidism or an overactive thyroid gland.

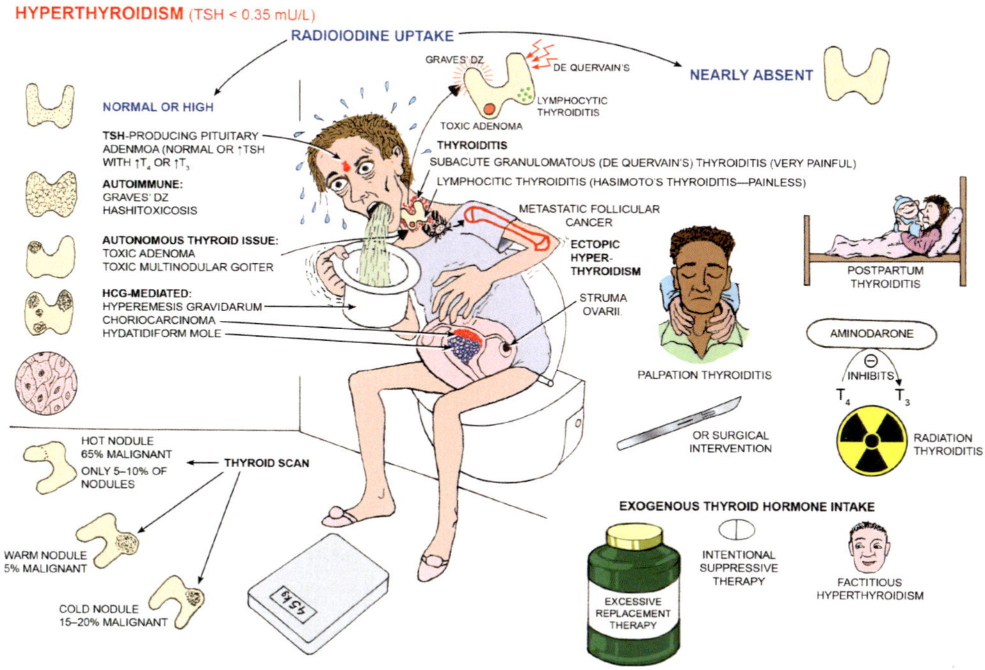

HYPERTHYROIDISM (TSH < 0.35 mU/L)
RADIOIODINE UPTAKE
NORMAL OR HIGH
TSH-PRODUCING PITUITARY ADENMOA (NORMAL OR ↑TSH WITH ↑T4 OR ↑T3
AUTOIMMUNE:
GRAVES' DZ
HASHITOXICOSIS
AUTONOMOUS THYROID ISSUE:
TOXIC ADENOMA
TOXIC MULTINODULAR GOITER
HCG-MEDIATED:
HYPEREMESIS GRAVIDARUM
CHORIOCARCINOMA
HYDATIDIFORM MOLE
GRAVES' DZ
DE QUERVAIN'S
LYMPHOCYTIC THYROIDITIS
TOXIC ADENOMA
NEARLY ABSENT
THYROIDITIS
SUBACUTE GRANULOMATOUS (DE QUERVAIN'S) THYROIDITIS (VERY PAINFUL)
LYMPHOCITIC THYROIDITIS (HASIMOTO'S THYROIDITIS—PAINLESS)
METASTATIC FOLLICULAR CANCER
ECTOPIC HYPER-THYROIDISM
STRUMA OVARII
POSTPARTUM THYROIDITIS
PALPATION THYROIDITIS
AMINODARONE
INHIBITS
T4
T3
OR SURGICAL INTERVENTION
RADIATION THYROIDITIS
HOT NODULE
65% MALIGNANT
ONLY 5–10% OF NODULES
THYROID SCAN
WARM NODULE
5% MALIGNANT
COLD NODULE
15–20% MALIGNANT
45 kg
EXOGENOUS THYROID HORMONE INTAKE
INTENTIONAL SUPPRESSIVE THERAPY
FACTITIOUS HYPERTHYROIDISM
EXCESSIVE REPLACEMENT THERAPY

"The darkest hour is just before dawn."

Serbian proverb

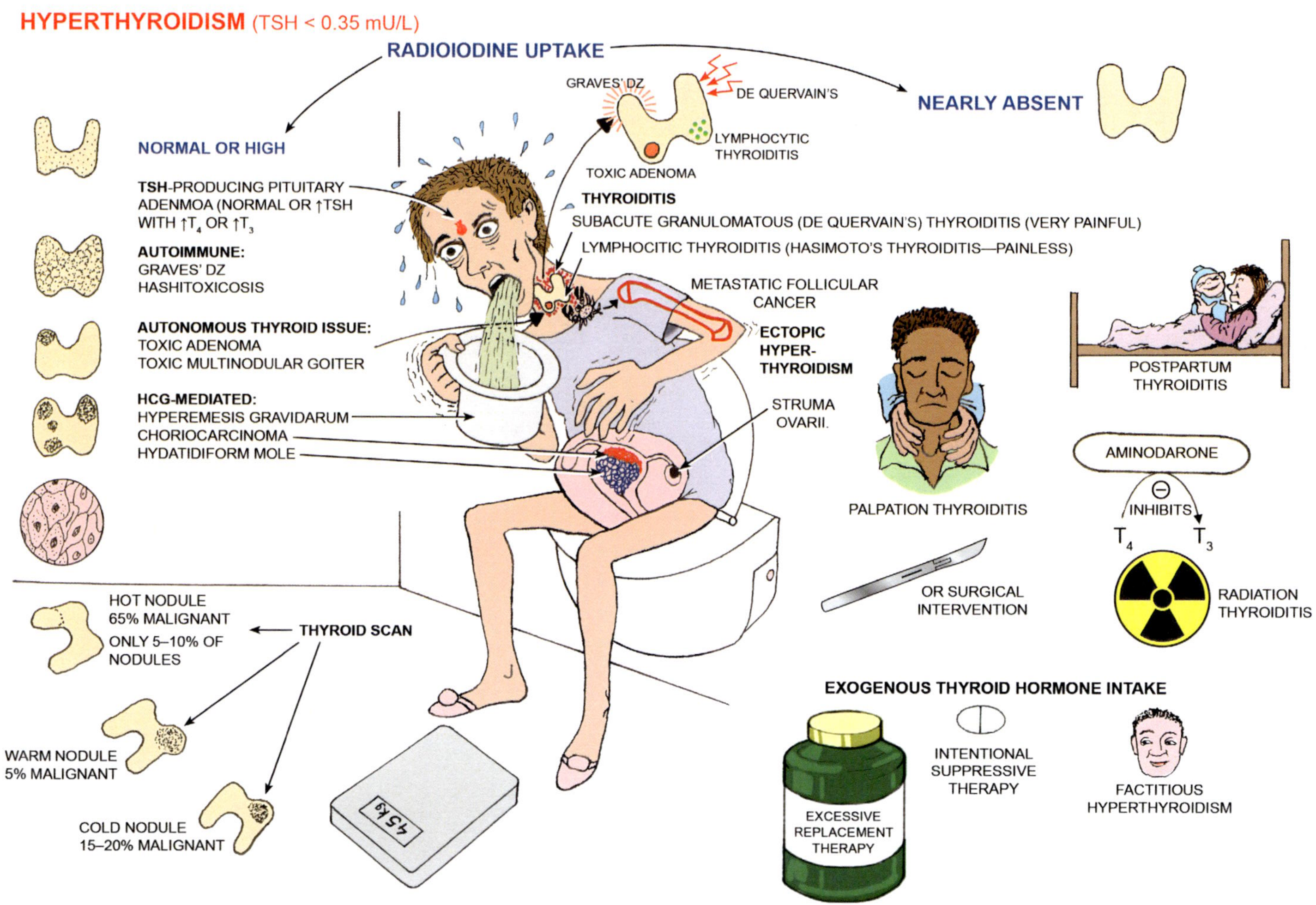
HYPERTHYROIDISM (TSH < 0.35 mU/L)
RADIOIODINE UPTAKE
NORMAL OR HIGH
NEARLY ABSENT
GRAVES' DZ
DE QUERVAIN'S
LYMPHOCYTIC THYROIDITIS
TOXIC ADENOMA
TSH-PRODUCING PITUITARY ADENMOA (NORMAL OR ↑TSH WITH ↑T4 OR ↑T3
AUTOIMMUNE:
GRAVES' DZ
HASHITOXICOSIS
AUTONOMOUS THYROID ISSUE:
TOXIC ADENOMA
TOXIC MULTINODULAR GOITER
HCG-MEDIATED:
HYPEREMESIS GRAVIDARUM
CHORIOCARCINOMA
HYDATIDIFORM MOLE
THYROIDITIS
SUBACUTE GRANULOMATOUS (DE QUERVAIN'S) THYROIDITIS (VERY PAINFUL)
LYMPHOCITIC THYROIDITIS (HASIMOTO'S THYROIDITIS—PAINLESS)
METASTATIC FOLLICULAR CANCER
ECTOPIC HYPER-THYROIDISM
STRUMA OVARII.
POSTPARTUM THYROIDITIS
PALPATION THYROIDITIS
OR SURGICAL INTERVENTION
AMINODARONE
INHIBITS
T4
T3
RADIATION THYROIDITIS
HOT NODULE
65% MALIGNANT
ONLY 5–10% OF NODULES
THYROID SCAN
WARM NODULE
5% MALIGNANT
COLD NODULE
15–20% MALIGNANT
45 kg
EXOGENOUS THYROID HORMONE INTAKE
EXCESSIVE REPLACEMENT THERAPY
INTENTIONAL SUPPRESSIVE THERAPY
FACTITIOUS HYPERTHYROIDISM

SUBCLINICAL HYPERTHYROIDISM

Subclinical hyperthyroidism is defined biochemically as **normal serum free thyroxine (T4) and triiodothyronine (T3)** concentrations in the presence of a **subnormal thyroid-stimulating hormone (TSH)** (<0.5 mU/L), confirmed on repeated measurement over a **three-** to **six-month** period. The term overt hyperthyroidism refers to patients with elevated levels of free T4, T3, or both and a subnormal TSH concentration. Both subclinical and overt hyperthyroidism are biochemical definitions since hyperthyroid symptoms are nonspecific and may be present in patients with subclinical disease and absent in those with overt disease, especially older adults.

Subclinical hyperthyroidism is a condition where the thyroid gland produces thyroid hormones, which are not detected as elevated, but which cause suppression of TSH. Such patients may not have any noticeable symptoms. This condition has been associated with an increased risk of cardiovascular disease, **especially in patients who already have cardiovascular risk factors**, and with an increased risk of osteoporosis, especially in **postmenopausal women**.

The excess thyroid hormone can cause tachycardia, atrial fibrillation, heart failure, pulmonary hypertension, and angina. Over time, this can also increase the risk of stroke. The excess thyroid hormone can increase the rate of bone catabolism, leading to osteoporosis and an increased risk of fractures. Therefore, it is important to treat subclinical hyperthyroidism in patients with cardiovascular risk factors and risk of osteoporosis.

In hyperthyroidism, **TSH < 0.1** mU/L should be treated. If **TSH < 0.5** mU/L **and fT4 is elevated**, it needs to be treated. If **TSH 0.1-0.5** mU/L it should be treated if the patient is older than 65 years, has low bone density, has cardiovascular disease, there are pronounced symptoms, or if there is no autonomous nodus seen on the scintigram (technetium 99-Tc99 thyroid scan. It is a question of treatment of subclinical hyperthyroidism: **TSH <0.5** mU/L **with normal fT4 and fT3**.

Not everyone needs to be treated, but it is necessary to determine the potential consequences and based on them, decide on individual therapy. The consequences of untreated subclinical hyperthyroidism might include:

- Progression in hyperthyroidism (the risk is 0.5-8% depending on the cause)
- Osteoporosis (thyroid hormones increase bone resorption, suppress bone formation, increase the risk of fracture [less in lumbar bone]). Bone density decreases especially in postmenopausal women, where menopause-decreased estrogen levels are a factor in reducing cortical-rich bones.
- Increased risk for atrial fibrillation, cardiac insufficiency, pulmonary hypertension and coronary disease
- There is a positive correlation between reduced TSH level and increased mortality
- Dementia
- Reduced quality of life

(Addendum for the picture of Subclinical Hypothyroidism: It should be noted that T4 substitution can contribute to changes in insulin resistance in people over 65 years of age. It can also increase the tendency for weight gain and disruption in a normal sleep cycle.

T4 substitution in people older than 65, with regular fT4 and elevated TSH of 5-9 is not required because there are no proven benefits and may increase the risk for atrial fibrillation and osteoporosis.)

T4 substitution in subclinical hypothyroidism is necessary if there is an elevated cardiovascular risk in conditions of elevated LDL and if there is a very pronounced clinical picture (e.g., fatigue).

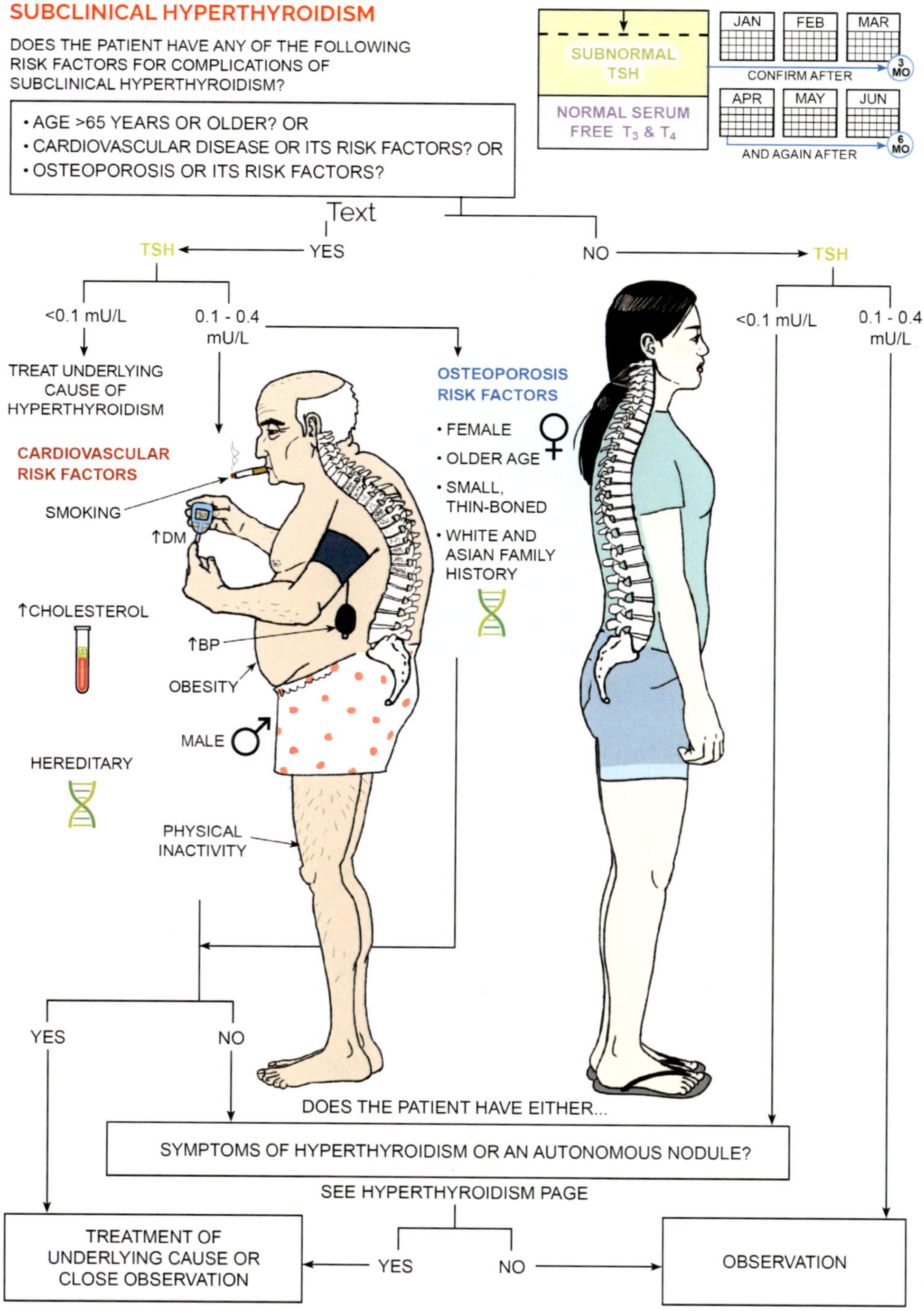
SUBCLINICAL HYPERTHYROIDISM
DOES THE PATIENT HAVE ANY OF THE FOLLOWING RISK FACTORS FOR COMPLICATIONS OF SUBCLINICAL HYPERTHYROIDISM?
• AGE >65 YEARS OR OLDER? OR
• CARDIOVASCULAR DISEASE OR ITS RISK FACTORS? OR
• OSTEOPOROSIS OR ITS RISK FACTORS?
SUBNORMAL TSH
NORMAL SERUM FREE T_3 & T_4
JAN
FEB
MAR
CONFIRM AFTER
3 MO
APR
MAY
JUN
AND AGAIN AFTER
6 MO
Text
YES
TSH
<0.1 mU/L
0.1 - 0.4 mU/L
TREAT UNDERLYING CAUSE OF HYPERTHYROIDISM
NO
TSH
<0.1 mU/L
0.1 - 0.4 mU/L
CARDIOVASCULAR RISK FACTORS
SMOKING
↑DM
↑CHOLESTEROL
↑BP
OBESITY
MALE
HEREDITARY
PHYSICAL INACTIVITY
OSTEOPOROSIS RISK FACTORS
• FEMALE
• OLDER AGE
• SMALL, THIN-BONED
• WHITE AND ASIAN FAMILY HISTORY
YES
NO
DOES THE PATIENT HAVE EITHER...
SYMPTOMS OF HYPERTHYROIDISM OR AN AUTONOMOUS NODULE?
SEE HYPERTHYROIDISM PAGE
YES
NO
TREATMENT OF UNDERLYING CAUSE OR CLOSE OBSERVATION
OBSERVATION

HYPOTHYROIDISM

TSH	T4	Interpretation
Normal	Normal	Normal thyroid function
Elevated	Low	Overt hypothyroidism
Normal/low	Low	Central hypothyroidism
Elevated	Normal	Subclinical hypothyroidism

Iodine is an essential element for the production of thyroid hormones. The thyroid gland uses iodine from the diet to produce hormones such as thyroxine (T4) and triiodothyronine (T3). In areas where there is insufficient iodine in the diet, the thyroid gland may become enlarged as it tries to compensate for the lack of iodine. However, most cases of hypothyroidism in the developed countries are caused by autoimmune disorders such as Hashimoto's thyroiditis.

Thyroid peroxidase (**TPO**), an enzyme normally found in the thyroid gland, plays an important role in the production of thyroid hormones. A **TPO** test detects antibodies against **TPO** in the blood. Anti-TPO antibodies are commonly found in individuals with autoimmune thyroid disorders such as Hashimoto's thyroiditis. Lymph nodes can also become enlarged in response to inflammation or infection in the thyroid gland or surrounding tissue.

In pregnancy, subclinical hypothyroidism is defined as a TSH **between 2.5 and 10 mIU/l** with a normal thyroxine level, while those with TSH above 10 mIU/l are considered to be overtly hypothyroid even if the thyroxine level is normal.

Importantly, TSH often oscillates, especially with Hashimoto thyroiditis, so TSH should be repeated after 3 months. If it is still greater than 7 mIU/l, therapy should be introduced. Most authors agree that TSH ≥ 9.0 is an indication for substitution therapy. When introducing Levothyroxine (LT4) of 50 mcg/day, a TSH follow-up should be done in 6 weeks. Eventual dose correction should be considered in **people >65 years**, satisfying TSH is up to 4.0 mIU/l. In **people under 65 years** of age, in most authors, the value of TSH of 7.0 mIU/l and above is an indication for treatment. (TSH should be repeated after 2-3 months.) The TSH of 7.0 mIU/l is a cutoff for the introduction of therapy except for a very pronounced clinical picture, like elevated LDL, menstrual cycle disorder, and if conception is planned. Then, the upper limit is 4.0 mIU/l with negative ATPO and Anti thyroglobulin antibody (ATG). If ATPO and ATG are positive, the limit of TSH is 2.5 mIU/l for people in preconception or for a history of recurrent, early abortions. Then Levothyroxine substitution should be started. **If the TSH is 2.5-4 mIU/l and the antibodies are negative, no substitute therapy is given.**

Resistance to TSH or thyroid hormone — An elevated TSH concentration may rarely be due to resistance to TSH secondary to alterations in the TSH receptor. Many of these patients are euthyroid, while others are hypothyroid. Serum-free T4 and triiodothyronine (T3) concentrations are typically normal or low. In some cases of resistance to thyroid hormone, the T3 and T4 values may be elevated (shown in the picture) or normal despite the patient experiencing symptoms of hypothyroidism or hyperthyroidism.

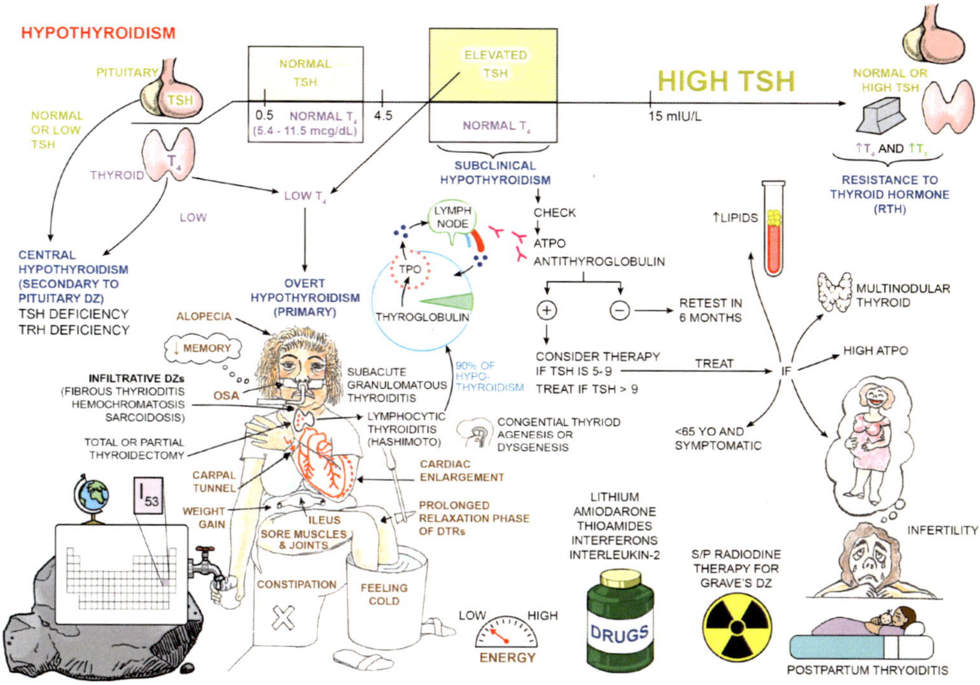
HYPOTHYROIDISM
PITUITARY
TSH
NORMAL OR LOW TSH
THYROID
LOW
CENTRAL HYPOTHYROIDISM (SECONDARY TO PITUITARY DZ)
TSH DEFICIENCY
TRH DEFICIENCY
NORMAL TSH
0.5
NORMAL T4 (5.4 - 11.5 mcg/dL)
4.5
ELEVATED TSH
NORMAL T4
SUBCLINICAL HYPOTHYROIDISM
HIGH TSH
15 mIU/L
NORMAL OR HIGH TSH
↑T4 AND ↑T3
RESISTANCE TO THYROID HORMONE (RTH)
LOW T4
OVERT HYPOTHYROIDISM (PRIMARY)
LYMPH NODE
TPO
THYROGLOBULIN
90% OF HYPO-THYROIDISM
CHECK
ATPO
ANTITHYROGLOBULIN
RETEST IN 6 MONTHS
CONSIDER THERAPY IF TSH IS 5-9
TREAT IF TSH > 9
TREAT
IF
↑LIPIDS
MULTINODULAR THYROID
HIGH ATPO
<65 YO AND SYMPTOMATIC
INFERTILITY
POSTPARTUM THRYOIDITIS
ALOPECIA
↓ MEMORY
OSA
INFILTRATIVE DZs
(FIBROUS THYRIODITIS
HEMOCHROMATOSIS
SARCOIDOSIS)
TOTAL OR PARTIAL THYROIDECTOMY
SUBACUTE GRANULOMATOUS THYROIDITIS
LYMPHOCYTIC THYROIDITIS (HASHIMOTO)
CONGENTIAL THYRIOD AGENESIS OR DYSGENESIS
CARDIAC ENLARGEMENT
CARPAL TUNNEL
WEIGHT GAIN
ILEUS
SORE MUSCLES & JOINTS
PROLONGED RELAXATION PHASE OF DTRs
CONSTIPATION
FEELING COLD
I 53
LOW
HIGH
ENERGY
LITHIUM
AMIODARONE
THIOAMIDES
INTERFERONS
INTERLEUKIN-2
DRUGS
S/P RADIODINE THERAPY FOR GRAVE'S DZ

“A still tongue makes a wise head.”

Folk saying

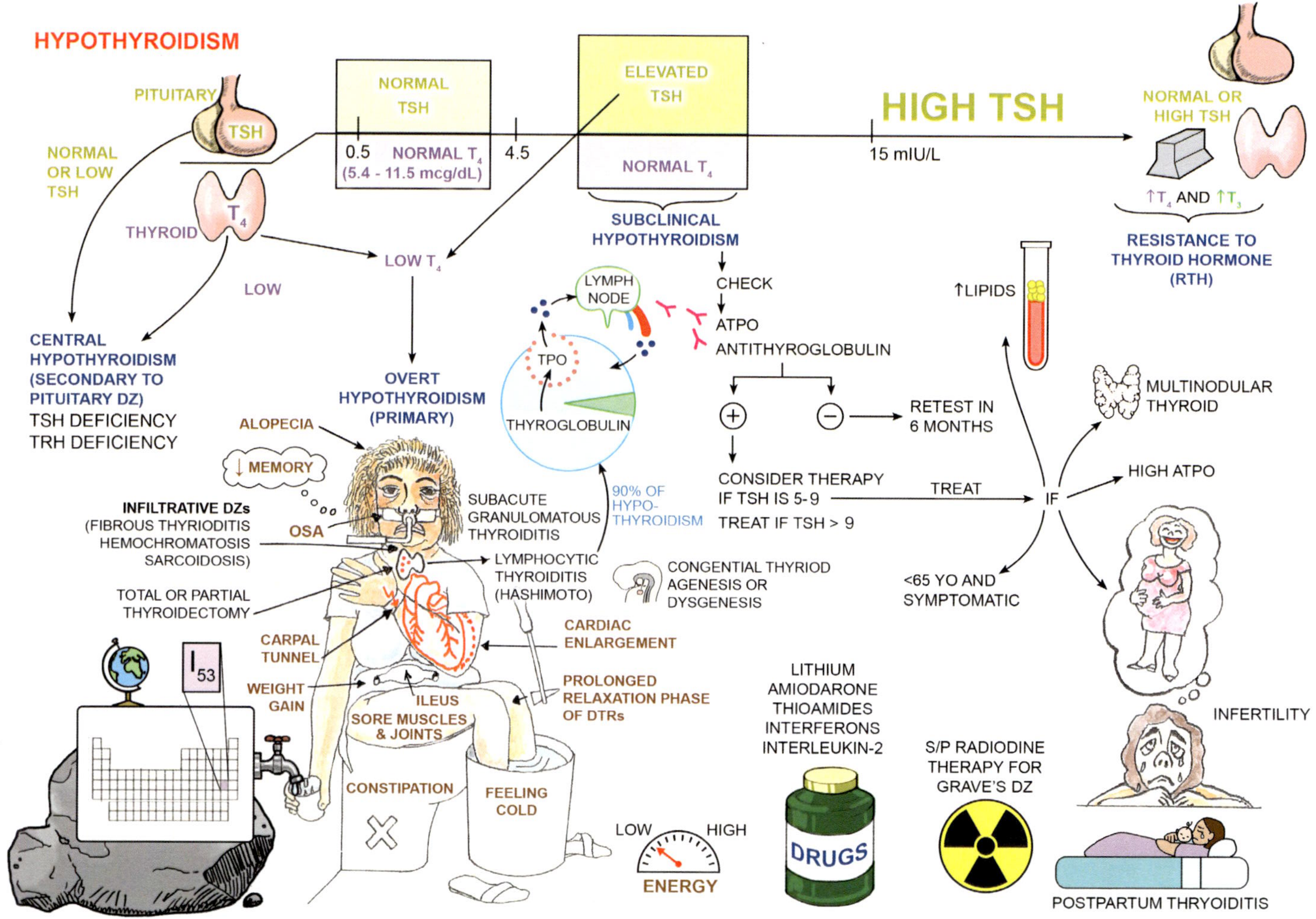
HYPOTHYROIDISM
PITUITARY
TSH
NORMAL OR LOW TSH
THYROID
T_4
LOW
CENTRAL HYPOTHYROIDISM (SECONDARY TO PITUITARY DZ)
TSH DEFICIENCY
TRH DEFICIENCY
NORMAL TSH
0.5
NORMAL T_4 (5.4 - 11.5 mcg/dL)
4.5
LOW T_4
OVERT HYPOTHYROIDISM (PRIMARY)
ELEVATED TSH
NORMAL T_4
SUBCLINICAL HYPOTHYROIDISM
HIGH TSH
15 mIU/L
NORMAL OR HIGH TSH
↑T_4 AND ↑T_3
RESISTANCE TO THYROID HORMONE (RTH)
CHECK
ATPO
ANTITHYROGLOBULIN
+
−
RETEST IN 6 MONTHS
CONSIDER THERAPY IF TSH IS 5-9
TREAT IF TSH > 9
TREAT
IF
↑LIPIDS
MULTINODULAR THYROID
HIGH ATPO
<65 YO AND SYMPTOMATIC
INFERTILITY
POSTPARTUM THRYOIDITIS
LYMPH NODE
TPO
THYROGLOBULIN
90% OF HYPO-THYROIDISM
ALOPECIA
↓ MEMORY
OSA
INFILTRATIVE DZs (FIBROUS THYROIDITIS HEMOCHROMATOSIS SARCOIDOSIS)
TOTAL OR PARTIAL THYROIDECTOMY
SUBACUTE GRANULOMATOUS THYROIDITIS
LYMPHOCYTIC THYROIDITIS (HASHIMOTO)
CONGENTIAL THYRIOD AGENESIS OR DYSGENESIS
CARPAL TUNNEL
WEIGHT GAIN
ILEUS
SORE MUSCLES & JOINTS
CARDIAC ENLARGEMENT
PROLONGED RELAXATION PHASE OF DTRs
CONSTIPATION
FEELING COLD
I_{53}
LOW
HIGH
ENERGY
LITHIUM
AMIODARONE
THIOAMIDES
INTERFERONS
INTERLEUKIN-2
DRUGS
S/P RADIODINE THERAPY FOR GRAVE'S DZ

"Carpe diem (Seize the day)."

Latin proverb

LAB TESTS CONT.

1. BLEEDING DISORDERS
2. BLEEDING DISORDERS CONT. WITH THROMBOCYTOPENIA
3. HYPERCOAGULABLE STATES
4. HYPERLIPIDEMIA
5. IRON METABOLISM (FE, TIBC, FERRITIN)
6. VITAMIN B12 (SEE LEUKOPENIA)

BLEEDING DISORDERS

There are three types of **PT/PTT abnormalities**:

1) **Increased PT/normal PTT** (Warfarin therapy, liver disease, Vit K deficiency, factor VII deficiency, early DIC)
2) **Increased PT/increased PTT** (Warfarin overdose, severe liver disease, severe Vit K deficiency, factors II, V or X deficiency, severe DIC)
3) **Normal PT/increased PTT** (antiphospholipid antibodies, coagulation factor deficiency, coagulation factor inhibitor)

The patient's necklace represents coagulation factors in the calculation cascade.

The skin lesions in the patient's right leg represent petechiae which result from blood vessel bleeding into the skin, the sign of widespread clothing in the early DIC.

The skin lesions in the patient's left leg represent purpura which is caused by bleeding under the skin in the severe DIC.

Vitamin K efficiency occurs due to low consumption or absorption or a metabolism issue. Since vitamin K is lipid soluble to the diseases affective lipid metabolism will reduce its level.

Broad-spectrum **antibiotic therapy** (illustrated in the picture as an antibiotic in the patient's rectum) potentially leads to intestinal microflora dysbiosis and restriction of vitamin K-producing bacterial populations, resulting in decreased vitamin K levels. (Cephalosporin antibiotics inhibit vitamin K function.)

Prothrombin time (PT) (the time taken for the plasma to clot after the tissue factory is added) measures the time for clothing through the extrinsic and common pathways. PT is used to monitor warfarin therapy.

Partial thromboplastin time (PTT) measures the time it takes for blood to clot through the increasing and common pathways. Elevated levels of PTT signify a missing or defective clothing factor. PTT is used to monitor heparin therapy. (Heparin increases the activity of antithrombin.) A **mixing study** is a laboratory test performed on blood plasma to distinguish between factor deficiencies and factor inhibitors.

The most common are:

1. **Lupus Anticoagulant (LA)**: This is a misnomer. Although it is called anticoagulant, it is associated with propensity for coagulation. Clots can form anywhere in the body, leading to serious complications like stroke, heart attack, and gangrene.
2. **Anticardiolipin Antibody (aCL)**: Often found together with the lupus anticoagulant but can also be detected alone. Its presence is associated with clotting risk.
3. Other antiphospholipid antibodies include **anti-beta 2 glycoprotein 1 (anti-ß2 GPI)**, **anti-prothrombin**, and the "false-positive" test for syphilis.

BLEEDING DISORDER

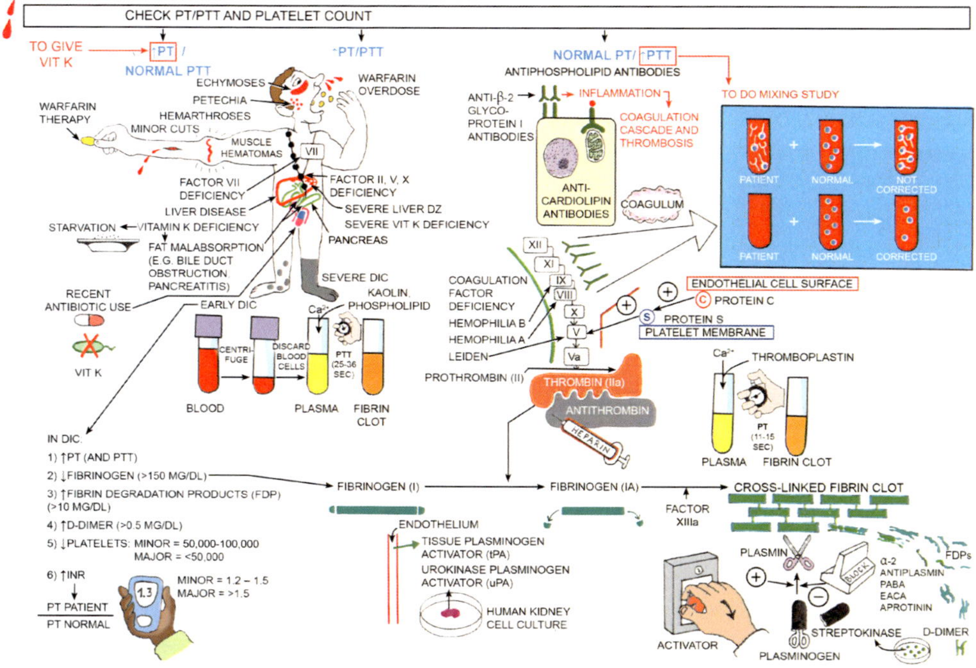

"There were so many things in life that we were afraid of,
but we shouldn't have, we should have lived."

Ivo Andric

BLEEDING DISORDER

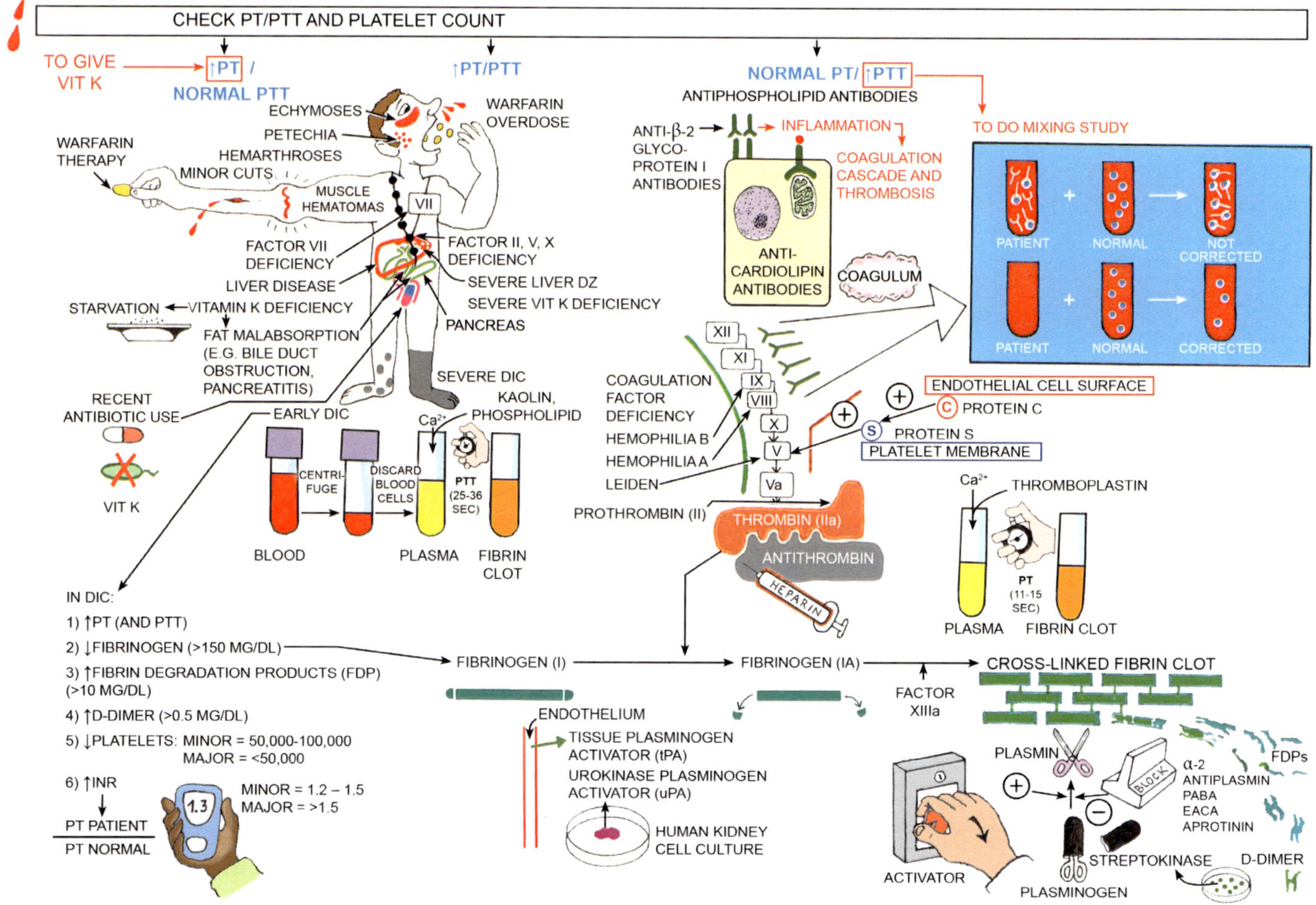

BLEEDING DISORDERS CONT. WITH THROMBOCYTOPENIA

If the platelet count and Prothrombin time/ Partial thromboplastin time (PT/PTT) are normal, the next step in the patient with a suspected bleeding disorder is to obtain a **bleeding time.** If the bleeding time is prolonged with the platelet count over 90,000 cells/µl, **platelet dysfunction** is implicated.

Acquired platelet dysfunction is usually systemic, due to **severe renal disease** (i.e., uremia), **severe liver disease**, **malignancy, and auto antibodies** (e.g., caused by β antibiotics, idiopathic thrombocytopenic purpura [ITP], **DIC, acquired storage pool disease, and aspirin**). The bleeding time may be prolonged with aspirin or NSAIDS but will only become abnormal if another underlying cause of platelet dysfunction is present.

Inherited platelet dysfunction disorders involve problems with **platelet adherence** (von Willebrand's disease [vWD]) and with **platelet aggregation (Bernard-Soulier syndrome,** due to loss in the platelet receptor for vWF glycoprotein Ib), **Glanzmann's thrombasthenia,** due to loss of the IIa-IIIb glycoprotein platelet receptor, which leads to decrease fibrinogen binding and therefore defective platelet aggregation, and **storage pool disease** (due to defective release of platelet granules, especially ADP, which results in decrease platelet aggregation).

See THROMBOCYTOPENIA for the right part of the picture. [23]

23 Abbreviations: GP Ib: **Glycoprotein Ib**, also known as **CD42**, is a component of the **GPIb-V-IX complex on platelets**. The GPIb-V-IX complex binds **von Willebrand factor**, allowing platelet adhesion and platelet plug formation at sites of vascular injury. GPIb functions as a receptor for von Willebrand factor (VWF); GP IIb/IIIa: a glycoprotein IIb/IIIa (GPIIb/IIIa, also known as integrin αIIbβ3) is an **integrin complex** found on platelets. It is a transmembrane receptor for **fibrinogen** and **von Willebrand factor,** and aids platelet activation*:* ADP: Adenosine Diphosphate.

BLEEDING DISORDERS CONT.

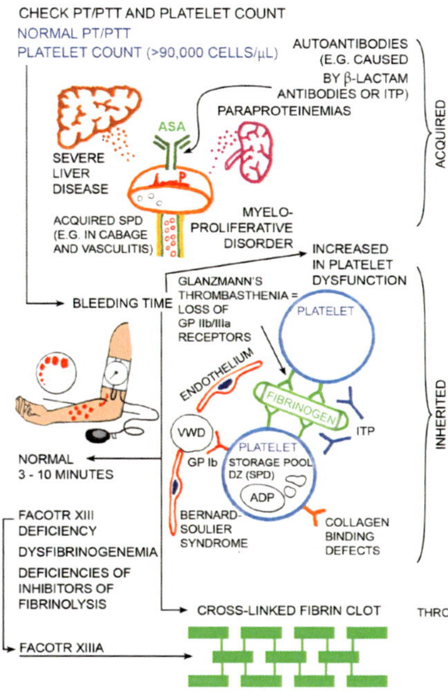

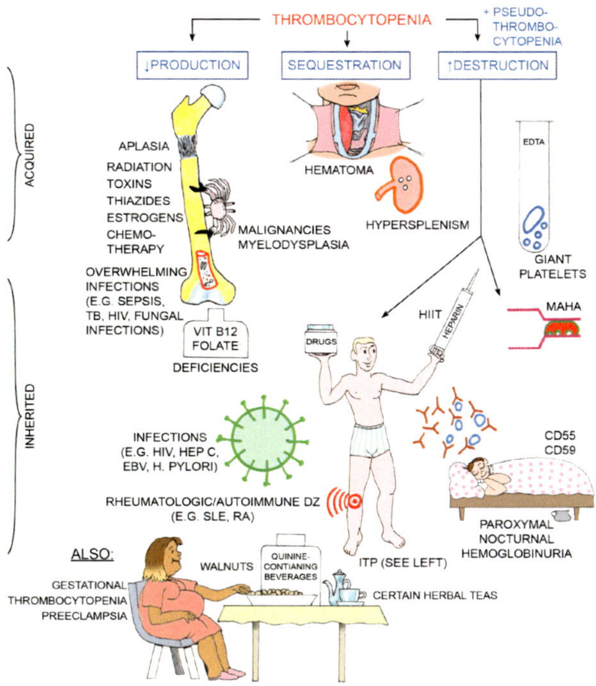

"It's strange how little people need to be happy, and it's even stranger how often they lack that little."

Ivo Andric

BLEEDING DISORDERS CONT.

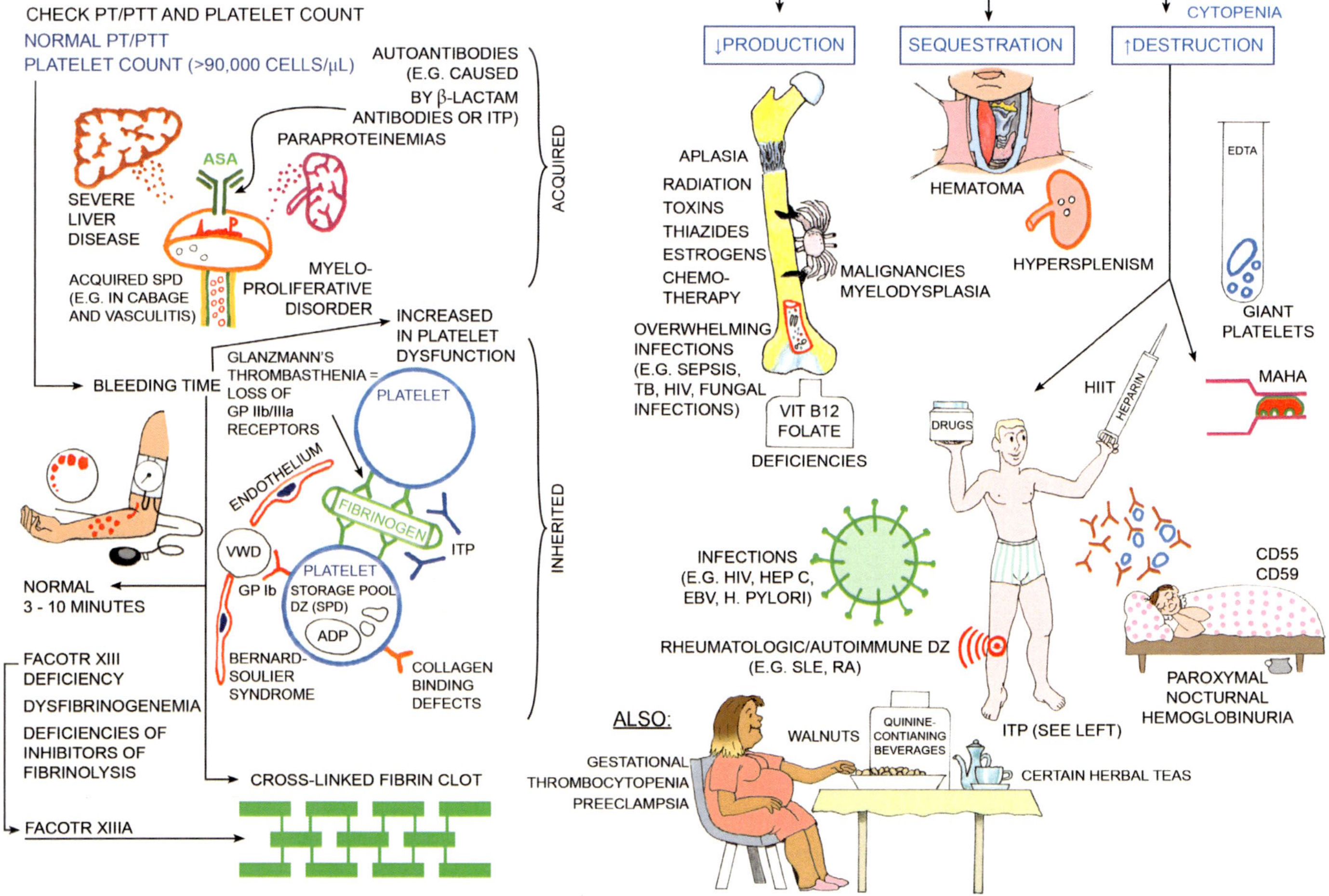

HYPERCOAGULABLE STATES

An inherited hypercoagulable state should be suspected in a patient who develops **thrombosis without predisposing factors** (which are shown in the right side of the picture), develops **multiple or recurring clots in unusual locations** (e.g., the upper extremities, mesenteric vessels, arteries, cerebral vein, renal vein thrombosis), and **thromboembolic disease at an early age**. Thrombophilia has been linked to recurrent **miscarriage**, and possibly various complications of pregnancy such as intrauterine growth restriction, stillbirth, severe pre-eclampsia and abruptio placentae.

When dealing with **hypercoagulable states**, it's essential to consider the appropriate anticoagulation therapy. The syringe near the patient on the left illustrates the fact that heparin and warfarin are generally not the best treatment options for treatment resistant or **recurrent thrombosis** (as well as patients with arterial thrombosis, thrombosis caused by cancer, microvascular thrombosis, and patients with a history of heparin-induced thrombocytopenia.

[HIT]). Patients with an underlying protein C deficiency who are placed on warfarin may be susceptible to the transient hypercoagulable state, leading to coumadin necrosis. Coumadin necrosis could be avoided by administering heparin along with warfarin.

Activated Protein C has demonstrated antithrombotic, anti-inflammatory, and profibrinolytic properties. Its antithrombotic activity is particularly important in microcirculation, and Protein C deficiency is associated with microvascular thrombosis.

When checking proteins C and S levels, serum should be drawn before warfarin therapy is initiated. Warfarin reduces protein C levels before those all-other vitamin K-dependent factors because protein C has the shortest half-life. Therefore, warfarin can lead to falsely low results or protein S assay.

Elevated homocysteine levels are associated with an increased risk for blood clots in the veins. Causes of elevated homocysteine levels in the blood include, low levels of thyroid hormone, kidney disease., psoriasis, some medicines (e.g., methotrexate, a disease-modifying antirheumatic drug (DMARD), cholesterol-lowering medication), and anticonvulsant medications.

Red dots on the patient's hands represent **rheumatoid arthritis** (RA).

In **nephrotic syndrome,** damage to the glomerular membrane results in increased filtration of small proteins such as antithrombin III, plasminogen, protein C, and protein S, and this in turn leads to increased coagulability.

Inflammatory Bowel Disease (IBD), Crohn's disease and **ulcerative colitis** promote **thrombosis**. The exact cause of this disequilibrium is multifactorial and not fully understood.

Heparin-induced thrombocytopenia (HIT) can occur in up to 5% of patients exposed to heparin products. HIT causes an extremely hypercoagulable state, where up to 50% of patients develop thromboembolic complications, associated with a mortality rate of up to 30%. **TTP** and **HUS** can cause thrombosis due to a deficiency in the activity of the ADAMTS13 enzyme, which normally breaks down the von Willebrand factor (vWF). In **PNH**, the absence of CD55 and CD59 leads to the complement system attacking and destroying erythrocytes (instead of foreign invaders such as bacteria), which releases microparticles that increase the risk of thrombosis.

HYPERCOAGULABLE STATES (THROMBOPHILIA)

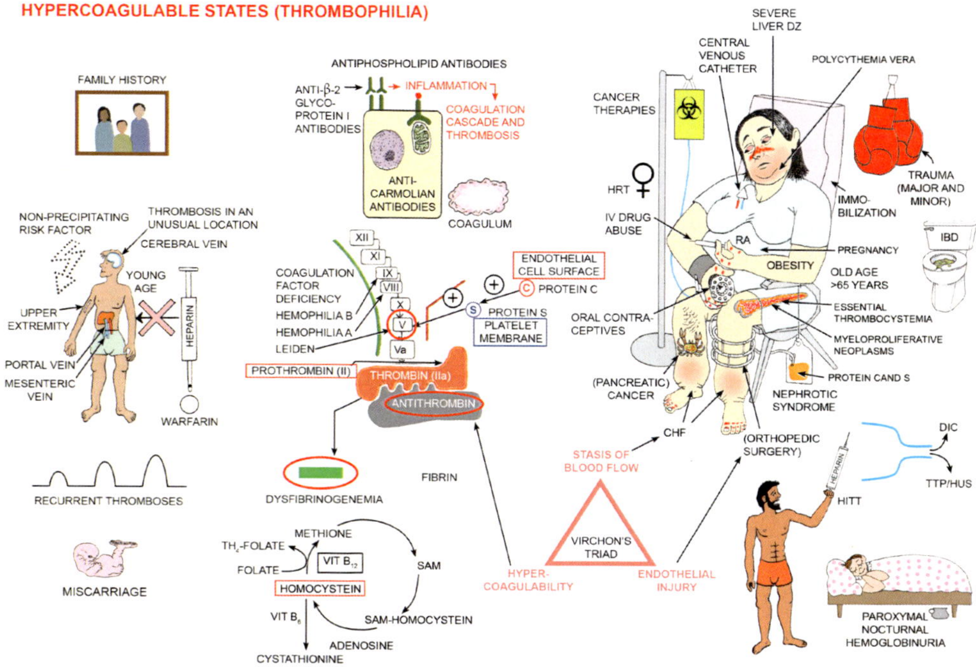

“The giving hand is above the receiving hand.”

African proverb

HYPERCOAGULABLE STATES (THROMBOPHILIA)

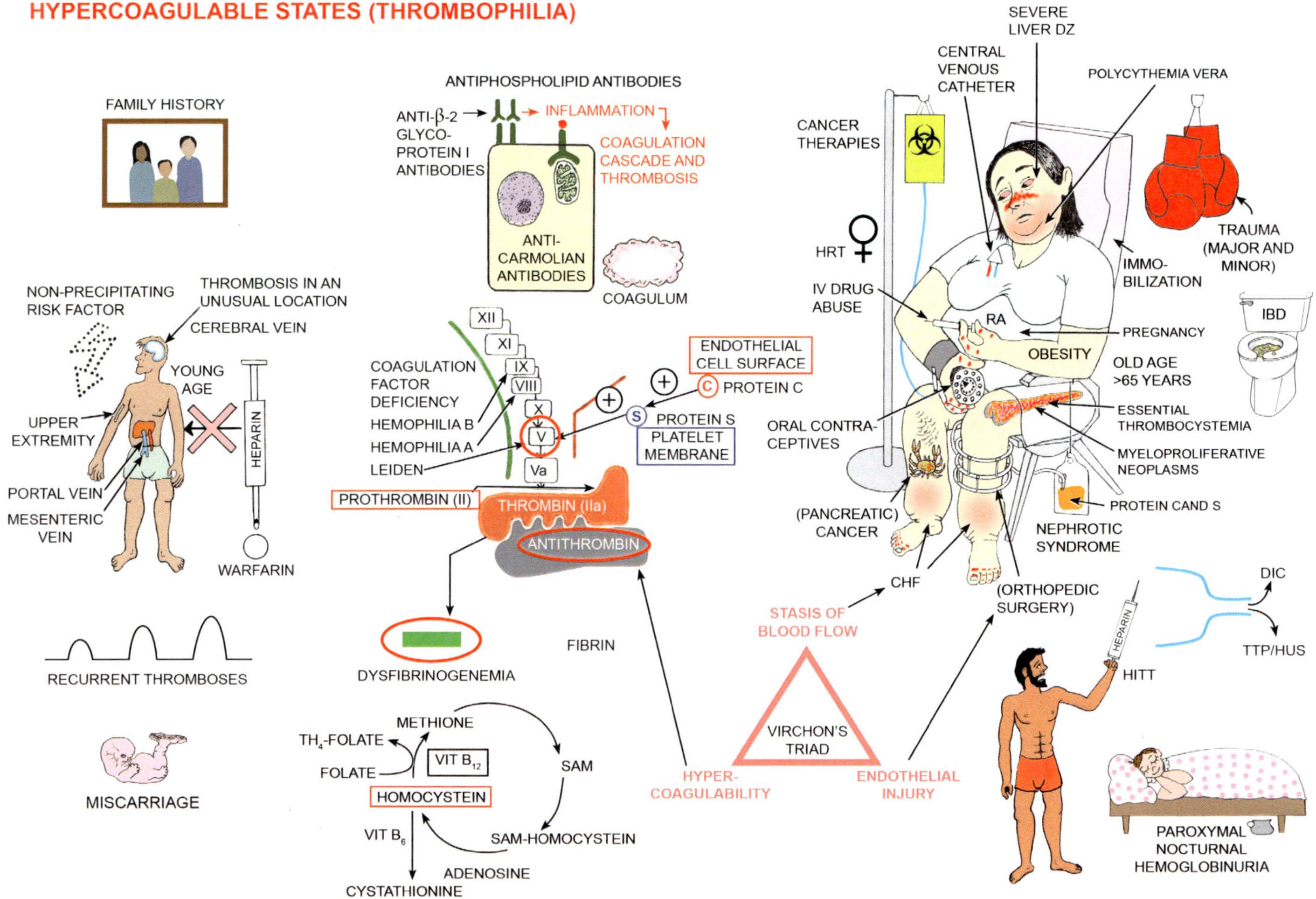

HYPERLIPIDEMIA

A test tube on the left shows a sample of hyperlipidemic blood. If left to settle for 4 hours without centrifugation, the lipids separate into the top fraction.

Hyperlipidemias could be classified as either familial (**primary**) when caused by specific genetic abnormalities (shown on the left side of the picture) or acquired (**secondary**) when resulting from another underlying disorder. Also, hyperlipidemia may be **idiopathic** (without a known cause).

Types of **Lipid abnormality**:

Type I **Elevated triglycerides (TG).** It presents in childhood with eruptive xanthomata and abdominal colic. Complications include retinal vein occlusion, acute pancreatitis, steatosis, organomegaly, and lipemia retinalis.

Type II is by far the most common form. (It occupies the left half of the circle). It is further classified into types IIa and IIb, depending on whether only LDL cholesterol is elevated (**Type IIa**), or whether elevation in the triglyceride level occurs in addition to LDL cholesterol (**Type IIb**).

Type III Elevated intermediate-density lipoprotein (**IDL**). It is also known as broad **beta disease** or **dysbetalipoproteinemia,** characterized by the early onset of cardiovascular disease and peripheral vascular disease.

Type IV Elevated **triglycerides** and **VLDL cholesterol.** (Pancreatitis usually does not occur in hyperlipidemic patients until their serum triglyceride level exceeds 1000 mg/dl.)

Type V Elevated **chylomicrons** and **VLDL cholesterol,** known as **mixed hyperlipoproteinemia familial** or **mixed hyperlipidemia.** (Almost 1 in 5 individuals who develop coronary heart disease before the age of 60 has this disorder).

Increased TG with **low albumin in the blood** and **increased protein in urine** are suggestive of **nephrotic syndrome.** The type of protein that is typically found in the urine in the **hepatic disease** is **albumin**. Unlike in hepatic disease, the type of proteins typically found in the urine of **nephrotic syndrome** is not limited to albumin, but could be also **globulins**.

If **increased TG is** coupled with **hyperglycemia**, DM is the most likely diagnosis. If **increased TG** is coupled with **hypoglycemia**, insulinoma or glycogen storage disease are possibilities.

Cigarette smoking modestly **lowers** the serum **HDL** cholesterol concentrations and HDL atheroprotective properties. (The "good" cholesterol HDL is like policemen, while the "bad" cholesterol LDL is like thieves. If there are a lot of thieves, a lot of policemen must be present. An elevated LDL is not a problem, as long as there is enough HDL to compensate for it. However, the problem happens if HDL is low.)

Excessive **alcohol** consumption **and ingestion of carbohydrates, especially concentrated (white flavor, sweets, potato, rice, pasta and fruits [all with glycemic index > 70])** can **raise triglyceride levels**.

Hypothyroidism reduces catabolism of lipids, leading to **an increase in LDL** and **triglycerides**. Polycystic ovary syndrome (**PCOS**) can lead to hyperlipidemia through hormonal imbalances and insulin resistance. Excessive **cortisol** in **Cushing syndrome** increases the production of lipids in the liver and causes **insulin resistance**.

Chronic renal failure decreases clearance of lipids from the bloodstream, alters lipid synthesis and metabolism and decreases expression of LDL receptors in the liver.

HYPERLIPIDEMIA

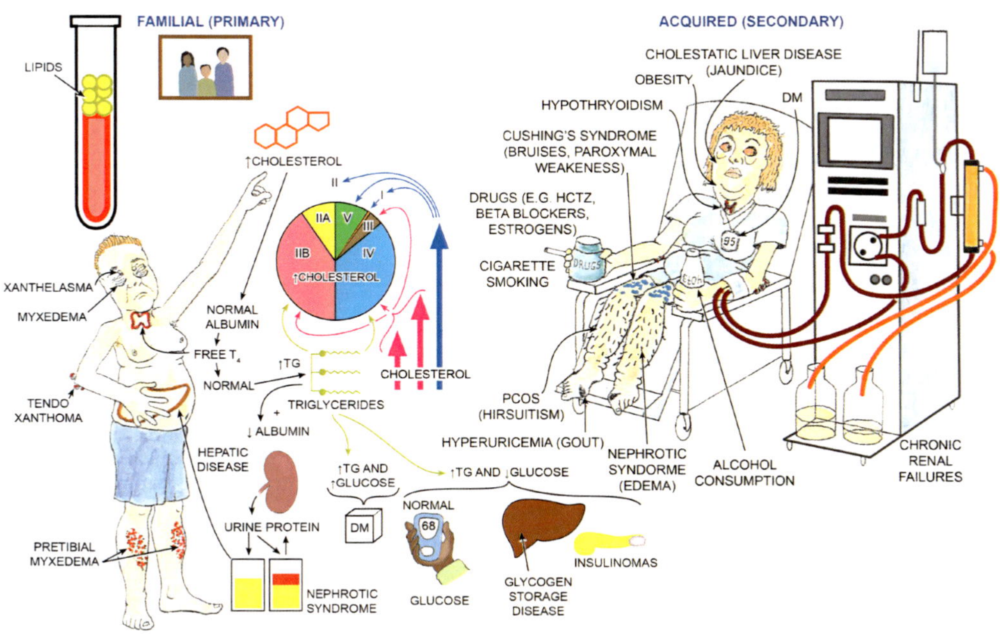

“Repetitio est mater studiorum. (Repetition is the matter of learning.)”

Latin proverb

HYPERLIPIDEMIA

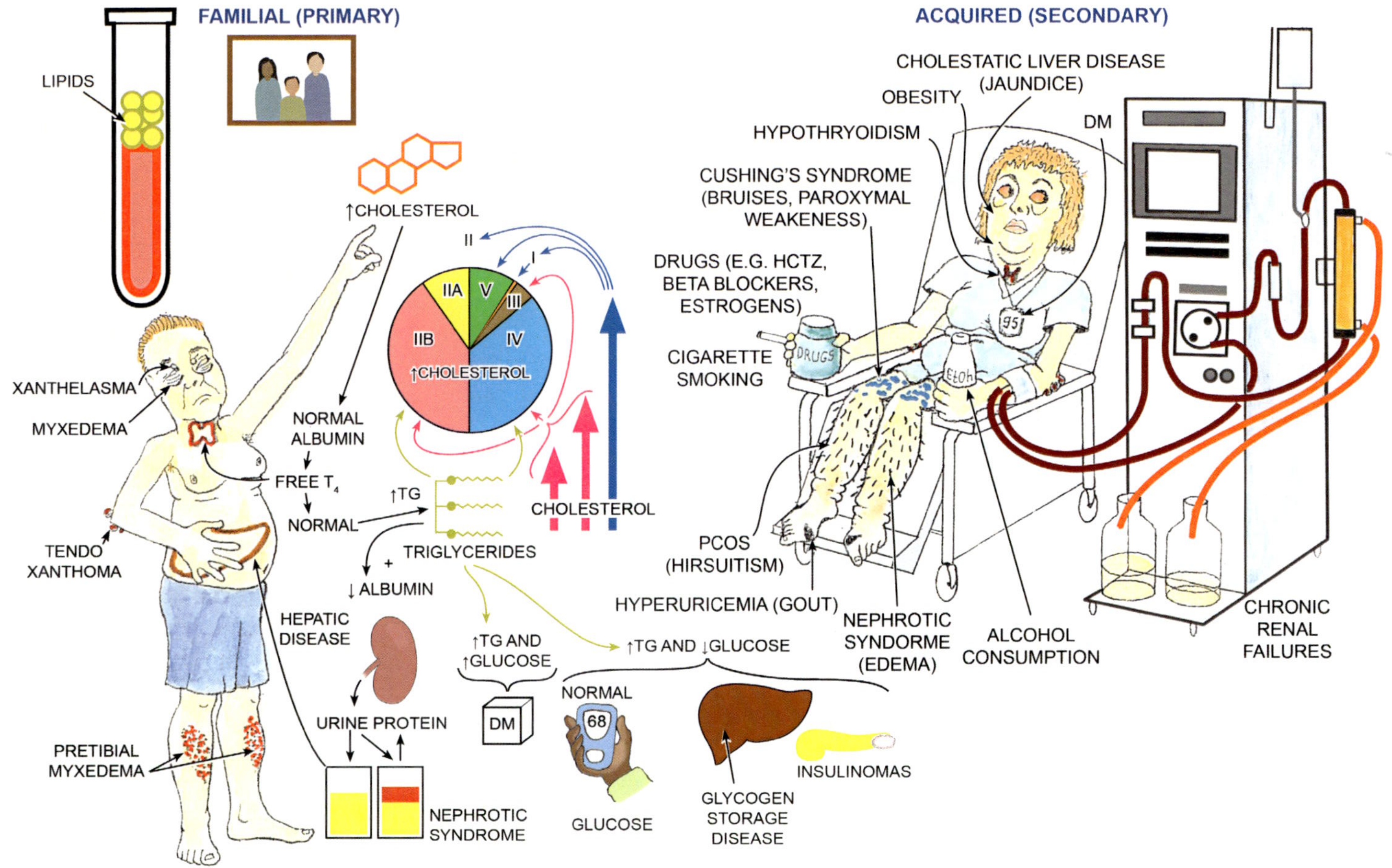

HIGH IRON

The magnet, which attracts iron, symbolizes increased iron in the body. The symptoms on the African American woman represent the consequences of increased iron in the body, while the diagnoses on the African American man represents the conditions which can lead to increased ferritin. (For example, metabolic syndrome is associated with insulin resistance which can lead to increased iron absorption in the body. Additionally, inflammation and oxidative stress, which are common in metabolic syndrome, can also lead to elevated ferritin levels.) Their beer drinking illustrates African iron overload (also called Bantu syndrome or **Bantu siderosis**) in which homemade beer contains excess iron leached from iron barrels. **Hemin** is an iron-containing medication used to treat certain porphyrias.

In response to inflammation or infection, the production of the cytokine **Interleukin-6 (IL6)** increases and stimulates the liver to produce more ferritin. This is because ferritin is an acute phase reactant, in response to inflammation to store excess iron and prevent it from being used by pathogens. Elevated serum ferritin levels may be a useful biomarker for detecting acute inflammation, although other factors, such as iron overload or liver disease, can also cause increased serum ferritin levels. If the patient is in the midst of an acute infection or inflammation, it may be prudent to delay iron studies testing until the acute event has resolved. A normal C-reactive protein (CRP) is inconsistent with inflammation or infection and in most cases eliminates these as an explanation for the increased ferritin.

A high **transferrin saturation (TSAT)** (≥45 percent in males or ≥40 percent in females) often occurs with iron overload. A TSAT below these levels is good evidence that the patient does not have iron overload, even if the ferritin is elevated.

The hormone **hepcidin** regulates the amount of iron absorbed from the diet by controlling iron export from cells that store it, such as macrophages and hepatocytes. It does this by binding to ferroportin, a protein that exports iron from these cells, and causing it to be degraded and removed. When hepcidin levels are high, less iron is released into the circulation from these cells, resulting in lower serum iron levels. On the other hand, when hepcidin levels are low, more iron is released into the circulation. The purpose of hepcidin's regulatory role is to maintain iron homeostasis in the body. This means that hepcidin helps to prevent iron overload, which can lead to tissue damage, as well as iron deficiency, which can result in anemia.

Ferritin is a protein that binds to iron inside cells and acts as a storage form of iron (particularly in the liver, spleen and bone marrow). When the body needs iron, ferritin releases the stored iron for use. **Transferrin** is a protein produced by the liver. Its primary role is to **bind to iron** and transport it throughout the body. It has two binding sites for iron. Transferrin levels can decrease during inflammatory processes. **TIBC** is a measurement of the **amount of iron** that can be bound by transferrin. While almost all of the iron in blood is bound to transferrin, there is a very small amount of free or unbound iron in the blood. This is because the body needs to maintain a delicate balance of iron, using it where it is needed and storing the excess. Free iron can be toxic to the body, so it is carefully regulated by proteins like transferrin.

However, under certain conditions, such as infections or inflammation, the amount of free iron in the blood may increase. This can be problematic as it can trigger the production of free radicals and cause oxidative stress. There are millions of transferring molecules in the blood. However, for the sake of simplicity, to illustrate the concept of TIBC, in this 1 dl of blood in the picture, there are only 12 of them. Four are saturated, while 8 and not. Therefore, one-third of transferrin is saturated in the healthy person. High TIBC levels may indicate **low iron levels** (iron deficiency) because more transferrin is available to bind iron. Conversely, low TIBC levels may suggest **excess iron** in the body.

IRON, FERRITIN, TIBC OVERLOAD

OVERLOAD → ↑SERUM FERRITIN (>200-300 MG/L IN MALE OR >150-200MG/L IN FEMALE)
↑TSAT (≥45%)

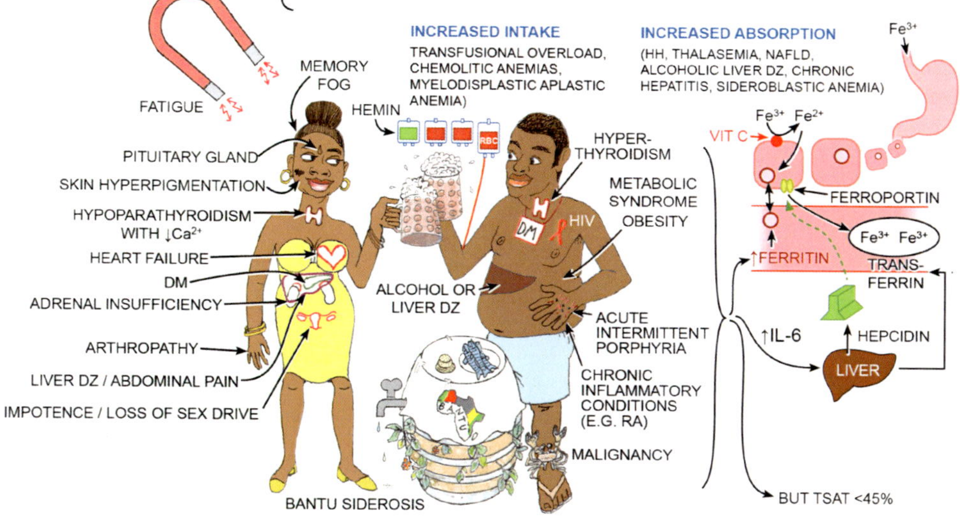

A candle loses nothing by lighting another candle.

Folk Saying

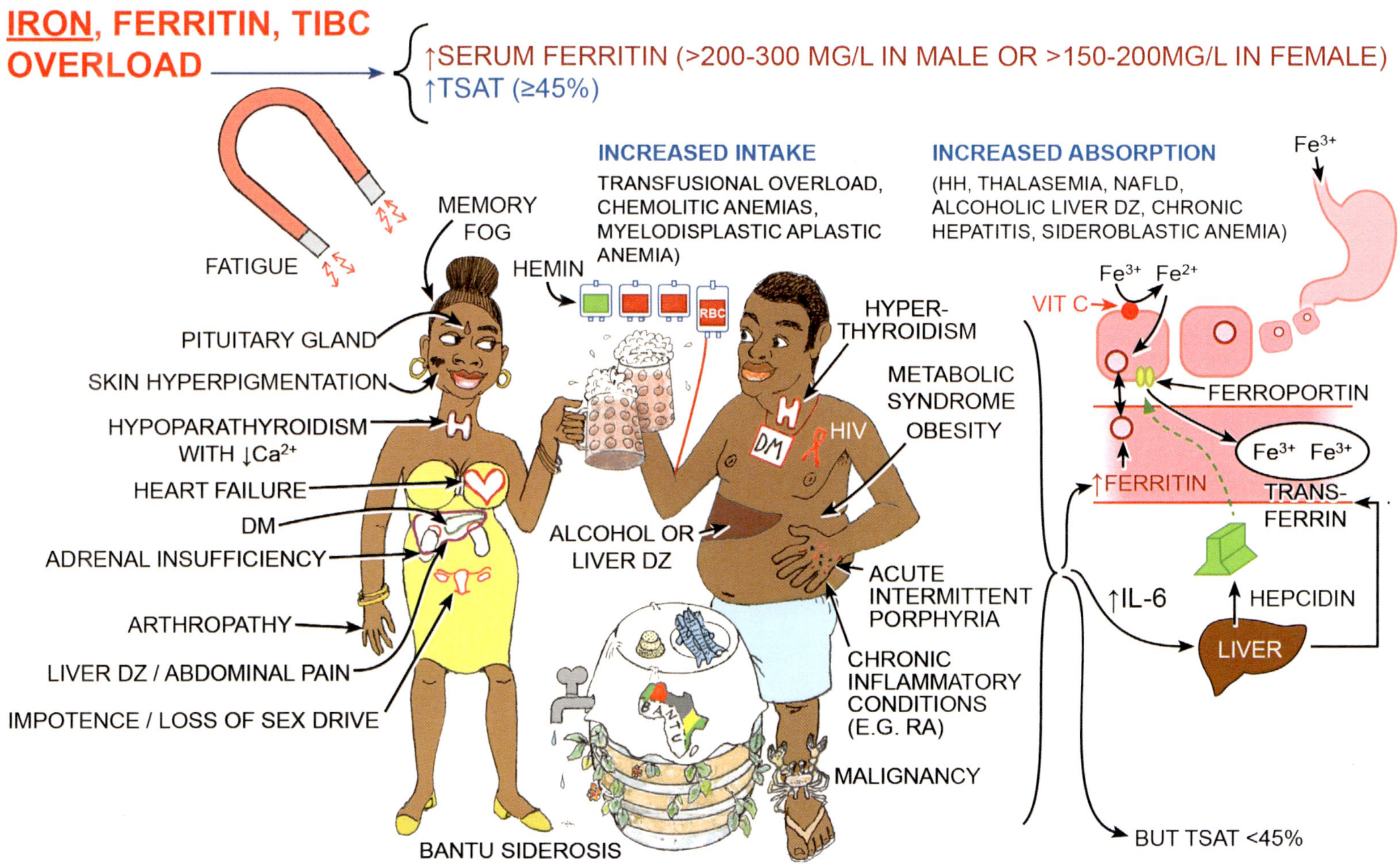

IRON, FERRITIN, TIBC OVERLOAD
↑SERUM FERRITIN (>200-300 MG/L IN MALE OR >150-200MG/L IN FEMALE)
↑TSAT (≥45%)
FATIGUE
MEMORY FOG
PITUITARY GLAND
SKIN HYPERPIGMENTATION
HYPOPARATHYROIDISM WITH ↓Ca2+
HEART FAILURE
DM
ADRENAL INSUFFICIENCY
ARTHROPATHY
LIVER DZ / ABDOMINAL PAIN
IMPOTENCE / LOSS OF SEX DRIVE
BANTU SIDEROSIS
HEMIN
RBC
INCREASED INTAKE
TRANSFUSIONAL OVERLOAD, CHEMOLITIC ANEMIAS, MYELODISPLASTIC APLASTIC ANEMIA)
ALCOHOL OR LIVER DZ
BANTU
DM
HIV
HYPER-THYROIDISM
METABOLIC SYNDROME
OBESITY
ACUTE INTERMITTENT PORPHYRIA
CHRONIC INFLAMMATORY CONDITIONS (E.G. RA)
MALIGNANCY
INCREASED ABSORPTION
(HH, THALASEMIA, NAFLD, ALCOHOLIC LIVER DZ, CHRONIC HEPATITIS, SIDEROBLASTIC ANEMIA)
Fe3+
VIT C
Fe3+ Fe2+
FERROPORTIN
Fe3+ Fe3+
↑FERRITIN
TRANS-FERRIN
↑IL-6
HEPCIDIN
LIVER
BUT TSAT <45%

LOW IRON

The **infertile** woman in the picture is dreaming about pregnancy and having a baby. Low iron in the bod can have a negative impact on fertility in both men and women. Iron plays a vital role in the production of healthy eggs and sperm. In women, low iron levels can cause menstrual irregularities, which can make it more difficult to predict ovulation and time intercourse. Iron deficiency can also lead to a lack of energy, making it harder to get in the mood for sex. In men, low iron levels can lead to reduced sperm production and motility, which can affect fertility.

The patient scraped off part of the paper wall and is eating it as a sign of **pica** which frequently accompanies iron deficiency

The most common hematologic manifestation of **idiopathic pulmonary hemosiderosis** is iron deficiency anemia.

Any **physical activity** that results in increased sweating can lead to a loss of essential minerals including iron. Additionally, playing a musical instrument like the **conga drums** can be physically demanding and may require a lot of energy, which could contribute to iron deficiency if a person's diet is not adequate.

Restless leg syndrome (RLS) is a condition characterized by the urge to move one's legs, especially when somebody is trying to relax or fall asleep. This can be accompanied by uncomfortable sensations like itching, tingling, or burning. Low iron levels may also affect dopamine production, which is important for movements.

Periodic limb movements in sleep (PLMS) involves involuntary movements of the legs during sleep, causing sleep disruption and daytime fatigue. They could also be caused by low iron level (ferritin).

Urinary hemosiderosis (**hemosiderinuria**), refers to the presence of hemosiderin in urine. This condition typically occurs due to chronic intravascular hemolysis, where excess hemoglobin is released from red blood cells into the bloodstream, surpassing the binding capacity of haptoglobin. Fortunately, most cases of renal hemosiderosis do not cause significant kidney damage. Organs may contain hemosiderin deposits, but the extent of damage depends on the iron accumulation.

There is a strong connection between the gastrointestinal tract and iron deficiency. Some common causes of gastrointestinal issues that can lead to iron deficiency include:

- Gastrointestinal hemorrhage, such as from ulcers or hemorrhoids
- Conditions that affect the small intestine, such as celiac disease or inflammatory bowel disease
- Surgeries that remove or bypass part of the stomach or small intestine[24]

24 Abbreviation: TSAT: transferrin saturation

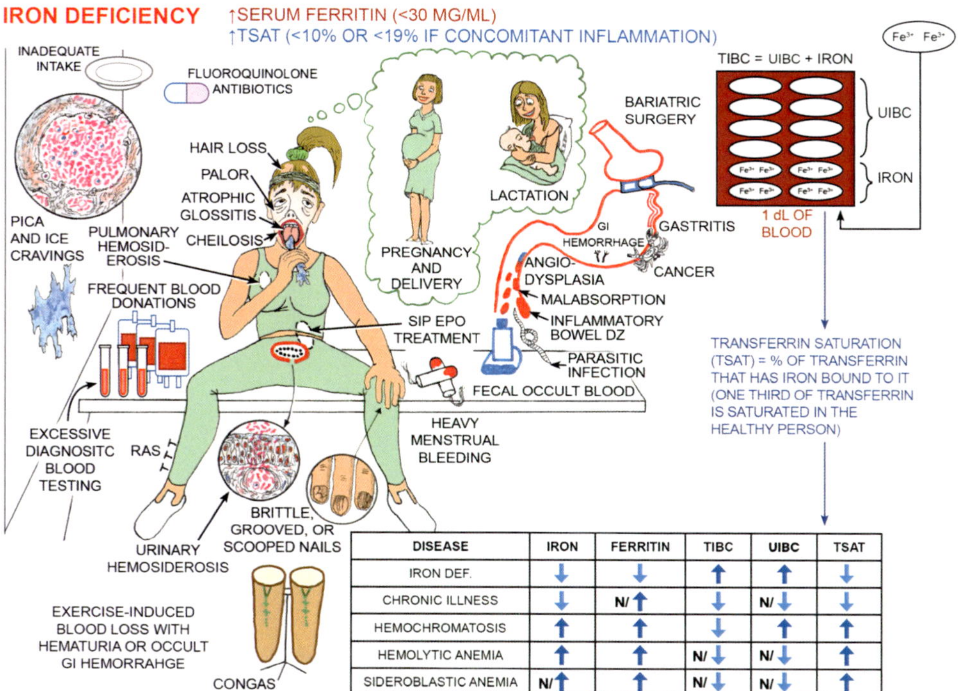

DISEASE	IRON	FERRITIN	TIBC	UIBC	TSAT
IRON DEF.	↓	↓	↑	↑	↓
CHRONIC ILLNESS	↓	N/↑	↓	N/↓	↓
HEMOCHROMATOSIS	↑	↑	↓	↑	↑
HEMOLYTIC ANEMIA	↑	↑	N/↓	N/↓	↑
SIDEROBLASTIC ANEMIA	N/↑	↑	N/↓	N/↓	↑
IRON POISONING	↑	N	N	↑	↑

Someone's sitting in the shade today because
someone planted a tree a long time ago.

African proverb

IRON DEFICIENCY

↑SERUM FERRITIN (<30 MG/ML)

↑TSAT (<10% OR <19% IF CONCOMITANT INFLAMMATION)

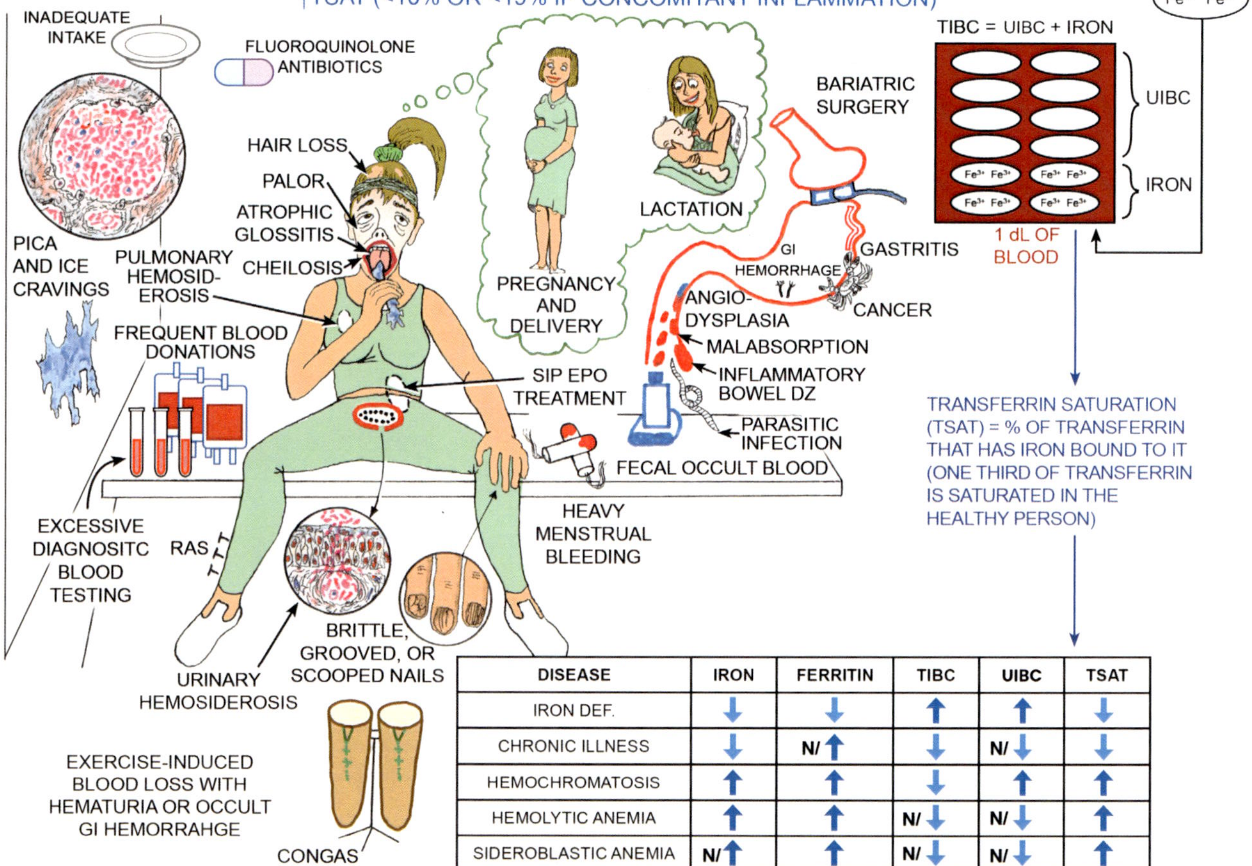

DISEASE	IRON	FERRITIN	TIBC	UIBC	TSAT
IRON DEF.	↓	↓	↑	↑	↓
CHRONIC ILLNESS	↓	N/↑	↓	N/↓	↓
HEMOCHROMATOSIS	↑	↑	↓	↑	↑
HEMOLYTIC ANEMIA	↑	↑	N/↓	N/↓	↑
SIDEROBLASTIC ANEMIA	N/↑	↑	N/↓	N/↓	↑
IRON POISONING	↑	N	N	↑	↑

"Little by little grow the bananas."

African proverb

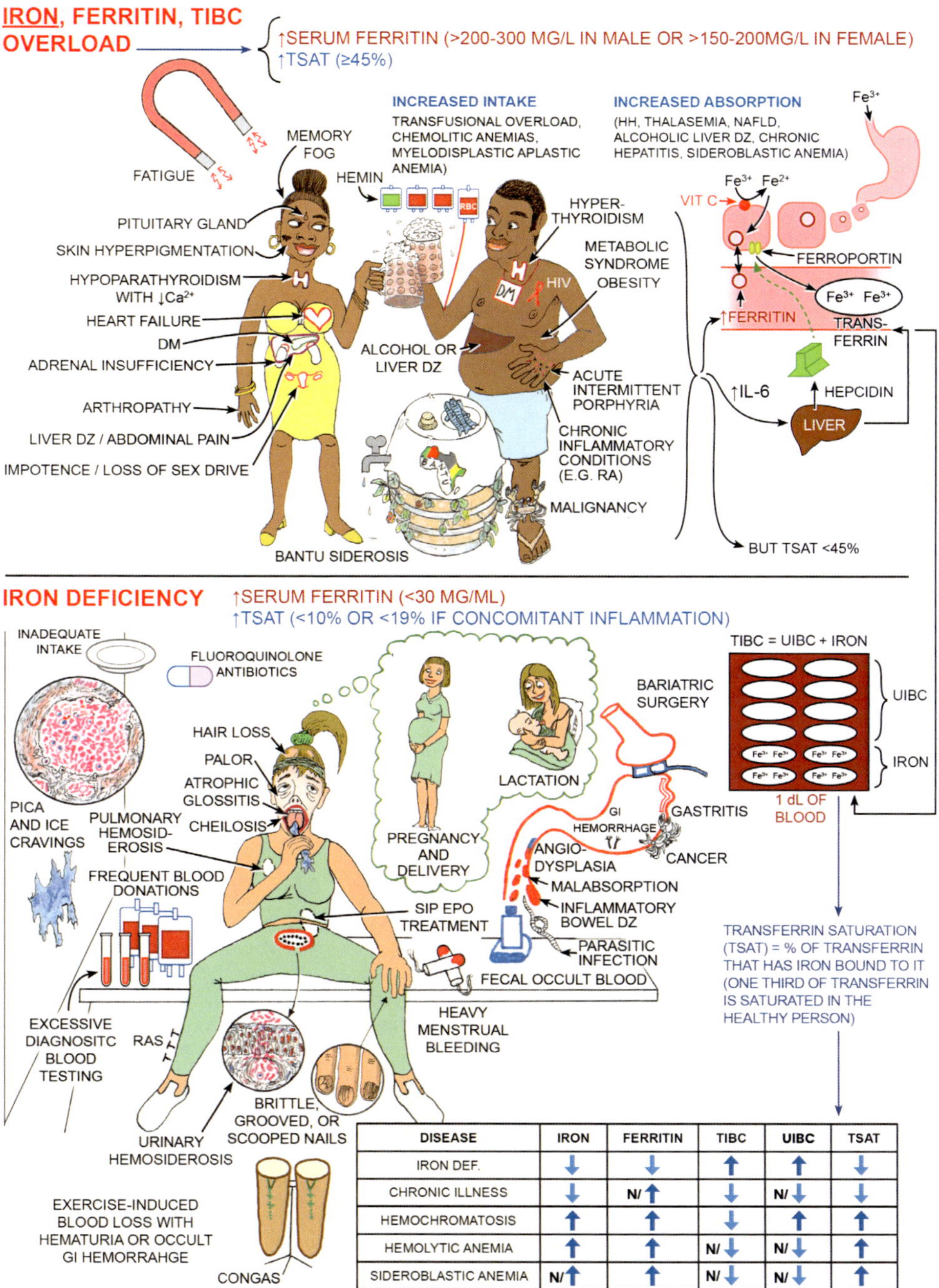

DISEASE	IRON	FERRITIN	TIBC	UIBC	TSAT
IRON DEF.	↓	↓	↑	↑	↓
CHRONIC ILLNESS	↓	N/↑	↓	N/↓	↓
HEMOCHROMATOSIS	↑	↑	↓	↑	↑
HEMOLYTIC ANEMIA	↑	↑	N/↓	N/↓	↑
SIDEROBLASTIC ANEMIA	N/↑	↑	N/↓	N/↓	↑
IRON POISONING	↑	N	N	↑	↑

"Per aspera ad astra.
(Through thorns [suffering] to the stars.)"

Latin proverb

COMMON SYMPTOMS

- HEMOPTYSIS
- ACUTE DIARRHEA
- ASCITES
- NEPHROTIC SYNDROME
- VERTIGO
- CIN VOMIT
- ILLUSTRATED APPROACH TO DIFFERENTIAL DIAGNOSES

HEMOPTYSIS

Hemoptysis, an expectoration of blood, could be **massive** (defined as > 200 ml of blood/24 hours) or **non-massive** (defined as < 200 ml of blood/24 hours). Massive hemoptysis requires immediate evaluation, while non-massive, which accounts for more than 90% of cases, usually does not necessitate admission of the patient to the hospital.

Bronchitis is the most common cause of hemoptysis, but rarely causes massive bleeding.

When **neovascularization** or the formation of new blood vessels occurs in the lungs, it may result in fragile, weak-walled vessels, which are prone to rupture and bleed. Inflammatory lung diseases, such as Wegener's granulomatosis or Goodpasture syndrome, have been associated with neovascularization and can also be a cause of hemoptysis. In some cases, lung tumors and infections, such as tuberculosis or fungal infections, or emphysema and sarcoidosis, can also lead to the development of neovascularization and hemoptysis.

Alveolar hemorrhage can be caused by autoimmune processes that also involve kidneys, like Goodpasture syndrome, and systemic lupus erythematosus (SLE). (Lupus is shown in the picture as a wolf because the word "lupus" (Latin for "wolf") is attributed to the thirteenth century physician Rogerius who used it to describe erosive facial lesions that were reminiscent of a wolf's bite.) Microscopic polyangiitis is a rare small-vessel vasculitis. **Arteritis,** like Churg-Strauss syndrome and Wegener's granulomatosis could also cause alveolar hemorrhage.

Mitral stenosis and **CHF** can cause hemoptysis due to increased pressure in the lungs due to stenosis and reduced ability to pump blood effectively, respectively. The increased pressure can cause a rupture in the thin wall capillaries in the lungs.

Tropical eosinophilia is illustrated with a palm tree whose trunk is made of eosinophils. It is a rare allergic disease caused by a chronic immune response to filaria parasites. Hemoptysis could be a symptom of tropical eosinophilia, although it is not common. It is mainly characterized by coughing, wheezing, breathing difficulties and splenomegaly (the spleen is drawn near the palm tree).

HEMOPTYSIS

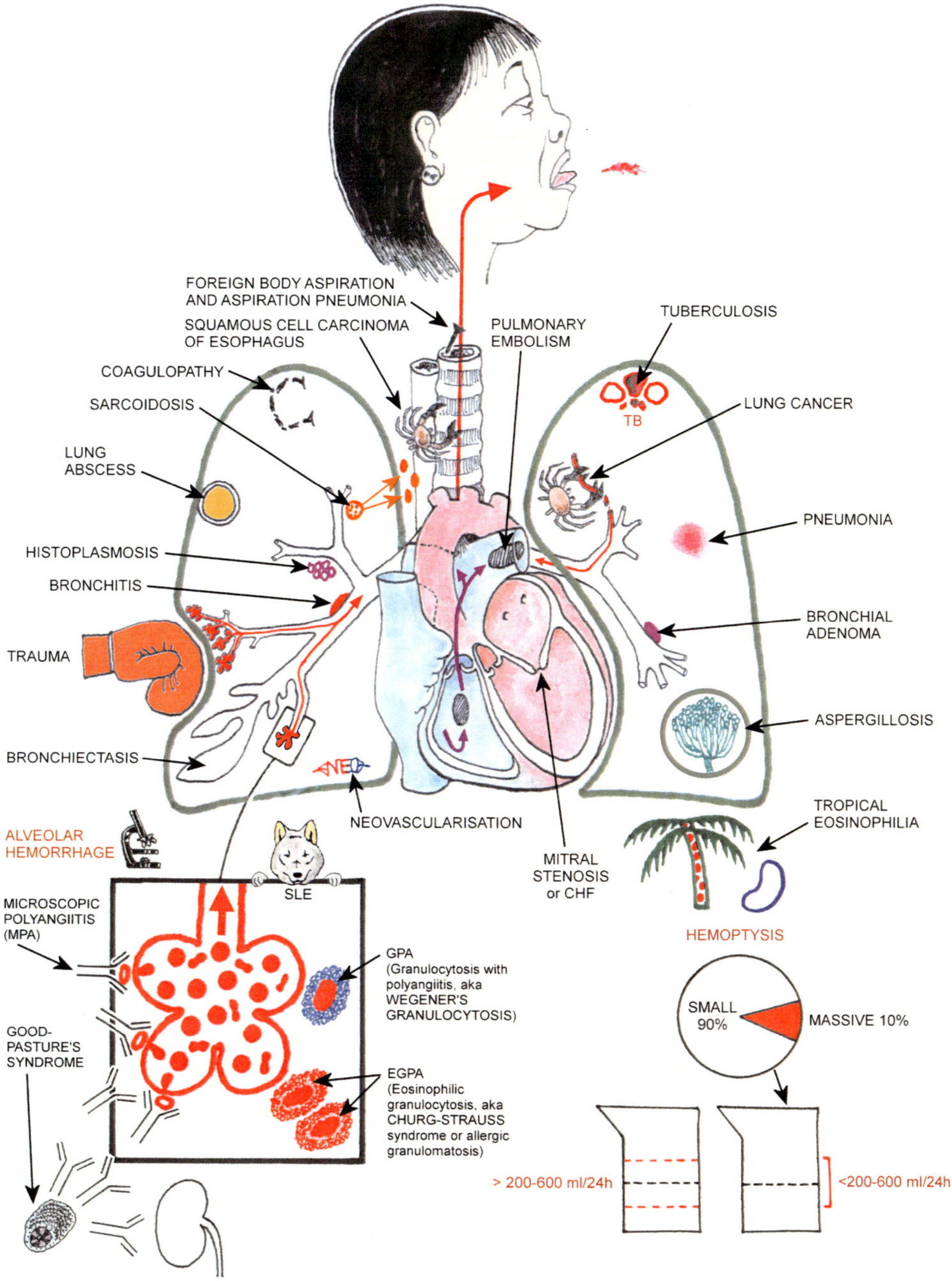

FOREIGN BODY ASPIRATION AND ASPIRATION PNEUMONIA
SQUAMOUS CELL CARCINOMA OF ESOPHAGUS
PULMONARY EMBOLISM
TUBERCULOSIS
TB
COAGULOPATHY
SARCOIDOSIS
LUNG CANCER
LUNG ABSCESS
PNEUMONIA
HISTOPLASMOSIS
BRONCHITIS
BRONCHIAL ADENOMA
TRAUMA
ASPERGILLOSIS
BRONCHIECTASIS
NEOVASCULARISATION
TROPICAL EOSINOPHILIA
ALVEOLAR HEMORRHAGE
MITRAL STENOSIS or CHF
SLE
MICROSCOPIC POLYANGIITIS (MPA)
HEMOPTYSIS
GPA (Granulocytosis with polyangiitis, aka WEGENER'S GRANULOCYTOSIS)
SMALL 90%
MASSIVE 10%
GOOD-PASTURE'S SYNDROME
EGPA (Eosinophilic granulocytosis, aka CHURG-STRAUSS syndrome or allergic granulomatosis)
> 200-600 ml/24h
<200-600 ml/24h

ACUTE DIARRHEA

Diarrhea is excretion of more than 200 g of stool per day. It can be classified as **acute** (< 3 three weeks in duration) or **chronic** (> 3 weeks in duration).

Causes of acute diarrhea include:

1. **Infection** -> pointing toward the toilet in the picture.
2. **Inflammation** -> pointing toward the patient's intestines with Crohn's disease and ulcerative colitis.
3. **Drugs**
4. **Toxins**

Most cases of acute infectious diarrhea are self-limited and do not need workup, but only supportive care. An algorithmic approach to acute diarrhea, shown on the right side of the picture, can help to differentiate which patients need a diagnostic workup and which patients need antimicrobial treatment.

If ova and parasites are negative, the cause of diarrhea could be a **virus, Escherichia coli:** enterohemorrhagic E. coli (serotype O157:H7) (**EHEC**) and entero invasive E. coli (**EIEC**), and **Vibrio species**. Observe and start general therapy, but if severe or persistent diarrhea is present, consider stool culture, Clostridium difficile toxin, flexible sigmoidoscopy with biopsy, and/or EGD.

If the test for ova and parasites is positive, the causes could be **Giardia**, **Amoeba** and **Cryptosporidium**. (A stool for Giardia antigen can also be done.)

Serologic studies will not be of much help in acute conditions, but they may help later or in cases of salmonellosis and amebiasis. A methylene blue smear for leukocytes should be done with wet saline preparation of the stool. Leukocytes on a smear suggest a bacterial cause and a culture should be done.

If there is a history of antibiotic use, stool should be tested for Clostridium difficile toxin. **Clostridium difficile toxin** is a potent enterotoxin causing pseudomembranous colitis. Risk factors for C. difficile infection include antibiotic treatment, which can disrupt normal intestinal microbiota and lead to colonization of C. difficile bacteria. **Severe vomiting** could also accompany **botulism**. Symptoms of foodborne botulism typically begin 12 to 36 hours after the toxin gets into the body. But depending on how much toxin was consumed, the start of symptoms may range from a few hours to a few days. (The other symptoms of foodborne botulism include: trouble swallowing or speaking, xerostomia, facial weakness on both sides of the face, diplopia, drooping eyelids, trouble breathing, stomach cramps and paralysis.)

Symptoms of wound botulism appear about 10 days after the toxin enters the body. **Amebiasis** (amoebic dysentery) may cause diarrhea, nausea, stomach cramps without fever. (Shigella, salmonella and campylobacter infections go with fever.) In osmotic diarrhea (which happens due to ingestion of poorly absorbed solutes), the pH may be lower than 5 due to the fermentation of these solutes by gut bacteria, resulting in the production of organic acids which can decrease the pH of intestinal contents.

A stool osmotic gap is a **measurement of the difference in solute types between serum and feces.** It is used to distinguish between different causes of diarrhea. The formula to calculate stool osmotic gap is: Stool osmolarity - 2 x (stool Na + stool K). The stool osmolarity is usually assumed to be between 290–300 mOsm/kg. A normal stool osmotic gap is less than 125 mOsm/kg, usually less than 50 mOsm/kg.

ACUTE DIARRHEA

(<3 WEEKS IN DURATION)

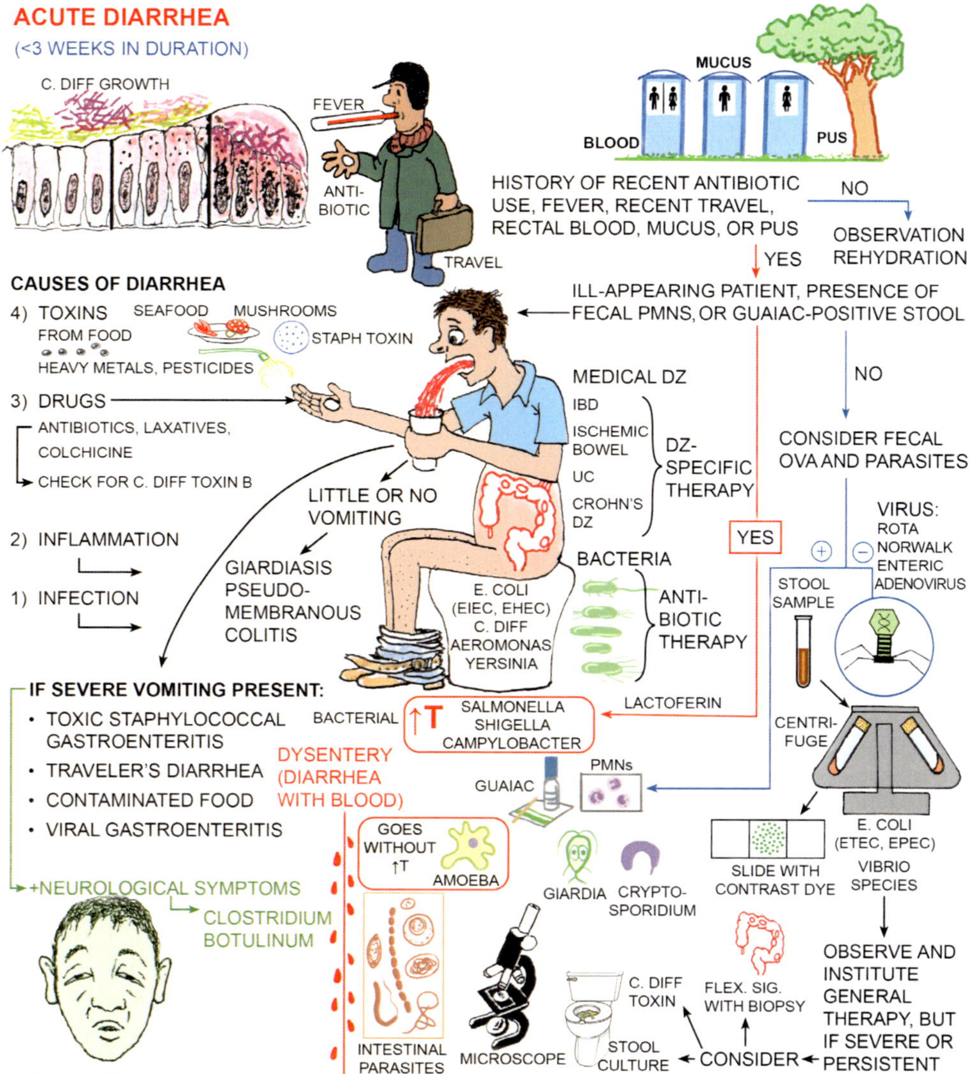

TYPES OF DIARRHEA

SECRETORY (BACTERIAL TOXINS, E.G. CHOLERA, VIRION, CARCINOID, GASTRINOMA, 2ES	OSMOTIC → (LACTOSE DEFICIENCY, COELIAC DZ, PANCREATIC INSUFFICIENCY	EXUDATIVE (CROHN DZ, UC, TB, E. COLI, 157:H7)	MOTILITY (DIABETIC NEUROPATHY, SIBO, IBS, HYPERTHYROIDISM, GASTRIC INTESTINAL RESECTION)
LARGE STOOL VOLUME (>1L/DAY), WATERY STOOL, NO BLOOD, PUS, OR MUCUS	VOLUME <299 mL/DAY NO BLOOD OR PUS	BLOOD AND PUS PRESENT	
PERSISTANT DIARRHEA DESPITE 24-48 HOUR FAST	DIARRHEA TYPICALLY STOPS WHEN PATIENT FASTS	PERSISTENT DURING FASTING	
pH >6	pH <5		PSEUDO DIARRHEA → OVERUSE OF LAXATIVES, BULIMIA, MUNSCHAUSEN
STOOL NA+ >70 mEq/L STOOL OSMOTIC GAP <50 mOsm/kg	STOOL NA+ <70 mEq/L USUALLY >125 mOsm/kg	STOOL OSMOTIC GAP <50 mOsm/kg	PARADOXICAL DIARRHEA (FECAL IMPACTION)

ASCITES

Ascites is the accumulation of excess fluid within the peritoneal cavity. It could occur as a part of **anasarca** (generalized edema) or as an **isolated fluid collection**. The causes of an anasarca could be remembered as a "**osis group**" – **nephrosis, cirrhosis, cardiosis**, and **hypothyroidosis.**

There are three primary mechanisms of ascites production:

1. **Increase hydrostatic pressure** (**cardiac –** right-sided heart failure and constrictive pericarditis**,** and **hepatic – postsinusoidal** [Budd-Chiarri syndrome], **sinusoidal obstruction** [cirrhosis], and **presinusoidal obstruction** [schistosomiasis or portal vein thrombosis])
2. **Decreased oncotic pressure** (starvation, severe liver disease, nephrotic syndrome, protein losing enteropathy)
3. **Increase capillary permeability** (**infection** [e.g., tuberculosis] or **malignancy**)

Miscellaneous causes can increase **hypothyroidism**, **pancreatitis**, **lymphatic obstruction** from trauma, and tumor or infection may cause **chylous ascites**.

Kwashiorkor leads to ascites due to decreased production of albumin, increased capillary permeability, and impaired lymphatic drainage.

Spontaneous bacterial peritonitis (SBP) is a bacterial infection that can occur in the ascitic fluid in patients with liver cirrhosis and ascites. It is known as "spontaneous" because the infection occurs without an apparent source of infection outside of the body. Common symptoms of SBP include abdominal pain, fever, and altered mental status. It can rapidly progress to sepsis and can be life-threatening.

The serum-ascites albumin gradient (SAAG) can help to determine the underlying cause of ascites. The calculation involves subtracting the albumin level in the ascitic fluid from the albumin level in the blood serum. If the **SAAG is 1.1 g/dL or greater**, it typically suggests that the ascites is due to **portal hypertension**, most commonly from cirrhosis, congestive heart failure, or hepatic vein thrombosis. On the other hand, if the **SAAG is less than 1.1 g/dL**, the ascites is likely due to other causes, such as peritoneal malignancy, tuberculosis, or pancreatitis.

If portal hypertension is accompanied by another disorder that produces increased capillary permeability, the gradient will usually remain greater than or equal to 1.1. SBP usually occurs in patients with portal hypertension, therefore the gradient is usually greater than or equal to 1.1 in these patients. SBP is unlikely if SAAG is < 1.1 g/dL.

ASCITES

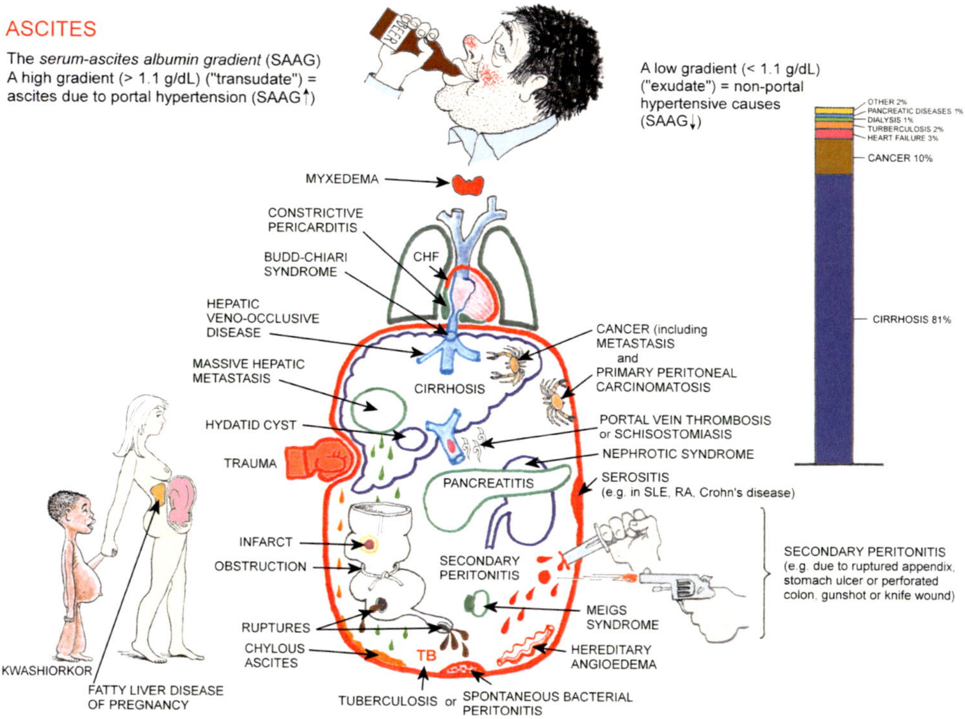
The *serum-ascites albumin gradient* (SAAG)
A high gradient (> 1.1 g/dL) ("transudate") = ascites due to portal hypertension (SAAG↑)
BEER
A low gradient (< 1.1 g/dL) ("exudate") = non-portal hypertensive causes (SAAG↓)
OTHER 2%
PANCREATIC DISEASES 1%
DIALYSIS 1%
TURBERCULOSIS 2%
HEART FAILURE 3%
CANCER 10%
CIRRHOSIS 81%
MYXEDEMA
CONSTRICTIVE PERICARDITIS
BUDD-CHIARI SYNDROME
CHF
HEPATIC VENO-OCCLUSIVE DISEASE
MASSIVE HEPATIC METASTASIS
CIRRHOSIS
CANCER (including METASTASIS and PRIMARY PERITONEAL CARCINOMATOSIS
HYDATID CYST
PORTAL VEIN THROMBOSIS or SCHISOSTOMIASIS
TRAUMA
NEPHROTIC SYNDROME
PANCREATITIS
SEROSITIS (e.g. in SLE, RA, Crohn's disease)
INFARCT
OBSTRUCTION
SECONDARY PERITONITIS
SECONDARY PERITONITIS (e.g. due to ruptured appendix, stomach ulcer or perforated colon, gunshot or knife wound)
MEIGS SYNDROME
RUPTURES
CHYLOUS ASCITES
TB
HEREDITARY ANGIOEDEMA
KWASHIORKOR
FATTY LIVER DISEASE OF PREGNANCY
TUBERCULOSIS or SPONTANEOUS BACTERIAL PERITONITIS

"Illustration has its own language, one that visually transcends boundaries of spoken or written language to evoke feelings and convey messages."

Anita Kunz

ASCITES

The *serum-ascites albumin gradient* (SAAG)
A high gradient (> 1.1 g/dL) ("transudate") = ascites due to portal hypertension (SAAG↑)

A low gradient (< 1.1 g/dL) ("exudate") = non-portal hypertensive causes (SAAG↓)

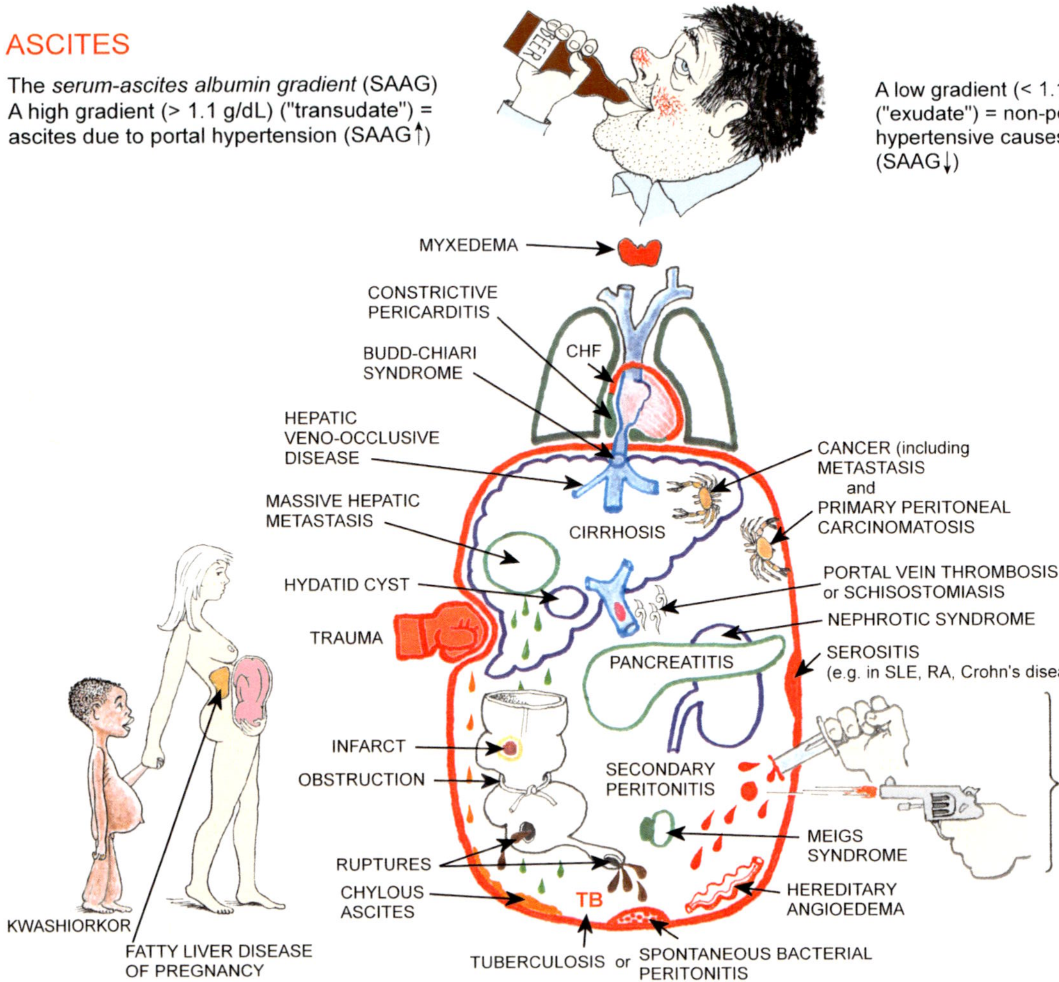

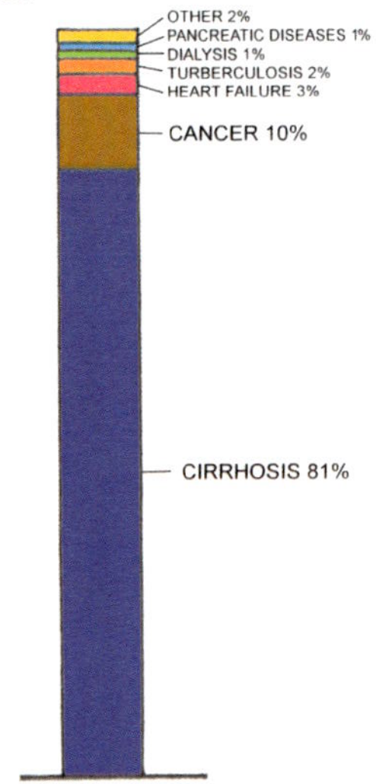

NEPHROTIC SYNDROME

In comparison to **nephritic** syndrome, which is caused by extensive inflammatory damage to the glomerulus capillaries, and which consists of

- Hematuria
- Proteinuria, ranging from sub-nephrotic (<3.5 g/day) to >10 g/day, although it is rarely above nephrotic range proteinuria levels
- Hypertension
- Blurred vision
- Azotemia
- Oliguria (low urine output <400 ml/day)
- Red blood cell casts
- Pyuria

Nephrotic syndrome consists of

- Large proteinuria (>3.5 g per day)
- Hypoalbuminemia (< 3.5 g/dl)
- Hyperlipidemia
- Edema (that begins in the face)

The anvil symbolizes **heavy metals**.

Many **cancers** can cause nephrotic syndrome. In elderly patients with unexplained nephrotic syndrome, an underlying malignancy should be suspected. Both hematological malignancies (lymphoma and leukemias) and solid tumor can cause nephrotic syndrome.

Heroin and its additives, as well as the other possibilities listed the picture, can cause glomerular damage with subsequent nephrotic syndrome.

NEPHROTIC SYNDROME

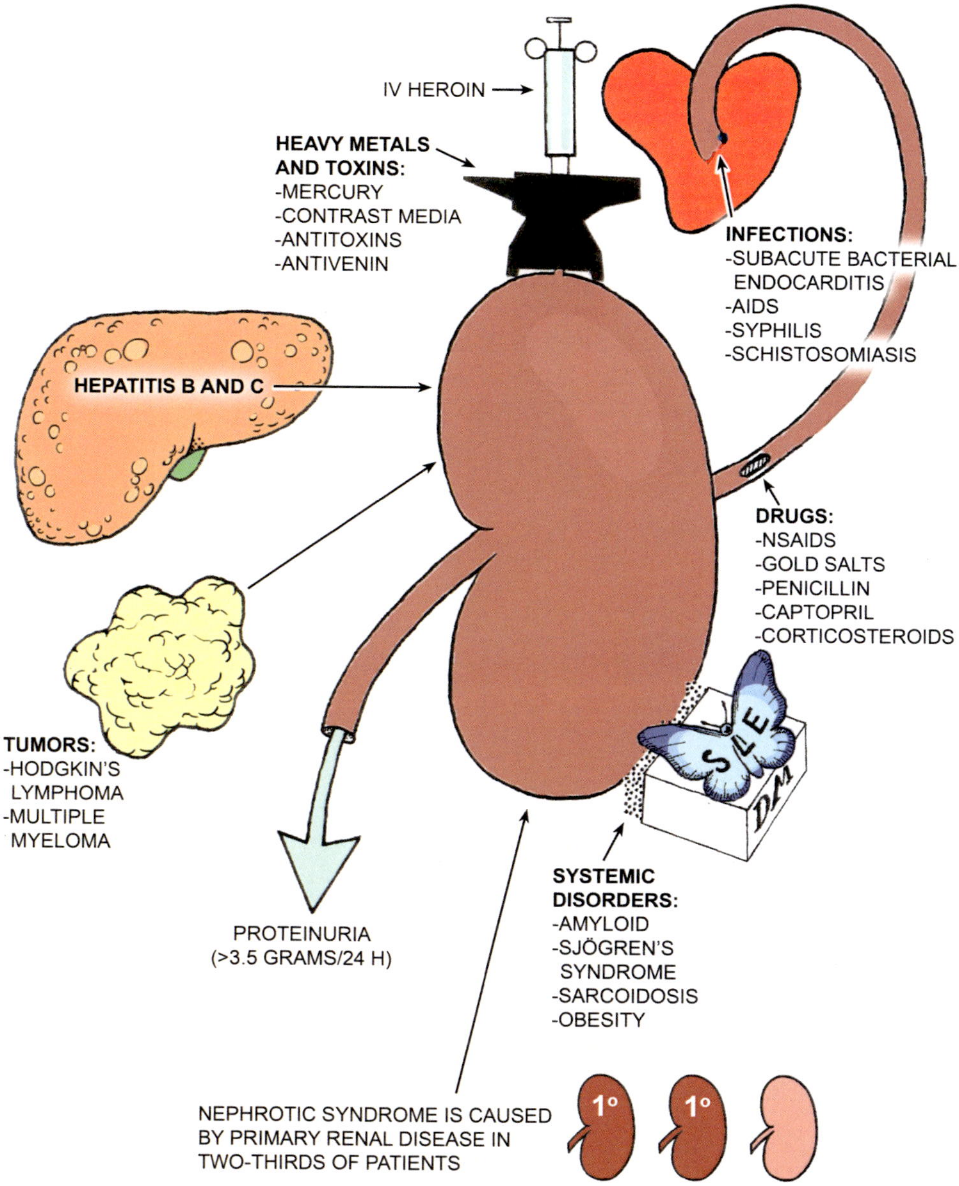

VERTIGO

Dizziness is a sensation of faintness, vertigo, or gait unsteadiness.

Faintness is usually described as a sense of lightheadedness and is typically caused by an insufficient supply of oxygen, blood or glucose to the brain. Faintness often occurs with hyperventilation, hypoglycemia, or just before a syncopal event.

Vertigo is the illusion of movement (usually spinning) **commonly caused by an inner ear problem**. The patient may report **feeling off balance** or describe the environment as moving while she remains stationary, or vice versa.

Vertigo is classified into either **peripheral** or **central** depending on the location of the dysfunction of the vestibular pathway. However, it can also be caused by **psychological factors** (such as **stress** or **anxiety**) or **systemic lesions** (drugs - anticonvulsants, hypnotics, antihypertensives, analgesics, tranquilizers, alcohol, [postural] hypotension, infectious disease—syphilis, other bacterial and viral infection, hypothyroidism, anemia, cardiac arrhythmia).

Common causes of vertigo are:

Benign Paroxysmal Positional Vertigo (BPPV): The most frequent cause of vertigo, where tiny crystals normally embedded in gelatinous matrices within the utricle and saccule become dislodged and float into one of the inner ear's semicircular canals. Specific head movements then trigger sudden, short episodes of vertigo. (The drawing depicts a shovel unloading a pebble, serving as a caricatured representation of the small crystals.)

The direction of nystagmus typically depends on which semicircular canal of the inner ear is affected. Most frequently, the posterior semicircular canal is involved. In that case, the nystagmus is torsional clockwise for the left side, counterclockwise for the right side (with the vertical updating component) during Dix-Hallpike positional testing.

Vestibular migraine: Vertigo, which can last from minutes to days, can occur synchronously or asynchronously with other typical migraine symptoms such as headache, sensitivity to light and sound, and nausea.

Labyrinthitis: Characterized by vertigo, hearing loss and tinnitus due to inner ear infection (such as from viruses) or inflammation. Vertigo typically lasts hours and days.

Ménière's Disease: Characterized by *fluctuating* hearing loss, tinnitus, vertigo and aural fullness. Vertigo typically lasts hours, and is associated with nausea and vomiting. Histologically, Ménière's disease is characterized by endolymphatic hydrops.

Vestibular neuronitis: Vertigo is sudden, severe, typically lasting days, often accompanied by nausea and vomiting; it is not associated with auditory symptoms. The condition is believed to arise from a viral infection or inflammation.

Other less common causes are perilymphatic fistula, cholesteatoma, otosclerosis, and stroke.

VERTIGO

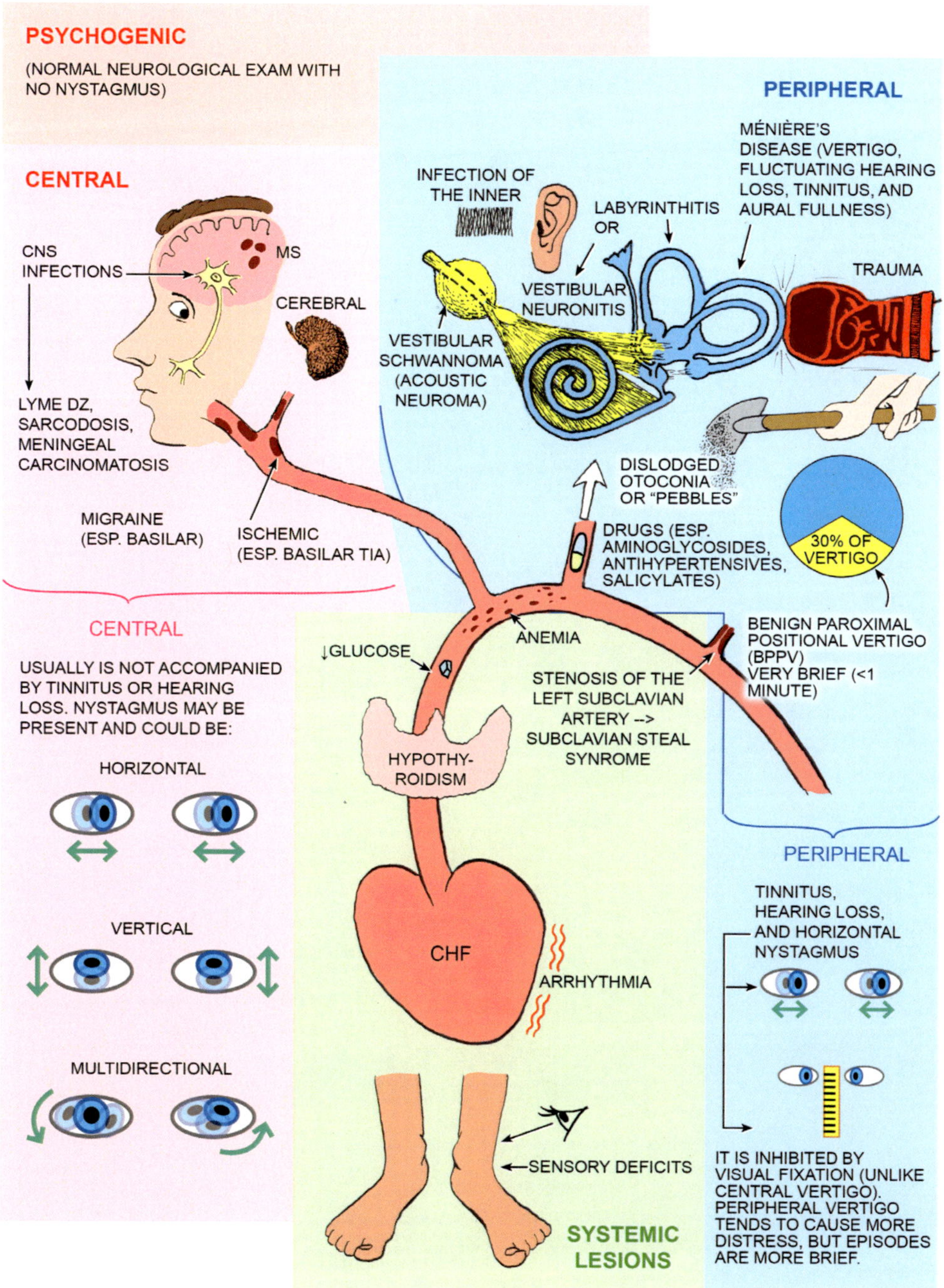

PSYCHOGENIC
(NORMAL NEUROLOGICAL EXAM WITH NO NYSTAGMUS)
CENTRAL
CNS INFECTIONS
MS
CEREBRAL
LYME DZ, SARCODOSIS, MENINGEAL CARCINOMATOSIS
MIGRAINE (ESP. BASILAR)
ISCHEMIC (ESP. BASILAR TIA)
CENTRAL
USUALLY IS NOT ACCOMPANIED BY TINNITUS OR HEARING LOSS. NYSTAGMUS MAY BE PRESENT AND COULD BE:
HORIZONTAL
VERTICAL
MULTIDIRECTIONAL
PERIPHERAL
MÉNIÈRE'S DISEASE (VERTIGO, FLUCTUATING HEARING LOSS, TINNITUS, AND AURAL FULLNESS)
INFECTION OF THE INNER
LABYRINTHITIS OR
VESTIBULAR NEURONITIS
TRAUMA
VESTIBULAR SCHWANNOMA (ACOUSTIC NEUROMA)
DISLODGED OTOCONIA OR "PEBBLES"
DRUGS (ESP. AMINOGLYCOSIDES, ANTIHYPERTENSIVES, SALICYLATES)
30% OF VERTIGO
BENIGN PAROXIMAL POSITIONAL VERTIGO (BPPV) VERY BRIEF (<1 MINUTE)
↓GLUCOSE
ANEMIA
STENOSIS OF THE LEFT SUBCLAVIAN ARTERY --> SUBCLAVIAN STEAL SYNROME
HYPOTHY-ROIDISM
CHF
ARRHYTHMIA
SENSORY DEFICITS
SYSTEMIC LESIONS
PERIPHERAL
TINNITUS, HEARING LOSS, AND HORIZONTAL NYSTAGMUS
IT IS INHIBITED BY VISUAL FIXATION (UNLIKE CENTRAL VERTIGO). PERIPHERAL VERTIGO TENDS TO CAUSE MORE DISTRESS, BUT EPISODES ARE MORE BRIEF.

CIN VOMIT

When physicians are not sure about the possible differential diagnosis of a medical problem, they have been relying on the classical mnemonic for potential etiologies:

C = congenital

I = infection, inflammation, iatrogenic

N = neoplasm

V = vascular

O = organ disease or "other"

M = metabolic

I = idiopathic

T = trauma

The following picture, after the traditional CIN VOMIT **verbal** mnemonic is an **illustrative** alternative approach.

MNEMONICS

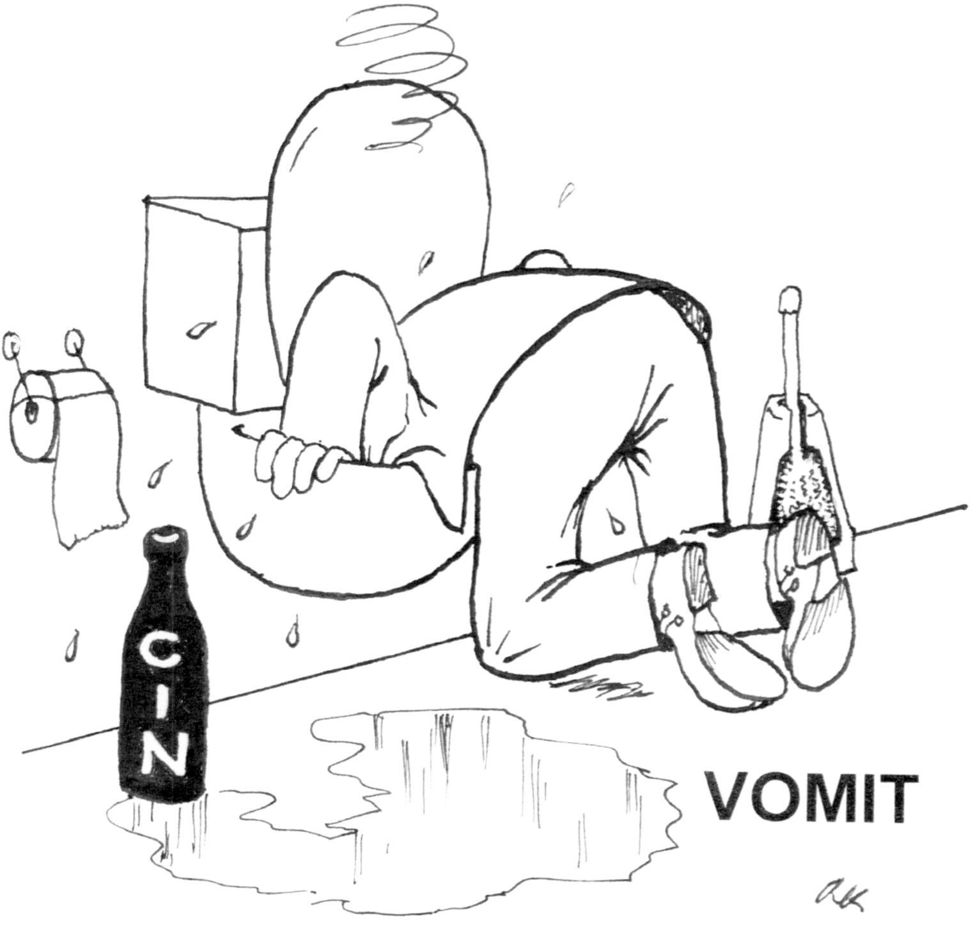

"Beauty will save the world."

Fyodor Mikhailovich Dostoevsky

ILLUSTRATED APPROACH TO DIFFERENTIAL DIAGNOSES

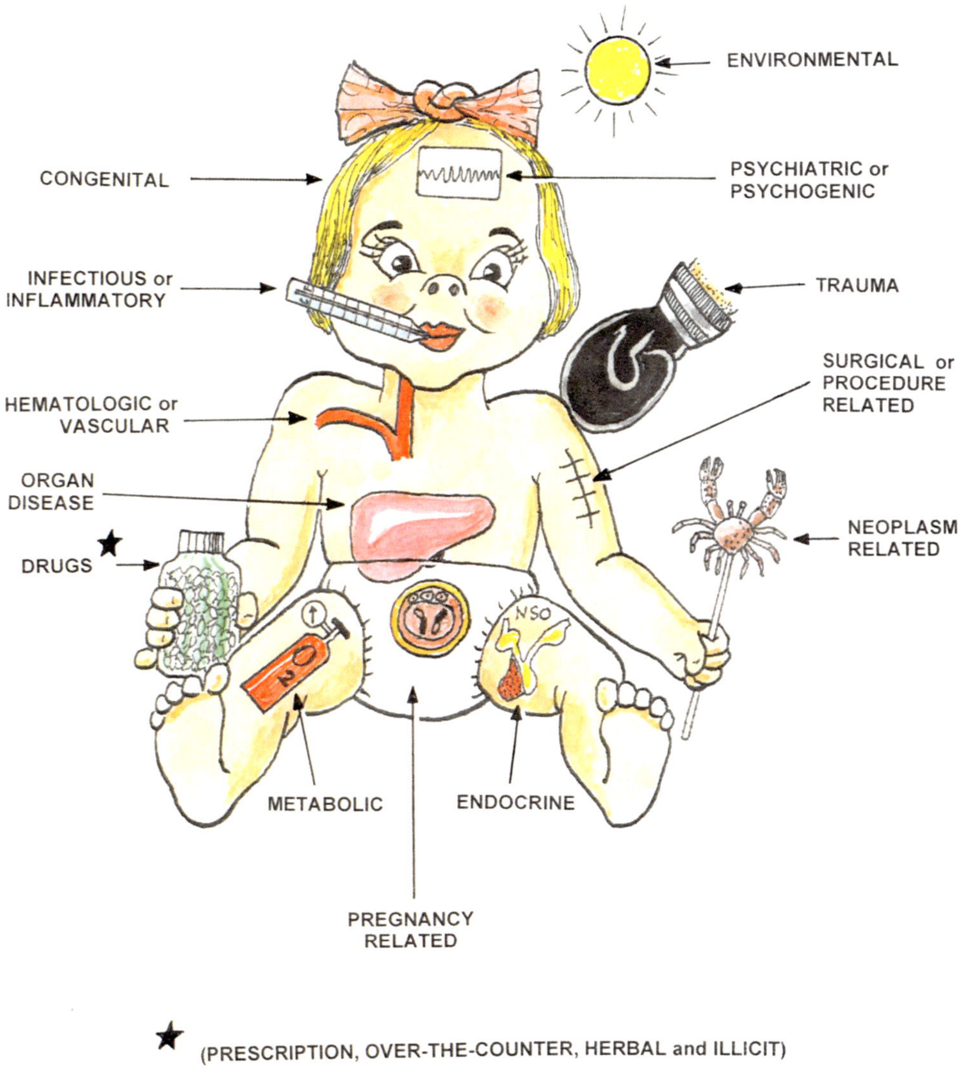

ACKNOWLEDGEMENTS:

I would like to express my special thanks to the following individuals and organizations.

Prof. Dr. Radivoj V. Krstic, Professor Emeritus of Histology and Embryology at the University of Lausanne, Switzerland for heroically bringing this book to fruition, despite facing challenges posed by his advanced age and medical problems.

Mrs. Ellen Weiss, a Seattle-based medical illustrator, animator, and artist, a 2017 graduate from the University of Illinois at Chicago with a Master of Science degree in Biomedical Visualization, for helping with illustrations when Prof. Dr. Krstic could no longer draw.

Dr. Sci. Blazenko Vukovic, a lifelong friend from earliest childhood days, a classmate through elementary school, a teammate in our bicycle racing team, a fellow student during medical school, a roommate during our refugee time in Serbia 1991-1993, and an endocrinologist at the Clinical Center of Banja Luka, Bosnia for reviewing the topic of *Hyper and Hypoglycemia*, *Hyper and Hypothyroidism, and Hyperlipidemia*.

Prof. Alan, Gilman, MD, a hematologist, oncologist and a teaching attending at Saint Joseph hospital in Chicago for his generosity, support and tremendous help during my internship.

Prof. Curtis Crock, MD, a pulmonologist and a teaching attending in the Internal Medicine residency program at the University of Illinois at Urbana Champaign IL for being an inspirational physician and serving as a role model.

Clinical Prof. Robert Healy, MD, a program director of the Internal Medicine residency program at the University of Illinois at Urbana Champaign IL for his kindness, guidance and the superb learning environment he created.

Prof. John Carey, MD and **Assistant Prof. Jenny Chen, MD, EDM** of Johns Hopkins University for their tender compassion and steadfast friendship during my brother's final months.

Our sister **Prof. Konstantina M. Stankovic, MD, PhD,** Chair of Otolaryngology-Head and Neck Surgery at Stanford University School of Medicine, and a member of the National Academy of Medicine, for reviewing the topic of *Vertigo*.

Ms. Donna Roberts for superb help with editing.

UpToDate company for permission to use their articles.

Elsevier publishing company for permission to use the clinical vignettes for the acid-base topic from the book "Fluid, Electrolyte, and Acid-base Balance: A Case Study Approach."

Wikipedia, a free encyclopedia for free access to many medical topics.

Hello AI for quick and simple access to assisted information.

“The whole is more than the sum of its parts.”

Aristotle

In the 52 illustrations shown on the next page, separated into 11 groups, is about 90% of differential diagnoses the general internist encounters in her or his practice.

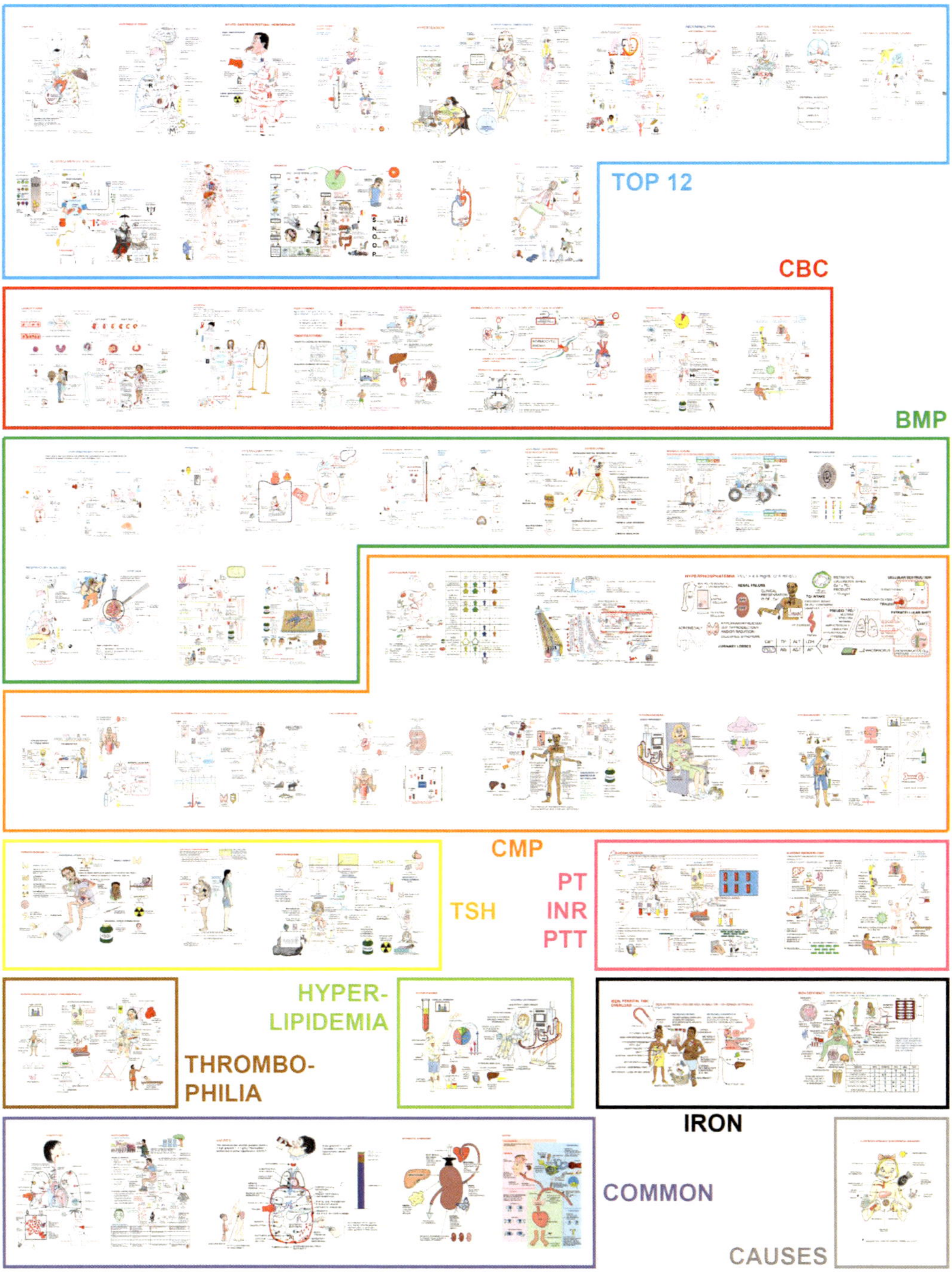
TOP 12
CBC
BMP
CMP
TSH
PT
INR
PTT
HYPER-
LIPIDEMIA
THROMBO-
PHILIA
IRON
COMMON
CAUSES

REFERENCES

VISUALIZATION OF DATA

[1]Miller, G. A. The magical number seven, plus or minus two: some limits on our capacity for processing information. *Psychological Review, 1956; 63(2), 81–97.*

[2]Why storytelling is so powerful in the digital era | Ashley Fell | TEDxUniMelb (https://mail.google.com/mail/u/0/#search/Ted+/QgrcJHsBqzNmKsHKVWZXtLdDxdQrcXTdSrl?projector=1)

[3]Moderate sleep deprivation produces impairments in cognitive and motor performance equivalent to legally prescribed levels of alcohol intoxication. *Occup Environ Med.* 2000;57(10):649-55.

CHEST PAIN

John R McConaghy, MD, CPE, FAAFP. Outpatient evaluation of the adult with chest pain. Mark D Aronson, MD, ed. UpToDate. Waltham, MA: UpToDate Inc. https://www.uptodate.com (Accessed on November 26, 2022.)

Sanjay Saint and Craig Frances. Chest Pain. In Siant-Frances guide to inpatient medicine. Lippincott Williams & Wilkins, 1997; 56-63.

Angina - Symptoms and causes - Mayo Clinic

Cardiac tamponade: Symptoms, causes, diagnosis and treatments (msn.com)

SHORTNESS OF BREATH

Azeemuddin Ahmed, MD, MBA and Mark A Graber, MD, MSHCE, FACEP. Approach to the adult with dyspnea in the emergency department. Korilyn S Zachrison, MD, MSc. ed. UpToDate. Waltham, MA: UpToDate Inc. https://www.uptodate.com (Accessed on November 26, 2022.)

Shortness of breath - Wikipedia

Sanjay Saint and Craig Frances. Acute dyspnea. In Siant-Frances guide to inpatient medicine. Lippincott Williams & Wilkins, 1997; 101-104.

Acute respiratory distress syndrome - Wikipedia

Blood Oxygen Level: What It Is & How To Increase It (clevelandclinic.org)

Oxygen Saturation and Dangerously Low Oxygen Levels (verywellhealth.com)

ACUTE GASTROINTESTINAL HEMORRHAGE

John R Saltzman, MD, FACP, FACG, FASGE, AGAF. Approach to acute upper gastrointestinal bleeding in adults. Mark Feldman, MD, MACP, AGAF, FACG, ed. UpToDate. Waltham, MA: UpToDate Inc. https://www.uptodate.com (Accessed on November 26, 2022.)

Gastrointestinal bleeding - Wikipedia

Sanjay Saint and Craig Frances. Acute gastrointestinal bleeding. In Siant-Frances guide to inpatient medicine. Lippincott Williams & Wilkins, 1997; 169-174.

ACUTE KIDNEY INJURY (AKI)

Pedram Fatehi, MD, MPH, and Chi-yuan Hsu, MD, MSc. Evaluation of acute kidney injury among hospitalized adult patients. Paul M Palevsky, MD, ed. UpToDate. Waltham, MA: UpToDate Inc. https://www.uptodate.com (Accessed on November 28, 2022.)

Acute kidney injury - Wikipedia

Sanjay Saint and Craig Frances. Acute renal failure. In Siant-Frances guide to inpatient medicine. Lippincott Williams & Wilkins, 1997; 205-216.

HYPERTENSION
Jan Basile, MD, Michael J Bloch, MD, FACP, FASH, FSVM, FNLA. Overview of hypertension in adults. George L Bakris, MD, William B White, MD , ed. UpToDate. Waltham, MA: UpToDate Inc. https://www.uptodate.com (Accessed on November 29, 2022.)
Hypertension - Wikipedia
Sanjay Saint and Craig Frances. Hypertension. In Siant-Frances guide to inpatient medicine. Lippincott Williams & Wilkins, 1997; 246-249.
HYPOTENSION
Geraldine Finlay, MD, David F Gaieski, MD, Mark E Mikkelsen, MD, MSCE. Evaluation of an initial approach to the adult patient with undifferentiated hypotension and shock. Polly E Parsons, MD, Korilyn S Zachrison, MD, MSc, ed. UpToDate. Waltham, MA: UpToDate Inc. https://www.uptodate.com (Accessed on September 9, 2023.)
Hypotension - Wikipedia
Part 10.4: Hypothermia | Circulation (ahajournals.org)
ABDOMINAL PAIN
Robert M Penner, BSc, MD, FRCPC, MSc, Mary B Fishman, MD. Evaluation of the adult with abdominal pain. Andrew D Auerbach, MD, MPH and Mark D Aronson, MD, ed. UpToDate. Waltham, MA: UpToDate Inc. https://www.uptodate.com (Accessed on September 9, 2023.)
Abdominal pain - Wikipedia
Sanjay Saint and Craig Frances. Abdominal pain. In Siant-Frances guide to inpatient medicine. Lippincott Williams & Wilkins, 1997; 155-161.
Familial Mediterranean fever | DermNet (dermnetnz.org)
Addison's disease - Symptoms and causes - Mayo Clinic
Carlos Tavares Bello, Miguel Franco Gago, Francelina Fernandes, Maria Manuela Oliveira. Abdominal Pain in Diabetic Ketoacidosis: Beyond the Obvious. *Journal of Endocrinology and Metabolism, 2018; 8 (2-3), 43-46.*
Porphyria - Symptoms and causes - Mayo Clinic
Brian Shian, MD, and Scott T. Larson, MD. Abdominal Wall Pain: Clinical Evaluation, Differential Diagnosis, and Treatment, *Am Fam Physician,* 2018;98(7):429-436.
Hello AI: "Why eating reduces duodenal ulcer pain?'
ALTERED MENTAL STATUS
Joseph Francis, Jr, MD, MPH, and G Bryan Young, MD, FRCPC. Diagnosis of delirium and confusional states. Michael J Aminoff, MD, DSc, Kenneth E Schmader, MD, and Janet L Wilterdink, MD, ed. UpToDate. Waltham, MA: UpToDate Inc. https://www.uptodate.com (Accessed on January 24, 2023.)
Sanjay Saint and Craig Frances. Altered mental status. In Siant-Frances guide to inpatient medicine. Lippincott Williams & Wilkins, 1997; 431-434.
Altered level of consciousness - Wikipedia
FEVER
David H Bor, MD. Approach to the adult with a fever of unknown origin. Denis Spelman, MBBS, FRACP, FRCPA, MPH, ed. UpToDate. Waltham, MA: UpToDate Inc. https://www.uptodate.com (Accessed on September 12, 2023.)
Sanjay Saint and Craig Frances. Approach to fever. In Siant-Frances guide to inpatient medicine. Lippincott Williams & Wilkins, 1997; 253-258.

Fever - Wikipedia

HEADACHE

Franz J Wippold II, MD, FACR, Mark A Whealy, MD, and Robert G Kaniecki, MD. Evaluation of headache in adults. Jerry W Swanson, MD, MHPE and Richard P Goddeau, Jr, DO, FAHA, ed. UpToDate. Waltham, MA: UpToDate Inc. https://www.uptodate.com (Accessed on January 25, 2024.)

Headache - Wikipedia

Diagnosis and treatment of idiopathic intracranial hypertension - PMC (nih.gov)

Management of Highly Elevated Intraocular Pressure | Ento Key

SYNCOPE

David Benditt, MD. Syncope in adults: Clinical manifestations and initial diagnostic evaluation. Peter Kowey, MD, FACC, FAHA, FHRS, Korilyn S Zachrison, MD, MSc, and Susan B Yeon, MD, JD, FACC, ed. UpToDate. Waltham, MA: UpToDate Inc. https://www.uptodate.com (Accessed on January 25, 2024.)

Syncope: Medications as Cause and Contributing Factors (uspharmacist.com)

Sanjay Saint and Craig Frances. Syncope. In Siant-Frances guide to inpatient medicine. Lippincott Williams & Wilkins, 1997; 30-33.

Syncope (medicine) - Wikipedia

FALLS

Douglas P Kiel, MD, MPH. Falls in older persons: Risk factors and patient evaluation. Kenneth E Schmader, MD and Jane Givens, MD, MSCE, ed. UpToDate. Waltham, MA: UpToDate Inc. https://www.uptodate.com (Accessed on January 25, 2024.)

Cataplexy - Wikipedia

LEUKOCYTOSIS

R. Douglas Collins. Leukocytosis. In. Algorithmic diagnosis of symptoms and signs: A cost-effective approach. Lippincott Williams & Wilkins, a Wolters Kluwer business, 2013; 300.

Sanjay Saint and Craig Frances. Leukocytosis. In Siant-Frances guide to inpatient medicine. Lippincott Williams & Wilkins, 1997; 327-329.

Hello AI: "Why is infectious mononucleosis called a kissing disease?'

Hello AI: "Which drugs cause eosinophilia?"

LEUKOPENIA

R. Douglas Collins. Leucopenia. In. Algorithmic diagnosis of symptoms and signs: A cost-effective approach. Lippincott Williams & Wilkins, a Wolters Kluwer business, 2013; 301.

Hello AI: "What is peudoleukopenia?"

POLYCYTHEMIA

Ayalew Tefferi, MD. Diagnostic approach to the patient with erythrocytosis/ polycythemia. Richard A Larson, MD and Alan G Rosmarin, MD, ed. UpToDate. Waltham, MA: UpToDate Inc. https://www.uptodate.com (Accessed on February 8, 2024.

R. Douglas Collins. Polycythemia. In. Algorithmic diagnosis of symptoms and signs: A cost-effective approach. Lippincott Williams & Wilkins, a Wolters Kluwer business, 2013; 375.

POEMS syndrome - Wikipedia

ANEMIA

Mind map - Wikipedia
Sanjay Saint and Craig Frances. Anemia. In Siant-Frances guide to inpatient medicine. Lippincott Williams & Wilkins, 1997; 317-322.

THROMBOCYTOSIS

Ayalew Tefferi, MD: Approach to the patient with thrombocytosis. Lawrence LK Leung, MD and Alan G Rosmarin, MD, ed. UpToDate. Waltham, MA: UpToDate Inc. https://www.uptodate.com (Accessed on February 12, 2024.)
Thrombocytosis - Symptoms and causes - Mayo Clinic
Essential Thrombocytosis - StatPearls - NCBI Bookshelf (nih.gov)
Correlation between thrombopoietin and inflammatory factors, platelet indices, and thrombosis in patients with sepsis: A retrospective study - PMC (nih.gov)
Hello AI: "What is the rebound effect after treatment of alcohol-induced thrombocytopenia?'
Hello AI: "How does treatment of Vitamin B12 deficiency lead to thrombocytosis?".

THROMBOCYTOPENIA

Sanjay Saint and Craig Frances. Thrombocytopenia. In Siant-Frances guide to inpatient medicine. Lippincott Williams & Wilkins, 1997; 309-314.
Donald M Arnold, MD, MSc and Adam Cuker, MD, MS: Diagnostic approach to thrombocytopenia in adults. Lawrence LK Leung, MD, Jennifer S Tirnauer, MD and Jane Givens, MD, MSCE, ed. UpToDate. Waltham, MA: UpToDate Inc. https://www.uptodate.com (Accessed on February 14, 2024.)
Heparin-Induced Thrombocytopenia - StatPearls - NCBI Bookshelf (nih.gov)
Drug-induced thrombocytopenia: MedlinePlus Medical Encyclopedia
Paroxysmal Nocturnal Hemoglobinuria (PNH) - Hematology and Oncology - MSD Manual Professional Edition (msdmanuals.com)
Giant platelet disorder - Wikipedia

HYPERNATREMIA

Hello AI: "Why are the patients with hypernatremia always hyperosmolar?"
Hello AI: "Why is hypervolemic hypernatremia associated with increased chloride?"
Hello AI: "Why is hypernatremia in Cushing syndrome associated with low chloride?"
Hello AI: "Why hypercalcemia leads to hypernatremia?"
Hello AI: "Why hypokalemia leads to hypernatremia?"
Hello AI: "Why does brain cancer lead to hypernatremia?"
R. Douglas Collins. Hypernatremia. In. Algorithmic diagnosis of symptoms and signs: A cost-effective approach. Lippincott Williams & Wilkins, a Wolters Kluwer business, 2013; 245.

HYPONATREMIA

Tammy L. Lin, John M. Mohart, and Kaori A. Sakurai. Electrolyte abnormalities. In The Washington manual internship survival guide. 2001; 72-73.
R. Douglas Collins. Hyponatremia. In. Algorithmic diagnosis of symptoms and signs: A cost-effective approach. Lippincott Williams & Wilkins, a Wolters Kluwer business, 2013; 261.
Hello AI: "How hyperproteinemia and hyperlipidemia cause hyponatremia?"
Hello AI: "How hypothyroidism causes hyponatremia?"

HYPERKALEMIA

Causes and evaluation of hyperkalemia in adults. Richard H Sterns, MD and John P Forman, MD, MSc, ed. UpToDate. Waltham, MA: UpToDate Inc. https://www.uptodate.com (Accessed on February 20, 2024.)

Hello AI: "What is psudohyperkalemia?"

Hello AI: "Exercising and hyperkalemia?"

Hello AI: "How does arginine cause hyperkalemia?"

HYPOKALEMIA

ToDate. Waltham, MA: UpToDate Inc. https://www.uptodate.com (Accessed on February 21, 2024.)

Laurie Gutmann, MD and Robin Conwit, MD: Hypokalemic periodic paralysis. Jeremy M Shefner, MD, PhD and Janet L Wilterdink, MD, ed. UpToDate. Waltham, MA: UpToDate Inc. https://www.uptodate.com (Accessed on February 21, 2024.)

Hello AI: "How does alkalosis cause hypokalemia?"

Hello AI: "How does Vitamin B12 deficiency cause hypokalemia?"

Hello AI: "How does GM-CSF cause hypokalemia?"

HYPERCHLOREMIA AND HYPOCHLOREMIA

Hello AI: "Medical causes of hyperchloremia"

Hello AI: "How does non-anion gap metabolic acidosis cause hyperchloremia?"

Hello AI: "How does respiratory alkalosis cause hyperchloremia?"

Hello AI: "How does infection cause hyperchloremia?"

Hello AI: "How does Addison's disease cause hyperchloremia?"

Hello AI: "Medical causes of hypochloremia"

Hello AI: "How does metabolic alkalosis cause hypochloremia?"

Hello AI: "How does respiratory acidosis cause hypochloremia?"

Hyperparathyroidism - Wikipedia

ACID-BASE BALANCE

https://en.wikipedia.org/wiki/Acid%E2%80%93base_homeostasis#/media/File:Acid-base_nomogram.svg

Acid-Base Disorders - Endocrine and Metabolic Disorders - Merck Manuals Professional Edition

01. Algorithm For Acid-Base Disorders | Hospital Handbook (ucsf.edu)

evaluation-of-acid-base-disorders.pdf (cuanschutz.edu)

Acid-base disorder - Wikipedia

RESPIRATORY ACIDOSIS

Sanjay Saint and Craig Frances. Respiratory failure. In Siant-Frances guide to inpatient medicine. Lippincott Williams & Wilkins, 1997; 144-146.

David J Feller-Kopman, MD and Richard M Schwartzstein, MD: The evaluation, diagnosis, and treatment of the adult patient with acute hypercapnic respiratory failure. James K Stoller, MD, MS and Geraldine Finlay, MD, ed. UpToDate. Waltham, MA: UpToDate Inc. https://www.uptodate.com (Accessed on February 24, 2024.)

geekymedics.com/type-1-vs-type-2-respiratory-failure/

Hypermagnesemia - Wikipedia

Pulmonary consequences of hypothyroidism - PMC (nih.gov)

Douglas C Johnson, MD: Respiratory function in thyroid disease. Douglas S Ross, MD and Jean E Mulder, MD, ed. UpToDate. Waltham, MA: UpToDate Inc. https://www.uptodate.com (Accessed on February 24, 2024.)

METABOLIC ACIDOSIS
Michael Emmett, MD and Harold Szerlip, MD, FACP, FCCP, FASN, FNKF: Approach to the adult with metabolic acidosis. Richard H Sterns, MD, Ellie Kelepouris, MD, FAHA, and John P Forman, MD, MSc. ed. UpToDate. Waltham, MA: UpToDate Inc. https://www.uptodate.com (Accessed on February 24, 2024.)
Evangelia Dounousi, Xanthi Zikou, Vasilis Koulouras, and Kostas Katopodis. Metabolic acidosis during parenteral nutrition: Pathophysiological mechanisms. *Indian J Crit Care Med. 2015; 19(5): 270–274.*
Autumn N Harris, P Richard Grimm, Hyun-Wook Lee, Eric Delpire, Lijuan Fang, Jill W Verlander, Paul A Welling, and I David Weiner. Mechanism of Hyperkalemia-Induced Metabolic Acidosis. *J Am Soc Nephrol. 2018; 29(5):1411-1425.*
Jon Tuchscherer, Habib Rehman. Metabolic acidosis in toluene sniffing. *CJEM. 2013;15(4):249-52.*
METABOLIC ALKALOSIS
Michael Emmett, MD and Harold Szerlip, MD, FACP, FCCP, FASN, FNKF: Causes of metabolic alkalosis. Richard H Sterns, MD and John P Forman, MD, MSc. ed. UpToDate. Waltham, MA: UpToDate Inc. https://www.uptodate.com (Accessed on February 24, 2024.)
Milk-alkali syndrome - Wikipedia
RESPIRATORY ALKALOSIS
Richard M Schwartzstein, MD, Jeremy B Richards, MD, MA, Jonathan A Edlow, MD, FACEP and Peter P Roy-Byrne, MD: Hyperventilation syndrome in adults. Mark D Aronson, MD, Korilyn S Zachrison, MD, MSc and Jane Givens, MD, MSCE, ed. UpToDate. Waltham, MA: UpToDate Inc. https://www.uptodate.com (Accessed on February 24, 2024.)
Sanjay Saint and Craig Frances. Hypoxemia. In Siant-Frances guide to inpatient medicine. Lippincott Williams & Wilkins, 1997; 113-116.
CLINICAL VIGNETTES
https://pubmed.ncbi.nlm.nih.gov/23997700/
Barry Kitch, MD, MPH, and Atul Malhotra, MD. Arterial Gas Interpretation. The 29th Annual Intensive Review of Internal Medicine by Harvard Medical School. Boston. July 16-22, 2006.
Mima M. Horne, Ursula Easterday Heitz, Pamela L. Swearingen. Fluid, Electrolyte, and Acid-base Balance: A Case Study Approach. Mosby, 1991, pp. 299-379.
Diagnostic predictors of obesity-hypoventilation syndrome in patients suspected of having sleep-disordered breathing. J Clin Sleep Med, 2013 Sep 15;9(9):879-84.
Kerry Brandis, MD. Acid-Base Physiology: Clinical Examples.
https://www.anaesthesiamcq.com/AcidBaseBook/ab9_6.php
BUN AND CREATININE
Lesley A Inker, MD, MS and Ronald D Perrone, MD: Assessment of kidney function. Richard H Sterns, MD and John P Forman, MD, MSc, MD, ed. UpToDate. Waltham, MA: UpToDate Inc. https://www.uptodate.com (Accessed on February 23, 2024.)
Urea-to-creatinine ratio - Wikipedia
Hello AI: "What is the connection between the pregnancy and reduced BUN?"
Hidden Causes of High or Low Blood Urea Nitrogen (BUN) - SelfDecode Labs
Lesley A Inker, MD, MS and Ronald D Perrone, MD: Drugs that elevate the serum creatinine concentration. Richard H Sterns, MD and John P Forman, MD, MSc, ed.

UpToDate. Waltham, MA: UpToDate Inc. https://www.uptodate.com (Accessed on February 23, 2024.)
Use of angiotensin-converting enzyme inhibitors in patients with heart failure and renal insufficiency: how concerned should we be by the rise in serum creatinine? - PubMed (nih.gov)

HYPERGLYCEMIA AND HYPOGLYCEMIA

https://en.wikipedia.org/wiki/Hyperglycemia
R. Douglas Collins. Hyperglycemia. In. Algorithmic diagnosis of symptoms and signs: A cost-effective approach. Lippincott Williams & Wilkins, a Wolters Kluwer business, 2013; 242.
Hello AI: "How does hypothermia lead to increased glucose levels in the blood?"
Adrian Vella, MD: Hypoglycemia in adults without diabetes mellitus: Clinical manifestations, causes, and diagnosis. Irl B Hirsch, MD, ed. UpToDate. Waltham, MA: UpToDate Inc. https://www.uptodate.com (Accessed on March 20, 2024.)
Insulin autoimmune syndrome: from diagnosis to clinical management - PMC (nih.gov)

LIVER FUNCTION TESTS

Sanjay Saint and Craig Frances. Liver Tests. In Siant-Frances guide to inpatient medicine. Lippincott Williams & Wilkins, 1997; 162-165.
Comparative Study of 5'-Nucleotidase Test in Various Liver Diseases - PMC (nih.gov)
Charcot's cholangitis triad - Wikipedia
Murphy's sign - Wikipedia
Murphy's sign • LITFL • Medical Eponym Library

HYPERCALCEMIA

Elizabeth Shane, MD: Diagnostic approach to hypercalcemia. Clifford J Rosen, MD and Jean E Mulder, MD, ed. UpToDate. Waltham, MA: UpToDate Inc. https://www.uptodate.com (Accessed on March 2, 2024.)
Sanjay Saint and Craig Frances. Hypercalcemia. In Siant-Frances guide to inpatient medicine. Lippincott Williams & Wilkins, 1997; 405-407.
Pibloktoq (hysteria) and Inuit nutrition: Possible implication of hypervitaminosis A - ScienceDirect
Hello AI: "What is the correlation between Vit A intoxication and hypercalcemia."

CALCIUM METABOLISM

Haden ST, Brown EM, Hurwitz S, et al. The effects of age and gender on parathyroid hormone dynamics. Clin Endocrinol, 2000; 52:329.
Bones, Calcium, Phosphate, and PTH in Kidney Failure | National Kidney Federation
Parathyroid Hormone: What It Is, Function & Levels (clevelandclinic.org)
Salman Bhai, MD, and Mazen M Dimachkie, MD. Rhabdomyolysis: Clinical manifestations and diagnosis. Ira N Targoff, MD, Jeremy M Shefner, MD, PhD, and John F Dashe, MD, PhD, ed. UpToDate. Waltham, MA: UpToDate Inc. https://www.uptodate.com (Accessed on February 24, 2024.)

HYPOCALCEMIA

David Goltzman, MD: Etiology of hypocalcemia in adults. Clifford J Rosen, MD and Jean E Mulder, MD, ed. UpToDate. Waltham, MA: UpToDate Inc. https://www.uptodate.com (Accessed on March 2, 2024.)

Sanjay Saint and Craig Frances. Hypocalcemia. In Siant-Frances guide to inpatient medicine. Lippincott Williams & Wilkins, 1997; 408-410.
Hungry Bone Syndrome: What It Is, Symptoms & Treatment (clevelandclinic.org)
Hello AI: "What is the correlation between high PTH and alkaline phosphatase."

HYPERMAGNESEMIA

Alan S L Yu, MB, BChir, Aditi Gupta, MD. Hypermagnesemia: Causes, symptoms, and treatment. Michael Emmett, MD, Richard H Sterns, MD, and Albert Q Lam, MD, ed. UpToDate. Waltham, MA: UpToDate Inc. https://www.uptodate.com (Accessed on February 24, 2024.)
Hello AI: "How primary hyperparathyroidism leads to hypermagnesemia."
standardofcare.com/hypermagnesemia/
www.sciencedirect.com/topics/medicine-and-dentistry/hypermagnesemia
www.ncbi.nlm.nih.gov/pmc/articles/PMC6024559/
www.ncbi.nlm.nih.gov/pmc/articles/PMC4133642/

HYPOMAGNESEMIA

Alan S L Yu, MB, BChir. Hypomagnesemia: Evaluation and treatment: Causes, symptoms, and treatment. Michael Emmett, MD, Richard H Sterns, MD, and Albert Q Lam, MD, ed. UpToDate. Waltham, MA: UpToDate Inc. https://www.uptodate.com (Accessed on February 24, 2024.)
Hello AI: "Hypomagnesemia and sugar cravings."
Hypomagnesemia: What It Is, Causes, Symptoms & Treatment (clevelandclinic.org)
www.ncbi.nlm.nih.gov/pmc/articles/PMC7803063/
Hypomagnesemia: Symptoms, Causes, Treatment, and More (verywellhealth.com)
ajcn.nutrition.org/article/S0002-9165(23)33246-5/fulltext
The Link Between Magnesium and RLS (healthline.com)
www.health.com/magnesium-deficiency-symptoms-7642391

HYPERPHOSPHATEMIA

Jason R Stubbs, MD and Alan S L Yu, MB, BChir. Overview of the causes and treatment of hyperphosphatemia. Michael Emmett, MD, Richard H Sterns, MD, and Albert Q Lam, MD, ed. UpToDate. Waltham, MA: UpToDate Inc. https://www.uptodate.com (Accessed on February 24, 2024.)
Hyperphosphatemia: Causes, Symptoms & Treatment (clevelandclinic.org)
Pseudohyperphosphatemia in a patient with relapsed multiple myeloma after bone marrow transplantation: A case report - PMC (nih.gov)
Hyperphosphatemia - StatPearls - NCBI Bookshelf (nih.gov)
Calcinosis Cutis - StatPearls - NCBI Bookshelf (nih.gov)
https://www.icliniq.com/articles/kidney-and-urologic-diseases/acute-phosphate-nephropathy
https://onlinelibrary.wiley.com/doi/full/10.1002/ccr3.2264
What Is a Match Head Made Of? | Sciencing

HYPOPHOSPHATEMIA

Jason R Stubbs, MD and Alan S L Yu, MB, BChir. Hypophosphatemia: Evaluation and treatment. Michael Emmett, MD, Richard H Sterns, MD, and Albert Q Lam, MD, ed. UpToDate. Waltham, MA: UpToDate Inc. https://www.uptodate.com (Accessed on March 6, 2024.)
Severe Hypophosphatemia in Respiratory Alkalosis (researchgate.net)

Incidence and determinants of hypophosphatemia in diabetic ketoacidosis: an observational study - PMC (nih.gov)
Hello AI: "How does hypoglycemia lead to hypophosphatemia."
Hello AI: "Why acute hypophosphatemia could be lethal?"

HYPERTHYROIDISM

Douglas S Ross, MD. Diagnosis of hyperthyroidism. David S Cooper, MD and Jean E Mulder, MD, ed. UpToDate. Waltham, MA: UpToDate Inc. https://www.uptodate.com (Accessed on March 23, 2024.)
Hello AI: "What is intentional suppressive therapy".
Hello AI: "What is factitious hyperthyroidism?".

SUBCLINICAL HYPERTHYROIDISM

Douglas S Ross, MD. Subclinical hyperthyroidism in nonpregnant adults. David S Cooper, MD and Jean E Mulder, MD, ed. UpToDate. Waltham, MA: UpToDate Inc. https://www.uptodate.com (Accessed on March 26, 2024.)
Hello AI: "Why does subclinical hyperthyroidism need to be treated in patients with cardiovascular risk and osteoporosis risk factors?

HYPOTHYROIDISM

Douglas S Ross, MD. Diagnosis of and screening for hypothyroidism in nonpregnant adults. David S Cooper, MD and Jean E Mulder, MD, ed. UpToDate. Waltham, MA: UpToDate Inc. https://www.uptodate.com (Accessed on March 25, 2024.)
https://en.wikipedia.org/wiki/Hypothyroidism
https://www.hyperthyroidismsymptomsx.com/normal-thyroid-levels
Hello AI: "What are T3 and T4 values in resistance to thyroid hormone?".
Hello AI: "What in resistance to thyroid hormone?".

VERTIGO

Sanjay Saint and Craig Frances. Vertigo. In Siant-Frances guide to inpatient medicine. Lippincott Williams & Wilkins, 1997; 440-443.
Vertigo - Wikipedia
Vertigo Causes and Risk Factors (everydayhealth.com)
https://www.ahajournals.org/doi/pdf/10.1161/01.str.11.3.301

BLEEDING DISORDERS

Sanjay Saint and Craig Frances. Bleeding disorders. In Siant-Frances guide to inpatient medicine. Lippincott Williams & Wilkins, 1997; 333-344.
Association of Broad-Spectrum Antibiotic Therapy and Vitamin E Supplementation with Vitamin K Deficiency-Induced Coagulopathy: A Case Report and Narrative Review of the Literature - PMC (nih.gov)
Difference Between PTT and PT | Difference Between
Antiphospholipid Antibodies: Johns Hopkins Lupus Center
GP1BA - Wikipedia
Glycoprotein IIb/IIIa - Wikipedia
Glanzmann's thrombasthenia - Wikipedia

BLEEDING DISORDERS CONT. WITH THROMBOCYTOPENIA

Sanjay Saint and Craig Frances. Thrombocytopenia. In Siant-Frances guide to inpatient medicine. Lippincott Williams & Wilkins, 1997; 309-314.

HYPERCOAGULABLE STATES

Kenneth A Bauer, MD, Gregory YH Lip, MD, FRCPE, FESC, FACC. Evaluating adult patients with established venous thromboembolism for acquired and

inherited risk factors. Jess Mandel, MD, MACP, ATSF, FRCP, James D Douketis, MD, FRCPC, FACP, FCCP and Geraldine Finlay, MD, ed. UpToDate. Waltham, MA: UpToDate Inc. https://www.uptodate.com (Accessed on March 15, 2024.)
Sanjay Saint and Craig Frances. Hypercoagulable states. In Siant-Frances guide to inpatient medicine. Lippincott Williams & Wilkins, 1997; 345-348.
Thrombophilia - Wikipedia
Inherited Thrombophilia: Genetics, Prevalence, Testing Guidelines - Bing video
Homocysteine Blood Test (medicinenet.com)
Heparin-Induced Thrombocytopenia - StatPearls - NCBI Bookshelf (nih.gov)
Hello AI: "How does PNH cause thrombosis."
Hello AI: "How do TTP and HUS cause thrombosis."

HYPERLIPIDEMIA

Hyperlipidemia - Wikipedia
Robert S Rosenson, MD. Secondary causes of dyslipidemia. Mason W Freeman, MD, Bernard J Gersh, MB, ChB, DPhil, FRCP, MACC, ed. UpToDate. Waltham, MA: UpToDate Inc. https://www.uptodate.com (Accessed on March 23, 2024.)
R. Douglas Collins. Hypertriglyceridemia. In. Algorithmic diagnosis of symptoms and signs: A cost-effective approach. Lippincott Williams & Wilkins, a Wolters Kluwer business, 2013; 250-251.

IRON METABOLISM (FE, TIBC, FERRITIN)

Janet L Kwiatkowski, MD, MSCE. Approach to the patient with suspected iron overload. Robert T Means, Jr, MD, MACP and Jennifer S Tirnauer, MD Jane Givens, MD, MSCE., ed. UpToDate. Waltham, MA: UpToDate Inc. https://www.uptodate.com (Accessed on March 11, 2024.)
Transferrin Saturation Calculator (mdapp. co)
Total iron-binding capacity - Wikipedia
TIBC (Total Iron-Binding Capacity) Test: What It Is & Results (clevelandclinic.org)
Iron Binding Capacity - StatPearls - NCBI Bookshelf (nih.gov)
Total Iron Binding Capacity (TIBC) Explained (youtube.com)
Transferrin Saturation Explained (youtube.com)
Hello AI: "Is all iron in the blood bound to transferrin?."
Hello AI: "What is the connection between interleukin 6 and transferrin?"
Hello AI: "What is the connection between hepcidin and transferrin?"
Hello AI: "How does metabolic syndrome lead to increased ferritin?
Hello AI: "How does low iron lead to infertility?"
Hello AI: "How does playing conga drums lead to iron deficiency?"
Periodic Limb Movement Disorder - StatPearls - NCBI Bookshelf (nih.gov)
Hello AI: "How does iron deficiency lead to restless legs?"
Hemosiderinuria - Wikipedia
Hello AI: "What is the connection between the gastrointestinal tract and iron deficiency?"

HEMOPTYSIS

Sanjay Saint and Craig Frances. Massive Hemoptysis. In Siant-Frances guide to inpatient medicine. Lippincott Williams & Wilkins, 1997; 105-108.
Hemoptysis - Wikipedia
The history of lupus | Lupus Foundation of America
Hello AI: "How does neovascularization in the lungs cause hemoptysis?"
Hello AI: "How do mitral stenosis and CHF cause hemoptysis?"

ACUTE DIARRHEA

Sanjay Saint and Craig Frances. Acute diarrhea. In Siant-Frances guide to inpatient medicine. Lippincott Williams & Wilkins, 1997; 166-168.

R. Douglas Collins. Diarrhea, acute. In. Algorithmic diagnosis of symptoms and signs: A cost-effective approach. Lippincott Williams & Wilkins, a Wolters Kluwer business, 2013; 115-116.

Botulism - Symptoms and causes - Mayo Clinic

Amebiasis (Amoebic Dysentery): Symptoms & Treatment (clevelandclinic.org)

Clostridium difficile toxin A - Wikipedia

Hello AI: “Why is ph < 5 in osmotic diarrhea?”

https://en.wikipedia.org/wiki/Stool_osmotic_gap

ASCITES

Sanjay Saint and Craig Frances. Ascites. In Siant-Frances guide to inpatient medicine. Lippincott Williams & Wilkins, 1997; 179-184.

Hello AI: “Serum-ascites albumin gradient (SAAG).”

Spontaneous Bacterial Peritonitis (SBP) - Internal Medicine Residency Handbook (vim-book.org)

Hello AI: “How does Kwashiorkor cause ascites).”

NEPHROTIC SYNDROME

Sanjay Saint and Craig Frances. Nephrotic syndrome. In Siant-Frances guide to inpatient medicine. Lippincott Williams & Wilkins, 1997; 179-184.

Nephritic syndrome - Wikipedia

Nephrotic syndrome - Wikipedia

ABBREVIATIONS

ACE angiotensin converting enzyme
ADH antidiuretic hormone
ADL activities of daily living
AG anion gap
AIHA autoimmune hemolytic anemia
AIN acute interstitial nephritis
ALL acute lymphocytic anemia
ALP alkaline phosphatase
ALS: amyotrophic lateral sclerosis
ALT alanine aminotransferase
AML acute myeloid leukemia
ARDS acute respiratory distress syndrome
AST aspartate aminotransferase
ATG anti thyroglobulin antibody
ATN acute tubular necrosis
ATPO anti-thyroid peroxidase antibody
Auto-PEEP Intrinsic positive end-expiratory pressure
BP blood pressure
BPH benign prostatic hyperplasia
BUN blood urea nitrogen
BZD benzodiazepine
CAD coronary artery disease
CASR calcium-sensing receptor
CCAH congenital central alveolar hypoventilation
CHF congestive heart failure
CLL chronic lymphocytic leukemia
CML chronic myeloid leukemia
CMV cytomegalovirus
CO carbon monoxide
COPD chronic obstructive pulmonary disease
CPAP continuous positive airway pressure
Cr creatinine
CVA cerebrovascular accident
DHT Dobhoff tube
DI diabetes insipidus
DIC disseminated intravascular coagulation
DKA diabetic ketoacidosis
DM I diabetes melitus Type I
DM II diabetes melitus Type II

DMARD disease-modifying antirheumatic drug

DTR deep tendon reflexes

DVT deep vein thrombosis

DZ disease

ECF extracellular fluid

eGFR estimated glomerular filtration rate

EHEC enterohemorrhagic E. coli (serotype O157:H7)

EIEC entero invasive E. coli

EPEC enteropathogenic E. coli

ERCP Endoscopic Retrograde Cholangiopancreatography

ESLD end-stage liver disease

ETEC enterotoxigenic E. coli

FeNa: fractional excretion of sodium

FHH familial hypocalciuric hypercalcemia

FHHNC Familial primary hypomagnesemia with hypercalciuria and nephrocalcinosis

FOU fever of unknown origin

GERD gastro esophageal reflux disease

GFR glomerular filtration rate

GGT gamma glutamine transpeptidase

GI gastrointestinal

GM-CSF Granulocyte-macrophage colony-stimulating factor

GP glycoprotein

G6PDD glucose 6 phosphate dehydrogenase deficiency

HAT heparin-associated thrombocytopenia

Hb hemoglobin

Hct hematocrit

HDL high density lipoprotein

HELLP hemolysis, elevated liver enzymes, and low platelet count syndrome

HF Hear failure

HH Hereditary hemochromatosis

HIT heparin-induced thrombocytopenia

HIV human immunodeficiency viruses

HRT hormone replacement therapy

HUS/TTP hemolytic uremic syndrome/thrombotic thrombocytopenic purpura

IAA insulin autoantibody

IAS insulin autoimmune syndrome

IBD Inflammatory Bowel Disease

ICF intracellular fluid

ICP intracranial pressure

IDL intermediate-density lipoprotein

IGF insulin-like growth factor
IIH Idiopathic intracranial hypertension
IL-6 Interleukin-6
IOP intraocular pressure
IRAbs insulin receptor autoantibodies
ITP idiopathic thrombocytopenic purpura
IVIG Intravenous immune globulin
LDH lactate dehydrogenase
LDL low density lipoprotein
LLQ left lower quadrant
LP lumbar puncture
LSD Lysergic acid diethylamide
LT4 Levothyroxine
LUQ left upper quadrant
MAHA microangiopathic hemolytic anemia
MAS Milk-alkali syndrome
MCV mean corpuscular volume
MEN multiple endocrine neoplasia
MI myocardial infarction
MPNs Myeloproliferative neoplasm
MS multiple sclerosis
NAFLD Nonalcoholic fatty liver disease
NG non anion gap
NGT nasogastric tube
NIPHS noninsulinoma pancreatogenous hypoglycemia syndrome
NO nitric oxide
NO3 nitrate
NSAIDs nonsteroidal anti-inflammatory drugs
5'-NT 5'-Nucleotidase
OP ocular pressure
PCP Phencyclidine
PE pulmonary embolism
PEEP positive end-expiratory pressure
PID pelvic inflammatory disease
PIMAX maximum inspiratory mouth pressure (also termed NIF = negative inspiratory force)
PLMS Periodic limb movements in sleep
PNH paroxysmal nocturnal hemoglobinuria
PP Periodic paralysis
preproPTH preproparathyroid hormone
PT prothrombin time

PTH parathyroid hormone
PTHrP PTH-related protein
PV polycythemia vera
RA rheumatoid arthritis
RAAS renin-angiotensin-aldosterone system
RLS Restless leg syndrome
RLQ right lower quadrant
RTA renal tubular acidosis
RUQ right upper quadrant
SBP Spontaneous bacterial peritonitis
SIBO small intestinal bacterial overgrowth
SIRS: systemic inflammatory response syndrome
SLE systemic lupus erythematosus
SOB shortness of breath
s/p LP status post lumbar puncture
SPEP Serum protein electrophoresis
SSRI selective serotonin reuptake inhibitors
T3 triiodothyronine
T4 thyroxine
TBI traumatic brain injury
TBIRS type B insulin resistance syndrome
TG elevated triglycerides
TIA transient ischemic attack
TMJ temporomandibular joint
TPN total parenteral nutrition
TPO Thrombopoietin
TSAT transferrin saturation
TSH thyroid-stimulating hormone
TTP Thrombotic thrombocytopenic purpura
TURP Transurethral resection of the prostate
UC ulcerative colitis
U/l units per liter
UNa: urine sodium concentration
UPEP urinary protein electrophoresis
VEGF vascular endothelial growth factor
V/Q ventilation (v) and perfusion (Q)
VTE Venous thromboembolism
vWD von Willebrand's disease
w/ with
WBC white blood cells

LIST OF PICTURES ACCORDING TO THE AUTHORS

Prof. Dr. Radivoj V. Krstic (RVK)
Mrs. Ellen Weiss (EW)
VISUALIZATION OF DATA - RVK, except female figures, which were drawn by EW CHEST PAIN- RVK
SHORTNESS OF BREATH - RVK
ACUTE GI HEMORRHAGE - RVK
ACUTE KIDNEY INJURY (AKI) - RVK
HYPERTENSION - RVK
HYPOTENSION - RVK
ABDOMINAL PAIN - RVK
ALTERED MENTAL STATUS- RVK
FEVER - RVK
HEADACHE – RVK, except the man in the middle of the picture ear, parotid gland, liver, stomach, intestine, the man with occipital headache, and SNOOP symbols including cancer, pregnancy, HIV, a head indicating neurological symptoms, an elderly man, and the woman with Vasava maneuver which were drawn by EW
SYNCOPE - RVK
FALLS – RVK, except symbols for dizziness, slips and trips, which were drawn by EW
LEUKOCYTOSIS - RVK
LEUKOPENIA - RVK
POLYCYTHEMIA - RVK
ANEMIA - RVK
THROMBOCYTOSIS - RVK
THROMBOCYTOPENIA - RVK
HYPERNATREMIA - RVK
HYPONATREMIA - RVK
HYPERKALEMIA - RVK
HYPOKALEMIA - RVK
HYPER AND HYPOCHLOREMIA – RVK except the hand at the top of the picture which was drawn by EW
RESPIRATORY ACIDOSIS - RVK
METABOLIC ACIDOSIS - RVK
METABOLIC ALKALOSIS - RVK
RESPIRATORY ALKALOSIS - RVK
CLINICAL VIGNETTES I - EW
CLINICAL VIGNETTES II - EW
CLINICAL VIGNETTES III - EW
CLINICAL VIGNETTES IV - EW

INCREASED AND REDUCED BUN AND CREATININE – RVK, except the dehydrated man on the left and the "High creatinine" part, and the man in the wheelchair and the man who is pushing him, as well as vegetables in the "Low creatinine" part, which were drawn by EW
HYPER AND HYPOGLYCEMIA - RVK
LIVER FUNCTION TESTS (LFT) – RVK, except the eyes, the gall blader, right upper quadrant of the abdomen and cells of the "hepatocellular" area, which were drawn by EW
LIVER FUNCTION TESTS (LFT) CONT. – RVK, except chemosis of the red blood cells and CAT scan of the abdomen in the right lower quadrant, which were drawn by EW
HYPERCALCEMIA - RVK
HYPOCALCEMIA - RVK
HYPERMAGNESEMIA – RVK, except the synapse in the right upper quadrant which was drawn by EW
HYPOMAGNESEMIA - RVK
HYPERPHOSPHATEMIA - RVK
HYPOPHOSPHATEMIA - RVK
HYPERTHYROIDISM - RVK
SUBCLINICAL HYPERTHYROIDISM - EW
HYPOTHYROIDISM - RVK
BLEEDING DISORDERS - RVK
BLEEDING DISORDERS CONT. WITH THROMBOCYTOPENIA - RVK
HYPERCOAGULABLE STATES – RVK, except the family picture on the left, which was drawn by EW
HYPERLIPIDEMIA - RVK, except the family picture on the left, which was drawn by EW
IRON METABOLISM (FE, TIBC, FERRITIN) - RVK
HEMOPTYSIS - RVK
DIARRHEA - RVK
ASCITES - RVK
NEPHROTIC SYNDROME -RVK, except the liver and tumor nodules and three small kidneys at the bottom of the picture, which were drawn by EW
VERTIGO - RVK, except pictures of nystagmus, which were drawn by EW
CIN VOMIT - RVK
ILLUSTRATED APPROACH TO DIFFERENTIAL DIAGNOSES - RVK

TESTIMONIALS

"What a delightful book based on a terrific idea: remembering facts and concepts can be made easier with pictures and drawings. In this easy-to-read book on differential diagnosis the authors help the reader approach common symptoms – like chest pain, fever, and confusion – and lab abnormalities – such as hyponatremia and acid-base disturbances – through the use of clever color illustrations. The drawings themselves are memorable and are accompanied by helpful text that orients the reader to the illustration. Doctors Trbovic and Trbovich should be commended on their wonderful book that will help physicians, advanced practice professionals, nurses, trainees, and others learn clinical medicine in a novel way!"

Sanjay Saint, MD, MPH, MACP
Chief of Medicine at the VA Ann Arbor Healthcare System & George Dock Professor of Internal Medicine at the University of Michigan

"As a family medicine program director, I recognize the challenges faced by medical students and residents to grasp complex pathological processes. The visual elements are particularly beneficial, as they allow learners to visualize processes that can often seem abstract in traditional texts.
Internal Medicine Differential Diagnoses Through Illustrations is an invaluable addition to any medical curriculum, and I look forward to incorporating this book into our residency training library. This illustrative medical book will certainly assist trainees to deepen their understanding of pathology in a practical and visually appealing manner."

Mercedez Bernard D.O.
Adjunct Professor for Oklahoma State University College of Health Sciences
Program Director
Family Medicine Residency
Comanche County Memorial Hospital
Lawton, Oklahoma

“This book stands out for its thoroughness and clarity in simplifying complex medical diagnoses. The illustrations in the book are highly relevant to common medical problems faced by post-surgical patients, such as hypotension, electrolyte imbalances, renal dysfunction, and altered mental status. Any surgical resident would greatly benefit from quick and easy access to this essential information.”

Bratislav Velimirovic, MD, PhD
Fellow of the American Association of Neurological Surgeons
Clinical Professor Neurosurgery Burrell College of Medicine
El Paso, Texas

“This book is very engaging from the first page, offering a refreshing and insightful perspective with the aid of illustrations. Additionally, it makes complex concepts interesting and easy to comprehend. Internal Medicine practitioners of all levels would benefit immensely from reviewing the book.”

Danish Mohammed Thameem, MD
Associate Professor of Medicine
Pulmonary and Critical Care
Carle Illinois College of Medicine

ABOUT AUTHORS

Sinisa M. Trbovic, M.D., Ph.D.

M.D. University of Belgrade School of Medicine, Serbia

Ph.D. in Pharmacology, University of Illinois at Chicago

Internal Medicine. University of Illinois at Urbana – Champaign

Sleep Medicine. University of Texas Southwestern Medical Center at Dallas

Psychiatry. Harvard

Adjunct Clinical Assistant Professor of Internal Medicine, Sleep Medicine and Psychiatry. Oklahoma State University Center for Health Sciences

---

Prof. Alexander M. Trbovich, M.D., Ph.D.

M.D. University of Belgrade School of Medicine, Belgrade, Serbia

Postdoctoral Fellowship in Reproductive Endocrinology, Massachusetts General Hospital, Boston, Massachusetts

Ph.D. in Pathology, Cellular and Molecular Biology. Boston University School of Medicine, Boston, Massachusetts

Professor of Pathophysiology. University of Belgrade School of Medicine, Belgrade, Serbia

While finishing this book, I had an unusual spiritual experience that brought everything full circle. When conceiving this book a few years ago, I was planning to start it with the words of Jesus Christ, “Come to me, all you who are weary and burdened, and I will give you rest,” explaining the main purpose of the book - to help the exhausted and sleep-deprived residents take care of their patients. At that time, I never imagined life would lead my ailing brother and me to the statue of Jesus at Johns Hopkins Hospital in Baltimore, where that quote is engraved.

Sinisa

“There are strange and inscrutable ways of God.”

Fyodor Mikhailovich Dostoevsky

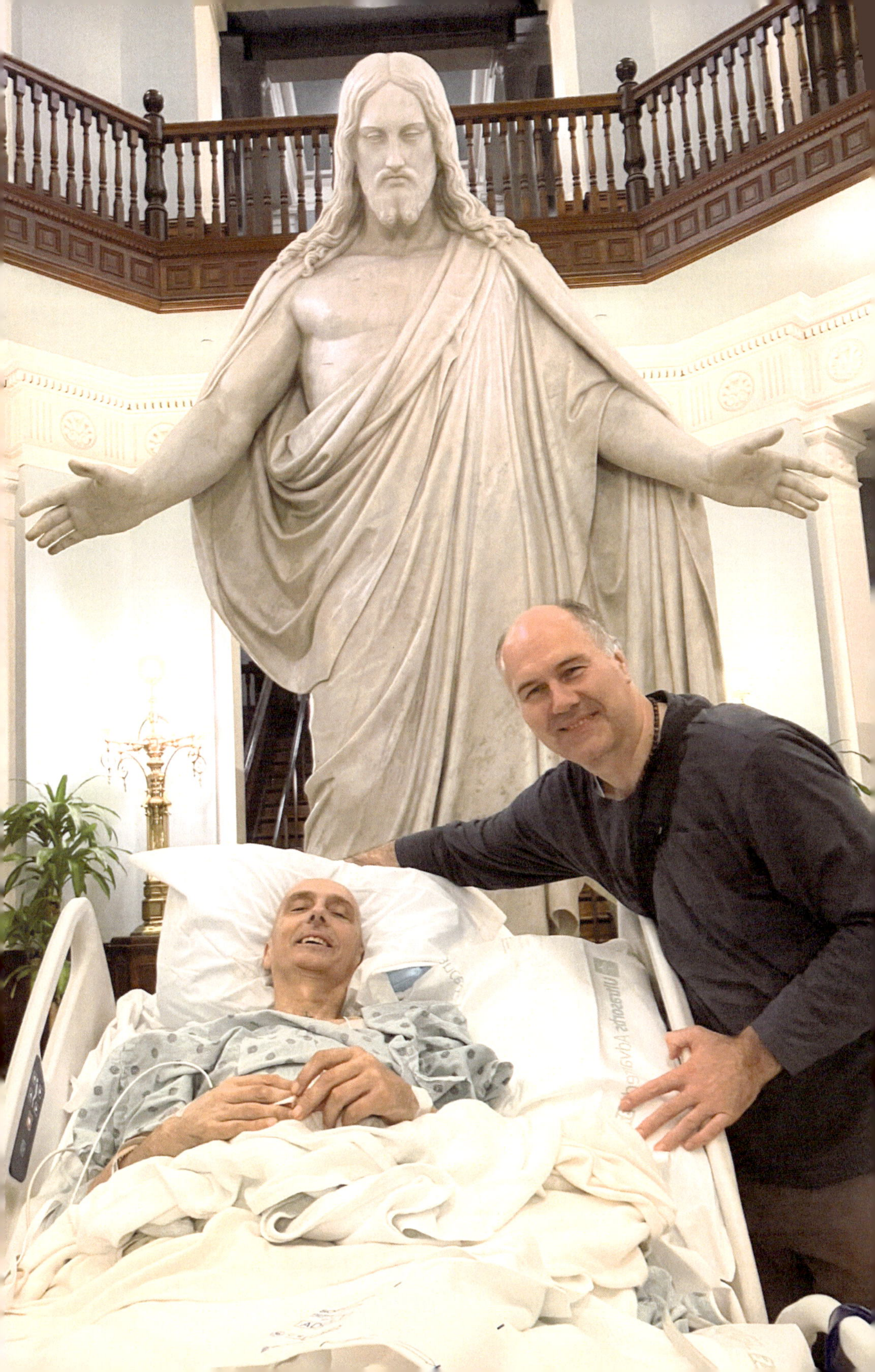

Johns Hopkins Hospital in Baltimore, Maryland
where my 57-year-old brother spent his last days fighting cancer.

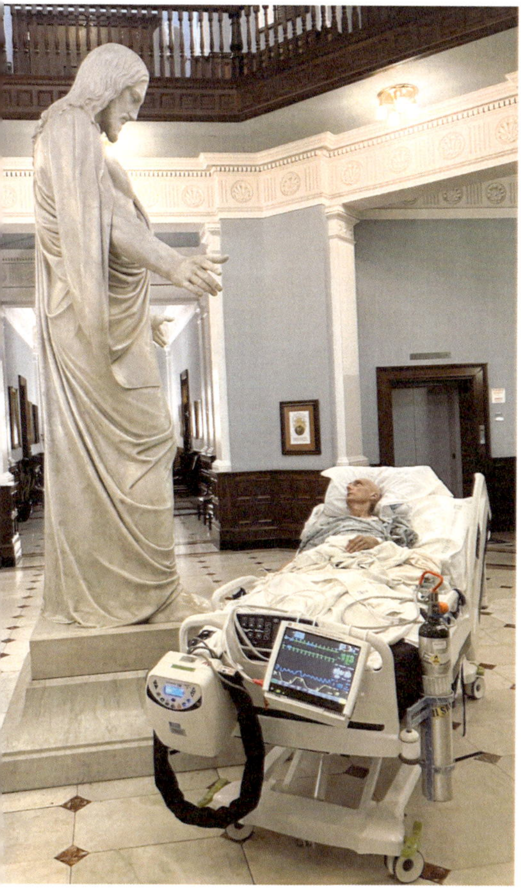

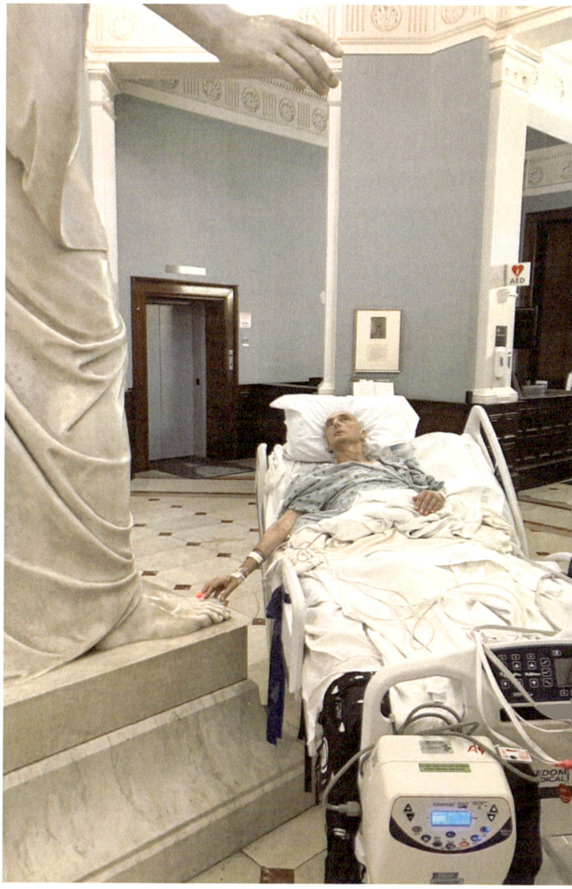
AED

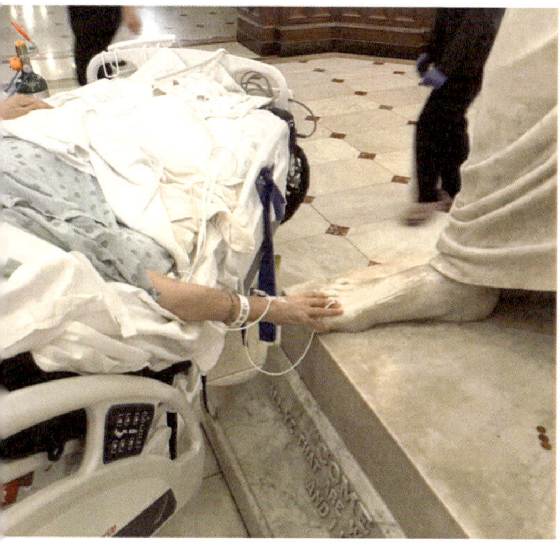

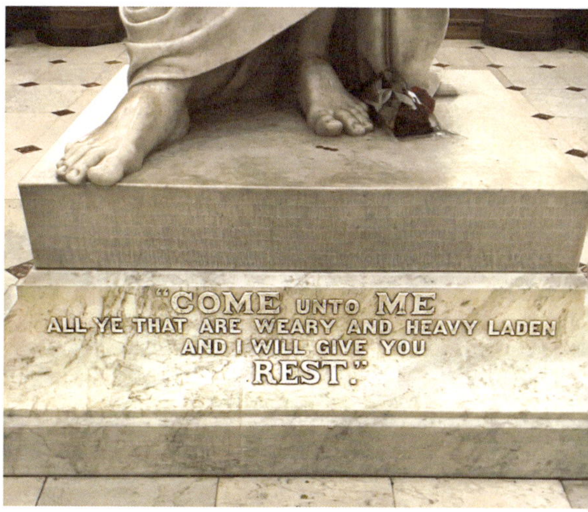
"COME UNTO ME
ALL YE THAT ARE WEARY AND HEAVY LADEN
AND I WILL GIVE YOU
REST."

www.ingramcontent.com/pod-product-compliance
Lightning Source LLC
LaVergne TN
LVRC080205220926
848482LV00007B/338

* 9 7 9 8 9 9 1 9 3 0 0 4 8 *